Toothpastes

Monographs in Oral Science

Vol. 23

Series Editors

M.C.D.N.J.M Huysmans Nijmegen
A. Lussi Bern
H.-P. Weber Boston, Mass.

Toothpastes

Volume Editor

Cor van Loveren Amsterdam

18 figures, 9 in color, and 20 tables, 2013

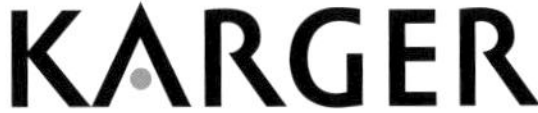

Basel · Freiburg · Paris · London · New York · New Delhi · Bangkok ·
Beijing · Tokyo · Kuala Lumpur · Singapore · Sydney

Cor van Loveren
Department of Preventive Dentistry
Academic Center for Dentistry Amsterdam (ACTA)
University of Amsterdam and VU University
Gustav Mahlerlaan 3004
NL–1081 LA Amsterdam (The Netherlands)

This volume received generous financial support from

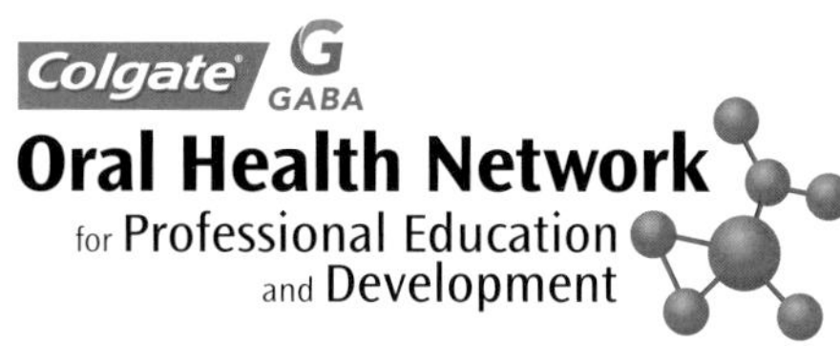

Library of Congress Cataloging-in-Publication Data

Toothpastes / volume editor, Cor van Loveren.
     p. ; cm. -- (Monographs in oral science, ISSN 0077-0892 ; vol. 23)
  Includes bibliographical references and indexes.
  ISBN 978-3-318-02206-3 (hard cover : alk. paper) -- ISBN 978-3-318-02207-0
(e-ISBN)
  I. Loveren, Cor van, editor of compilation. II. Series: Monographs in oral
science ; v. 23. 0077-0892
  [DNLM: 1. Toothpastes. 2. Tooth Diseases--therapy. 3. Toothbrushing.
W1 MO568E v.23 2013 / WU 113]
  RK60.7
  617.6'01--dc23
                                                        2013014780

Bibliographic Indices. This publication is listed in bibliographic services, including MEDLINE/Pubmed.

© Copyright 2013 by S. Karger AG, P.O. Box, CH–4009 Basel (Switzerland)
www.karger.com
Printed in Switzerland on acid-free and non-aging paper (ISO 9706) by Reinhardt Druck, Basel
ISSN 0077–0892
e-ISSN 1662–3843
ISBN 978–3–318–02206–3
e-ISBN 978–3–318–02207–0

Contents

Preface

The editors of the Monographs in Oral Science series asked me whether it would be worthwhile to produce a volume on toothpaste. I could only give a resounding 'Yes!' because I always notice that most dentists and many dental researchers are unaware of the complexity of toothpastes and the science that goes into them. Questions about the relative effectiveness of different toothpastes are often vaguely answered. Furthermore, the last comparable publication dated from 1992.

Although used for several thousand years, dentifrices have evolved rapidly over the last century from suspensions of crushed egg shells or ashes used by the ancient Egyptians and toothpowders of the 19th century to the complex toothpaste formulations of today. A landmark was the widespread mass-marketed introduction of fluoride in toothpaste in the 1950s. From then on, toothbrushing with fluoridated toothpaste became indispensable for good oral health. The use of toothpastes had no longer only a cosmetic but also a therapeutic effect. Fancy packaging, a variety of flavours and colours and commercials emphasising the benefits made oral hygiene attractive for consumers, with a pivotal role for toothpaste as it combines the delivery of active ingredients with the mechanical removal of dental plaque and food debris during use. Manufacturers have continuously improved formulations for better fluoride bioavailability, and also included other active 'therapeutic' ingredients to fight gum disease, malodour, calculus, erosion and dentin hypersensitivity. The cosmetic effect of toothpastes improved as a result of tailored abrasives to clean and whiten teeth, ingredients to facilitate removal and prevention of extrinsic stain, flavours for the purpose of breath freshening and dyes for better visual appeal. The development and promotion of these latter 'cosmetic' toothpastes fits into a switch in emphasis in dental practice and among patients to cosmetic dentistry and may therefore have an important function in stimulating consumers to use the pastes. However, this shift in emphasis from therapeutic toothpastes to ones marketed for their cosmetic benefits should not lead to the notion that such cosmetic benefits are more important than the therapeutic ones. Consumers should continue to realize that the first and global goal of using toothpaste is to fight caries: still the most prevalent oral disease. Other functions should not jeopardize this important task.

Toothpastes have become truly multi-functional due to the incorporation of a range of active ingredients that aim to combat a variety of oral diseases and conditions and to provide cosmetic benefits. To be effective, such ingredients need to be delivered to the mouth and ideally be retained at target sites for as long as possible. Effective toothpastes are those that are formulated for maximum bioavailability of their actives. This, however, can be challenging as compromises have to be made when several different actives are formulated in one phase. Toothpaste development is by no means complete as many challenges and especially sub-optimal oral substantivity of active ingredients are yet to be overcome. Therefore, transparent quality control of manufacture to confirm the bioavailability of the ingredients is essential to support the credibility of efficacy claims. In this respect, established brands may be preferred over generic products. The intra-oral retention or substantivity of active ingredients in toothpastes is not only influenced by product-related but also by user-related factors. The latter factors include biological aspects such as salivary flow and salivary clearance, and behavioural aspects, such as frequency and duration of brushing, amount of toothpaste used and post-brushing rinsing behaviour. Whilst product-related factors are fundamental to the intrinsic efficacy of toothpaste, the user-related factors have the potential to significantly enhance or reduce effectiveness.

Dentists are often asked about which toothpastes are the best or about the benefits of specific ingredients. Furthermore, dentists want to advise their patients on the best way to use toothpaste. After reading this book the dentist, and more generally all those who want to advise on the use of toothpaste, will be able to do so in an evidence-based manner. There are head-to-head comparisons of the effectiveness of toothpaste, but such comparisons are not available for all possible comparisons. It is not realistic to expect or demand head-to-head comparisons on all possible claims. Furthermore, head-to-head comparisons can be outdated because by the time the results are published manufacturers may have changed a poorly performing formulation. The limited number of such comparisons in relation to the large number of brands, types and claims of toothpastes implies that many answers will have to be given based on short-term clinical studies (e.g. 4-day plaque growth studies) or on model in vitro studies. A proper understanding of the wider validity of these outcomes is of paramount importance. For therapeutic claims that cannot be directly checked by consumers themselves, scientific evidence is essential; for cosmetic claims, subjective experience and appreciation may be overriding.

As editor of this monograph, I was lucky to find so many distinguished colleagues willing to contribute their time and expertise. On behalf of myself and all readers, I would like to thank them for their hard labour and their willingness to share their knowledge with us. The monograph is structured such that after a general introduction on the purpose, history and composition of toothpaste, six chapters deal mainly with the clinical evidence of effectiveness in caries prevention, in reducing and preventing plaque, gingivitis, and halitosis, in preventing calculus formation, in facilitating removal and prevention of extrinsic stain, and in preventing dentine hypersensitivity and erosion. Later chapters deal with important issues that contribute to our understanding of why toothpastes do what they do. The relevant topics are the abrasiveness of the pastes, the substantivity of active ingredients in the oral cavity and the possible models to study effectiveness when full-scale clinical trials are not possible. The last chapter focuses on two of the user-related factors that have been most widely studied: frequency of toothbrushing and post-brushing rinsing behaviour.

Whether for those new to the field or for the established worker, this monograph will prove to be a most valuable resource of the available knowledge on toothpaste effectiveness.

Finally, I would like to thank Colgate and GABA for supporting the release of this book.

Cor van Loveren, Amsterdam

van Loveren C (ed): Toothpastes. Monogr Oral Sci. Basel, Karger, 2013, vol 23, pp 1–14
DOI: 10.1159/000350456

An Introduction to Toothpaste – Its Purpose, History and Ingredients

Frank Lippert

Department of Preventive and Community Dentistry, Oral Health Research Institute, Indiana University School of Dentistry, Indianapolis, Ind., USA

Abstract

Toothpaste is a paste or gel to be used with a toothbrush to maintain and improve oral health and aesthetics. Since their introduction several thousand years ago, toothpaste formulations have evolved considerably – from suspensions of crushed egg shells or ashes to complex formulations with often more than 20 ingredients. Among these can be compounds to combat dental caries, gum disease, malodor, calculus, erosion and dentin hypersensitivity. Furthermore, toothpastes contain abrasives to clean and whiten teeth, flavors for the purpose of breath freshening and dyes for better visual appeal. Effective toothpastes are those that are formulated for maximum bioavailability of their actives. This, however, can be challenging as compromises will have to be made when several different actives are formulated in one phase. Toothpaste development is by no means complete as many challenges and especially the poor oral substantivity of most active ingredients are yet to overcome.

The following chapter will provide a brief overview about toothpaste – its history, ingredients and their purpose, delivery formats and issues relating to safety.

History

This section will provide an overview of the history of toothpastes and its much older relative, toothpowders. Due to the lack of (credible) scientific publications on the matter, a summary of information gathered from various (sometimes conflicting) sources [1–11] will be presented.

Toothpowders and toothpastes are by no means inventions of modern times. Around 3,000–5,000 BC, ancient Egyptians first developed a dental cream which contained powdered ashes from oxen hooves, myrrh, egg shells and pumice, primarily with the aim to remove debris from teeth. Most likely, water was added only at the time of use. Persians then added burnt shells of snails and oysters along with gypsum, herbs and honey around 1,000 BC. Some 1,000 years later, Greeks and Romans added more abrasives to the powder mixture, for example crushed bones and oyster shells. Romans appear also to be the first to add flavors, most likely to help with bad breath and to make their paste more palatable. This flavoring was more or less powdered charcoal and bark – distant relatives of nowadays flavors. Around the same time, China and India were using a powder/paste as well. The Chinese in particular were formulating their toothpastes with flavoring, such as ginseng, herbal mints, and salt, thereby resembling toothpastes which are not too dissimilar from those used nowadays. Most common issues with ancient toothpastes were the high level of abrasivity, poor taste and high cost, making it not the affordable mass-market product toothpastes are nowadays.

Little change happened until the dawn of the industrial age in the 18th century, when the use of toothpowders became more common. Doctors, dentists and chemists were responsible for the development of toothpowders for the sole purpose to clean teeth. These powders were very harsh to teeth, due to abrasives such as brick dust, crushed china, earthenware and cuttlefish. The still nowadays popular bicarbonate of soda was used as the body for most toothpowders. Borax powder (sodium borate) was added at the end of the 18th century to produce a favorable foaming effect – again, a sensory cue that has survived. Glycerin was added early in the 19th century to make the powders into a paste, more palatable and to prevent the paste from drying out. Strontium was introduced at this time as well, which was believed to strengthen teeth and reduce sensitivity. A dentist called Peabody became the first person to add 'soap' (salts of fatty acids such as sodium palmitate) to toothpowder in 1824 and chalk was added in the 1850s by John Harris. In 1873, toothpaste was first mass-produced in a jar by the then Colgate & Co. In 1892, Dr. Washington Sheffield of Connecticut was the first to put toothpaste into a collapsible tube.

In 1914 came undoubtedly one of the most important breakthroughs in the history of toothpastes – the introduction of fluoride. British Patent GB 3,034 (filed in 1914, patented in 1915) describes 'Improvements in or relating to dentifrices' and therein toothpaste formulations containing sodium fluoride among others. It is unclear, however, when the first fluoridated toothpaste was actually sold. Crest toothpaste, introduced by Proct-

er & Gamble in the USA in test markets in 1955 and across the entire USA in 1956, was likely to be first mass-marketed fluoride toothpaste in the world. This launch came after more than 10 years of caries research and largely due to a joint research project headed by Dr. Joseph Muhler at Indiana University. A new toothpaste containing 1,000 ppm fluoride as stannous fluoride and heat-treated calcium phosphate as abrasive was developed. This toothpaste was found to result in a significant reduction in caries occurrence in children in a clinical trial [12]. This was, however, not the first reported caries trial employing fluoride toothpaste. An earlier study by Bibby [13], evaluating the anticaries benefits of several 500 ppm fluoride as sodium fluoride-containing toothpastes in children and adolescents was unable to demonstrate a cariostatic benefit. It is worth noting that new introductions are often seen with a certain degree of skepticism – the American Dental Association (ADA) were initially opposed to fluoride, which can be understood given the poor understanding of fluoride's toxicity at the time. However, the ADA approved the use of fluoride salts in toothpastes in 1960, paving the way for a global roll-out of fluoride toothpastes.

Jumping back in time, the development of synthetic surfactants after World War II led to the introduction of sodium lauryl sulfate (SLS), which is still the most commonly used surfactant in toothpastes nowadays. But what else happened to toothpastes during the last century? Manufacturers have gradually improved formulations for better fluoride bioavailability, lower abrasivity, better stain removal and breath freshening. Furthermore, toothpastes have become 'multitaskers' due to the incorporation of active ingredients in the hope to combat a variety of oral diseases and conditions and to provide cosmetic benefits. Worth mentioning here are antiplaque agents which were largely introduced in the 1980s to control the formation of supragingival plaque and antitartar agents. Several other, more or less anecdotal, references about supposedly therapeutic toothpaste ingredients which have been tried and (most of them) forgotten about can be found elsewhere [14]. It must be noted though that enzymes can still be found in some toothpastes nowadays. Supposedly, enzymes support gingival health, whitening, and plaque removal, although there is little scientific evidence to support any of these functions. In Europe, a toothpaste containing glucose oxidase and amyloglucosidase to support the natural antimicrobial activity of saliva and plaque fluid has been successfully marketed.

The development of toothpastes, however, is far from complete. The biggest challenge yet to overcome is the generally poor intraoral substantivity of active agents and most importantly fluoride [15].

Toothpaste Ingredients and Delivery Formats

Toothpastes are perhaps the most complex healthcare product. Typically, an abrasive or mixture thereof is suspended in an aqueous humectant phase by means of a hydrocolloid. In this matrix, surfactants, active (i.e. therapeutic) ingredients, flavor compounds, sweeteners, colorings, preservatives and other excipients are embedded [16].

During brushing, toothpaste slurry will be formed with saliva as the slurry medium and the mechanical aid of the toothbrush. Slurry formation will not only aid in the dispersion of active ingredients in the oral cavity, it will also lower their concentration – the more dilute the slurry, the lower their concentration. Furthermore, saliva will also alter the slurry pH due to its buffering capacity (less so for strongly buffered toothpaste, e.g. $NaHCO_3$ pastes), increase its temperature and allow for saliva components (e.g. Ca, proteins) to react with toothpaste excipients. Why is all this important? An ideal scenario would be the immediate reaction of active ingredients with their specific target site(s) to allow for maximum efficacy. However, this does not occur with tooth-

pastes as the toothpaste needs to be dispersed first to release its active ingredients. And depending on the formulation and perhaps also the toothbrush head geometry and filaments and certainly the person's brushing technique, this process of distribution of active ingredients in the oral cavity is by no means straightforward. Furthermore, salivary secretion rates and composition further complicate the matter as these vary considerably between individuals [17].

Are toothpastes even the most efficacious means to deliver active ingredients? Most likely, no, they are not. Almost all active ingredients, esp. fluoride and antiplaque agents, are best delivered in a rinse delivery format as toothpaste formulation excipients typically lower their bioavailability. Perfect examples worth mentioning here are cetylpyridinium chloride and chlorhexidine digluconate – both are easily formulated in a rinse, but difficult to formulate into a paste format due to required presence of abrasives, viscosity and rheology modifiers and surfactants. Rinses can be specifically formulated for maximum stability and bioavailability of actives; the larger volume of an applied rinse vs. the mass of a full head of toothpaste also allow for a higher dose and concentration of an active to be applied; interactions with salivary components are comparatively limited as solutions reach their target site without the need of saliva, and, likewise, actives can be delivered at specific pH values as the dilution of rinses with saliva is largely insignificant. But one has to bear in mind that tooth brushing is the most common form of oral hygiene in the world and the most efficient means to physically remove plaque. Furthermore, toothpastes can be formulated in the absence of water, i.e. in a non-aqueous base, allowing excipients and active ingredients to be incorporated that cannot be incorporated into a rinse. Also, changing oral care habits by introducing pre- or postbrushing rinses would mean to revolutionize the world of oral care which will likely prove an improbable task, given the historic role of toothpastes. Hence, every effort should be taken to optimize the delivery of actives from toothpastes – from both manufacturers and researchers alike.

Active Ingredients
Therapeutic agents will be discussed in greater detail in the forthcoming chapters. Hence, the information provided here should be seen as a brief summary.

Fluorides
Depending on the country's or region's specific legislation, several fluoride compounds can be utilized and at various concentrations. As the legislation varies considerably between countries, only information from the EU [18] and the USA [19], as two important oral care markets, are presented here.

In the EU, fluoride compounds are regulated as a cosmetic, and a total of 20 different compounds are permissible (table 1). Mixtures of several fluoride compounds are allowed, providing the maximum concentration of fluoride does not exceed 1,500 ppm. Rather interestingly, several of the permissible fluoride compounds (e.g. CaF_2, MgF_2) are only sparingly soluble.

In the USA, fluoride compounds are regulated as a drug and far fewer compounds are permissible (table 2).

Mixtures of various fluoride compounds are not allowed, and unlike in the EU, toothpastes are required to contain a certain level of (bio) available fluoride which depends on the fluoride compound. The rationale behind these requirements is sound and reflects what is known about the effectiveness of fluoride – fluoride has cariostatic properties only when present in its ionic form. The differences in minimum concentrations between fluoride compounds are likely due to historic reasons (these guidelines were put together after a 25-year-long process in 1995) – abrasives were of poorer quality than nowadays and used to contain a certain level of metal impurities (e.g. Ca, Mg, Al) which will reduce the concentration of soluble fluoride in formulation over time and especially in those formulations containing NaF. Likewise, SnF_2 is not formulated in the presence of calcium pyrophosphate anymore due to the poor compatibility of both ingredients. Toothpastes containing Na_2PO_3F can be formulated with literally any abrasive due the excellent compatibility of the monofluorophosphate ion with e.g. Ca-containing abrasives. Consequently, the requirements for available fluoride for toothpastes containing Na_2PO_3F are somewhat stricter.

The Federal Drug Administration also introduced 'testing procedures for fluoride dentifrice drug products' which manufacturers of oral care products containing fluoride are required to adhere to. Any new fluoride toothpaste is required to be at least equivalent to its relevant United States Pharmacopeia reference standard in the animal caries reduction test, and either the enamel solubility reduction or the fluoride enamel uptake tests. While these tests provide some assurance of predicted clinical effectiveness, they can now be questioned for their scientific merit and should be replaced with more accurate surrogate measures of clinical efficacy, such as laboratory pH cycling models capable of demonstrating a fluoride dose-response as a minimum standard [see Tenuta and Cury, this vol.].

Legislative differences exist between maximum permissible fluoride concentrations in toothpastes for adults and children under the age of 6 years. In the EU, the latter can contain a maximum of 1,500 ppm fluoride, although fluoride concentrations vary considerably between toothpastes (250–1,500 ppm fluoride) intended to be used by children aged 6 years and lower. In the USA, the maximum permissible fluoride concentration is 1,150 ppm for ages 2 years and up with little variation in fluoride concentration among products from major brands due to the drug status of fluoride compounds in toothpastes.

In almost all other parts of the world, only three fluoride compounds can be found in tooth-

Table 1. Fluoride compounds approved for the use in cosmetic products in the EU (in alphabetical order by substance name) [18]

Substance	Linear formula	INCI[1]	IUPAC[1]
Amine fluoride 3-(N-hexadecyl-N-2-hydroxyethyl-ammonio) propylbis(2-hydroxy-ethyl) ammonium dihydrofluoride[2]	$C_{27}H_{59}N_2O_3F_2$	olaflur	olaflur
Aluminium fluoride[2]	AlF_3		
Ammonium monofluorophosphate	$(NH_4)_2PO_3F$	not listed	
Ammonium fluoride	NH_4F		
Ammonium fluorosilicate	$(NH_4)_2SiF_6$		ammonium hexafluorosilicate
Calcium fluoride	CaF_2		
Calcium monofluorophosphate	$CaPO_3F$		calcium fluorophosphate
Hexadecyl ammonium fluoride	$C_{16}H_{35}NHF$	cetylamine hydrofluoride	hetaflur
Magnesium fluoride	MgF_2		
Magnesium fluorosilicate	$MgSiF_6$		magnesium hexafluorosilicate
N,N′,N′-tris(polyoxyethylene)-N-hexadecyl-propylenediamine dihydrofluoride	n/a	not listed	
Nicomethanol hydrofluoride[2]	C_6H_8FNO	not listed	
Octadecenyl-ammonium fluoride	n/a	not listed	
Potassium fluoride[2]	KF		
Potassium fluorosilicate	K_2SiF_6		dipotassium hexafluorosilicate
Potassium monofluorophosphate	K_2PO_3F		dipotassium fluorophosphate
Sodium fluoride[2]	NaF		
Sodium fluorosilicate	Na_2SiF_6		disodium hexafluorosilicate
Sodium monofluorophosphate[2]	Na_2PO_3F		disodium monofluorophosphate
Tin difluoride[2]	SnF_2	stannous fluoride	

[1] INCI (International Nomenclature of Cosmetic Ingredients) and/or IUPAC (International Union of Pure and Applied Chemistry) names are only shown if different from the substance name.
[2] Substances which are presently being utilized in toothpastes sold in Europe.

Table 2. Fluoride compounds approved for the use in toothpastes in the USA (in alphabetical order by substance name) [19]

Substance	Permissible theoretical fluoride concentration, ppm	Minimum available fluoride concentration, ppm
Sodium fluoride	850–1,150	650
Sodium monofluorophosphate	850–1,150 or 1,500	800 or 1,275
Stannous fluoride	850–1,150	700 or 290 for products containing calcium pyrophosphate

pastes – NaF, Na_2PO_3F or SnF_2 – presumably because most markets are dominated by the same companies as in the EU and USA.

Antiplaque/Antigingivitis Agents

The most commonly used and scientifically supported antiplaque/antigingivitis agents in toothpastes are triclosan, stannous chloride/fluoride and zinc citrate/chloride.

Triclosan [IUPAC name: 5-chloro-2-(2,4-dichlorophenoxy)phenol] was introduced in combination with Gantrez® (copolymer of methylvinyl ether and maleic acid) with the latter claimed to enhance the intraoral substantivity of triclosan [20]. It is typically used at a concentration of 0.3% w/w and Gantrez at 2% w/w. Triclosan is classified as 'very toxic to aquatic life with long lasting effects' according to The Globally Harmonized System of Classification and Labelling of Chemicals and has, consequently, come under more scrutiny in recent years. The EU's Scientific Committee on Consumer safety, having reviewed the issue of antimicrobial resistance, supports the continued use of triclosan in cosmetics. Due to its chemical nature, triclosan can migrate into the plastic, thereby requiring good quality packaging material to sustain availability. Triclosan has also been reported to have a direct anti-inflammatory effect on the gingival tissues [21].

Stannous fluoride has been used extensively in the past and was revived several years ago and on a more holistic scale by two manufacturers. Formulations containing a combination of stannous fluoride and stannous chloride have been introduced with the aim to increase the stannous concentration as the amount of stannous from stannous fluoride is limited by the permissible fluoride concentration. The stannous chemistry is complex as several species form upon hydration of stannous fluoride or its reaction with the dental hard tissues. Due to the reactive nature of the tin(II) ion, it has to be stabilized in a formulation to prevent it from being oxidized [to tin(IV); i.e. stannic] and consequently become insoluble and ineffective. Stannous salts require low pH formulations and the presence of sodium gluconate and/or olaflur (amine fluoride), which will act as chelators, for optimum stability. Stannous has often been linked to extrinsic staining, but improved formulations (e.g. use of polyphosphates) have largely overcome this issue.

Zinc salts have been used in combination with triclosan or stannous salts or on their own. The two most commonly used salts are zinc citrate and zinc chloride. The citrate salt is only sparingly soluble, whereas the chloride is readily soluble. Zinc salts are astringent and their metallic taste is difficult to mask. Zinc chloride is typically formulated with molar excess of sodium citrate as it would be unpalatable otherwise. Zinc salts are incompatible with phosphates due to their poor solubility. Zinc citrate is used up to 2% w/w, whereas zinc chloride's upper limit is approx. 0.5% w/w.

More recently, o-cymen-5-ol (INCI name; IUPAC name: 4-isopropyl-m-cresol; systematic name: 4-isopropyl-3-methylphenol, or more commonly IPMP), an antimicrobial and anti-inflammatory agent, has been introduced by several manufacturers either alone or in combination with zinc salts.

Antimalodor Agents

Antimalodor agents typically rely on the chemical reaction with volatile sulfur compounds (VSCs) such as methyl mercaptan and hydrogen sulfide. The above-mentioned zinc salts are most commonly used as zinc does not only possess antimicrobial properties. Zinc is also capable to react with VSCs, thereby turning them into non-volatile zinc salts (zinc sulfide is one of the least soluble compounds) [22].

Antitartar/Anticalculus Agents

Calculus is defined as 'a concretion usually of mineral salts around organic material found especially in hollow organs or ducts' [23], whereas tartar is defined as 'an incrustation on the teeth consisting of plaque that has become hardened by the deposition of mineral salts' [24]. Hence, only the term tartar will be used hereafter. Antitartar agents are essentially apatite crystal growth inhibitors and aid in the removal and prevention of supragingival plaque. These agents basically act as 'crystal poisons' and prevent further growth of apatitic or other calcium phosphate phases [25]. The most common ones are condensed inorganic and organic phosphates, either linear or cyclic in structure. Among these, sodium or potassium salts of the pyrophosphate, tripolyphosphate or hexametaphosphate ion are most often found in toothpastes (used at 5–12% w/w). These formulations are typically high in pH to prevent hydrolysis of the condensed phosphate. Also, zinc salts are being utilized as well, but not in combination with condensed phosphates (the resulting zinc phosphate is insoluble and inactive), as these too act as crystal growth inhibitors. Antitartar formulations typically exhibit higher flavor contents to mask the taste of the condensed phosphate.

Whitening Agents
Formulation ingredients for enhanced extrinsic stain removal and prevention can be divided into mechanical, chemical and optical whitening agents, depending on their mode of action. Most chemical whitening agents are condensed phosphates (see above) with the exact same salts being utilized not only for antitartar benefits, but also for enhanced stain removal and prevention. It has been shown that these agents are capable of displacing pellicle proteins and pellicle-bound stains and prevent the de novo adhesion of new stain molecules [26–28]. Others worth noting are enzymes, such as papain and peroxides (see next paragraph), although the scientific evidence to support a whitening action for either delivered from toothpaste is somewhat dubious. Mechanical whitening agents rely on the physical removal of extrinsic stains. Here, most commonly abrasives with different morphology, mean particle size and hardness compared to conventional abrasives (see separate chapter) are being utilized.

Toothpaste formulations typically contain a combination of chemical and mechanical whitening agents due to (likely) synergistic effects. Recently, toothpaste containing blue covarine (a frequently used optical brightener) was launched. Blue covarine is said to adhere to the tooth surface, thereby changing the optical properties of the teeth and not only perceivably but also measurably whitening teeth [29].

Intrinsic stain removal is difficult to accomplish with toothpastes as the chemical as well as mechanical whitening agents are limited to the removal of surface-bound stains. While toothpastes with hydrogen peroxide (to bleach enamel, thereby oxidizing intrinsic stain molecules and consequently changing their absorption spectra to become invisible to the naked eye) have been marketed, their efficacy is debatable to say the least. Hydrogen peroxide is difficult to stabilize in toothpaste formulations and the concentrations found (approx. 1% w/w) combined with the short treatment period are unlikely to provide a significant intrinsic whitening benefit. Hence, these toothpastes often also contain chemical and mechanical whitening agents with the addition of hydrogen peroxide being more or less a marketing ploy. In Europe, only 0.1% H_2O_2 is allowed.

Agents for the Relief of Dentin Hypersensitivity
The relief of dentin hypersensitivity can be accomplished in different ways – through nerve desensitization and/or physical blockage ('plugging') of dentinal tubules (occlusion) [30]. Nerve desensitization can be accomplished by potassium salts, such as the citrate and nitrate. These salts are typically used at relatively high concentrations (approx. 5% w/w), which negatively impacts on the taste of toothpastes (bitterness). Despite their widespread use, the scientific evidence to support their efficacy is still being debated [31]. Several compounds are being used for tubule occlusion: strontium salts (acetate, chloride), stannous fluoride, and more recently calcium sodium phosphosilicate ('bioglass') and ar-

ginine bicarbonate in combination with calcium carbonate. While their mode of action is somewhat different, all these agents have been reported to occlude dentinal tubules [32–35]. However, several compromises have to be made when formulating these agents – strontium salts are being used at high concentrations (approx. 8% w/w), which limits fluoride bioavailability due to the low solubility of strontium fluoride (taste is another issue), stannous has already been discussed (see above), calcium sodium phosphosilicate requires a non-aqueous formulation, thereby limiting fluoride efficacy, and the arginine formulation requires the use of sodium monofluorophosphate due to the required presence of calcium carbonate.

Erosion Prevention Agents

Only recently, toothpastes claiming to combat dental erosion have been introduced. The lack of reliable clinical indices to measure the progression of erosion in vivo meant that these toothpastes were developed primarily using in vitro and in situ models with highly controlled, standardized and perhaps also biased conditions. The philosophy to combat erosion can almost be divided by manufacturer – some argue that an optimized delivery of sodium fluoride to enhance remineralization of an early erosive lesion is the best strategy [36, 37], whereas other manufacturers utilize the reactivity of stannous fluoride and/or chloride with the enamel and dentin surfaces to form a protective layer on the dental hard tissues [38–40]. While manufacturers have been able to produce encouraging data, the scientific evidence to support either strategy remains to be established in longitudinal in vivo studies and especially in populations most prone to this condition.

Other Noteworthy Active Ingredients

Several supposedly anticaries agents have and are being utilized in toothpastes. Among these are calcium glycerophosphate (CaGP) [41], xylitol [42], isomalt [43] nano-hydroxyapatite (primarily in Japan) [44], sodium trimetaphosphate [45] and co-called remineralizing agents (e.g. 'enamelon' technology, CPP-ACP) [46, 47] which will be addressed separately. CaGP and nano-hydroxyapatite cannot (or should not!) be formulated with sodium fluoride in a single-phase formulation due to poor fluoride bioavailability. Dual-phase formulations, i.e. two formulations which come in contact with another when dispersed, are one route to avoid ingredient incompatibilities, but are generally avoided by manufacturers due to considerably higher costs. Furthermore, the clinical benefit of co-delivery of incompatible actives from dual-phase formulations has not been fully investigated yet, although one study [see 55] highlighted some benefits.

Formulation Excipients

Whereas the above-discussed active ingredients are largely responsible for the therapeutic benefits of toothpaste, toothpaste would not be toothpaste without the below discussed excipients.

Abrasives

Abrasives are the most traditional toothpaste excipient and contribute secondarily to toothpaste rheology. During brushing, abrasive particles can become trapped between toothbrush bristles. As these particles are harder than the stain but softer than sound enamel, stain can be removed without causing significant damage to the tooth surface [48]. The abrasives used in toothpastes include hydrated silica, calcium carbonate, dicalcium phosphate dihydrate, calcium pyrophosphate, sodium metaphosphate, alumina, perlite, nano-hydroxyapatite and sodium bicarbonate. The abrasive cleaning process is affected by various key parameters, such as particle hardness, shape, size, size distribution, concentration and applied load during brushing. Furthermore, toothbrush filament diameter and shape also impact on how abrasive particles are being dragged across the hard tissue surface. The amount of abrasive to be used in a formulation does not only depend on the type but also on the level of cleaning ability one wants to achieve. Hydrated silica and calcium carbonate are the most common abrasives and are typically used at concentrations ranging between 8 and 20% w/w, whereas sodium bicarbonate can be used in excess of 50% w/w. While the latter is the least abrasive material for cleaning teeth, it adds a salty taste to toothpaste and negatively impacts on foaming. Dicalcium phosphate dihydrate and calcium pyrophosphate are also being utilized, but, in addition to calcium carbonate, cannot/should not be formulated with sodium fluoride due to poor fluoride bioavailability. Hydrated silica is the abrasive of choice in clear gel type formulations as a refractive index of approx. 1.45 of the final product is required. Alumina and perlite are polishing agents. Due to their high abrasivity on enamel, however, they are only used at low concentrations (approx. 1–2% w/w) and in combination with conventional abrasives and/or chemical whitening agents. The 'holy grail' for manufacturers of abrasives and toothpaste manufacturers alike is to make toothpastes that clean well while being virtually non-abrasive to the dental hard tissues and especially dentin.

Surfactants
Surfactants are not only responsible for the foaming action of toothpastes, they also aid in the intraoral dispersion of toothpaste and in the micellization of hydrophobic ingredients, such as flavor compounds and organic antiplaque/antigingivitis actives (e.g. triclosan). Depending on the nature of the hydrophilic part of the surfactant molecule, they can be classified as anionic, cationic, nonionic or amphoteric. This moiety also determines the surfactant's irritancy with, generally speaking, anionic and cationic surfactants being considerably more irritant than amphoteric and non-ionic ones which are the least irritant [see 49 for more detail]. Overall, very few different surfactants are being used by major toothpaste manufacturers, primarily due to taste and cost reasons. Surfactants are typically used at concentrations ranging from 0.5 to 2.5% w/w. The most commonly used surfactant in toothpastes, SLS (IUPAC name: sodium dodecyl sulphate) belongs to the group of anionic surfactants. Other anionic surfactants used in toothpaste formulations belong to the group of sarcosinates, e.g. sodium lauroyl sarcosinate (IUPAC name: sodium 2-[dodecanoyl(methyl)amino]acetate) and sodium cocoyl sarcosinate (IUPAC name: sodium 2-(methylamino)acetate). The most common amphoteric surfactant is cocamidopropyl betaine (IUPAC name: {[3-(dodecanoylamino)propyl] (dimethyl)ammonio}acetate), which has not been linked with canker sores but does not foam as well as SLS. Toothpastes containing amine fluoride such as olaflur typically do not contain added surfactants as the amine cation functions as surfactant molecule and therefore aids the intraoral dispersion of fluoride. Nonionic surfactants are currently not being utilized in toothpaste but in mouthwash formulations due to their poor foaming ability. Combinations of several different surfactants, most often SLS and cocamidopropyl betaine, are being used when an enhanced foaming action is desired (formation of mixed micelles) [50].

More recently, some manufacturers have moved away from SLS and introduced other, less irritant surfactants with similar foaming ability. Among those are the groups of non-ionic polyethylene glycol ethers of stearic acid (e.g. Steareth-30) and anionic alkyl sulfonates (e.g. sodium C14–16 olefin sulfonate, sodium C14–17 secondary alkyl sulfonate).

Viscosity and Rheology Modifiers
The primary function of viscosity and rheology modifiers is to produce a gel phase containing a homogeneous distribution of all toothpaste ingredients and to prevent the components from separating during long periods of storage. Separa-

tion is often referred to as syneresis which is defined as the spontaneous separation of a liquid from a gel or colloidal suspension [51]. The viscosity and rheology modifiers will also contribute to viscosity build and are responsible for an easy but not too rapid flow of toothpaste from the tube and a clear break rather than stringy appearance when applied to a toothbrush and a good ribbon stand-up. The most common viscosity and rheology modifiers are carboxymethylcellulose, hydroxyethylcellulose, carrageenan, xanthan gum, cellulose gum, and crosslinked polyacrylates which are being used at concentrations ranging between 0.5 and 2.0% w/w. Additionally, thickening silicas (used at approx. 10% w/w) are often being used to aid in viscosity build-up and as a processing aid. These silicas differ from those used as abrasives due to their higher structure and very low cleaning ability.

Humectants

Humectants are being used to avoid water separation and evaporation ('capping-off', i.e. drying out of paste at the dispensing point is one of the major issues), to provide a smooth and glossy appearance, and to provide a homogenous delivery system. Glycerin and sorbitol are the most commonly used compounds for this purpose and primarily based on their compatibility with other formulation excipients and raw material cost. Glycerin and sorbitol are used in combination as an all-sorbitol formulation would still suffer from 'capping-off' and a stringy appearance, whereas an all-glycerin formulation would not allow the use of rheology and viscosity modifiers, thereby raising the risk of separation of ingredients during long-term storage. Hence, manufacturers often settle for formulations containing water, glycerin and sorbitol. A non-aqueous formulation is not desirable due to the high cost and limitations in fluoride delivery/efficacy. Humectant concentrations in toothpastes are typically between 20 and 30% w/w with the majority being sorbitol. Toothpaste formulations in pumps rather than tubes contain higher humectant concentrations due to increased risk of 'capping-off'. In addition to glycerin and sorbitol, propylene glycol, xylitol, isomalt and erythritol are being used as humectants.

Flavors

Flavors are added primarily for cosmetic/palatable reasons. They mask the often unpleasant taste of surfactants, provide breath freshening and sensorial cues such as cooling, heating or tingling, depending on the flavor compound being used. Universally, mint flavors are most commonly used, but others such as herbal, cinnamon or lemon are also found in local markets. Flavors are the most expensive and most volatile excipient and can be used at concentrations between 0.3 and 2.0% w/w. Surfactants are primarily responsible for dispersion of flavors in toothpastes.

Sweeteners

Sweeteners are added to toothpastes to improve their taste. All commonly used sweeteners are artificial and the majority of toothpaste manufacturers utilize either sodium saccharin or, albeit rarely, sucralose. Typically, sweeteners are used at concentrations below 0.5% w/w. Xylitol (typically used at approx. 10% w/w) can also be considered a sweetener, although its main and still discussed purpose is caries prevention.

Coloring

The color of toothpaste is important for consumer acceptability. The majority of manufacturers desire a white paste which can be combined with various colored stripes to suggest multiple benefits. Whiteness is achieved by adding titanium dioxide (approx. 1% w/w), whereas artificial colorants (approx. 0.1% w/w) are added to realize colored stripes or a colored core.

Stripes can be introduced in different ways. The two most common forms are (a) filling a single compartment tube simultaneously with striped cores of the same paste, or (b) filling one or more striped core into different compartments of the tube. Different nozzle designs then allow for striped toothpaste of varying proportions of colored to white cores.

As mentioned above, clear toothpastes (refractive index of approx. 1.45) are achieved by the choice of abrasive (silica) and a certain humectant/water ratio which will also depend on other excipients.

Preservatives

Toothpaste formulations that do not contain an ionic surfactant are often formulated with preservatives (approx. 0.2% w/w) to prevent bacterial growth during long-term storage. The most commonly used preservatives are sodium benzoate, ethyl and methyl paraben. Few formulations contain preservatives nowadays, as growth of microorganisms is usually prevented in formulations with high humectant levels due to the high osmotic pressure in the aqueous phase. Furthermore, anionic surfactants are inherently antimicrobial and flavor compounds also contribute to stability.

Water

Undoubtedly, the cheapest excipient which manufacturers strive to maximize in toothpaste formulation – water – is an important solvent for inorganic active ingredients and most importantly fluorides. Water needs to be purified first to remove calcium and trace elements that could lower the stability and bioavailability of active ingredients. Non-aqueous formulations have the disadvantage that inorganic active ingredients are present in their solid state and need to be solubilized by saliva first before they can interact with their target tissue(s). Hence, water is an important excipient.

Other Excipients

Mica (part of the phyllosilicate mineral family) is used for its sparkle and polishing ability in toothpastes. Sodium hydroxide is used for pH adjustment, ethanol as a solvent and polyethylene and polypropylene glycols are used as humectants, dispersants and to keep xanthan gum uniformly dispersed in toothpastes. Other noteworthy excipients (which are often attributed 'efficacy' by some manufacturers despite being unsubstantiated due to the lack of credible evidence) are vitamins C and E as antioxidants and allantoin for 'gum health', enzymes (e.g. glucose oxidase, lactoferrin, lactoperoxidase, lysozyme) for the prevention of plaque growth and herbal extracts for their antimicrobial properties.

Delivery Formats

The most traditional toothpaste delivery format is the tube. Toothpaste in pumps is also available, but due to higher formulations and production costs and the greater likelihood of 'capping-off', pumps are not preferred among manufacturers. Formulations of lower viscosity are delivered in stand-up tubes for easier dispensing. Recently, one manufacturer introduced gel-to-foam products delivered in a can. The formulations contain isopentane which, because of its low boiling point, supposedly aids in the intra-oral dispersion of actives.

Almost all commercial toothpastes nowadays are sold in single-phase tubes. Dual- or multiple phase tubes can be utilized when several incompatible ingredients are to be used that would otherwise chemically react and lower an active's bioavailability in a single-phase tube. A typical example would be the co-delivery of calcium and fluoride salts.

Safety Issues Relating to Toothpaste Ingredients

Perhaps the biggest concern about fluoride toothpastes is fluoride toxicity through accidental or deliberate ingestion. The 'probably toxic dose' of fluoride has been estimated as 5 mg/kg body weight [52]. This would equate to 33.3 g 1,500 ppm fluoride toothpaste (roughly 1/3 of a 75 ml tube) for a child with a body weight of 10 kg. On the other end of the spectrum, one has to consider the 'upper limit for fluoride intake by children' [53] where accidental/deliberate swallowing of fluoride toothpaste during brushing is the main contributor to fluoride intake.

The American Academy of Pediatrics proposed a daily fluoride dose of between 0.05 and 0.07 mg fluoride/kg body weight/day as an upper limit [54], which would equate to 0.3 g 1,500 ppm fluoride toothpaste, not considering other sources of fluoride intake, of course. In adults, a tolerable upper intake level of 10 mg fluoride per day was recommended by the US Institute of Medicine (6.6 g 1,500 ppm fluoride toothpaste) [55]. A recent review [56] concluded that 'weak unreliable evidence that starting the use of fluoride toothpaste in children less than 12 months of age may be associated with an increased risk of fluorosis. The evidence for its use between the age of 12 and 24 months is equivocal. If the risk of fluorosis is of concern, the fluoride level of toothpaste for young children (under 6 years of age) is recommended to be lower than 1,000 ppm'.

A further safety concern is related to the most commonly used surfactant, SLS, which has been linked with the occurrence of aphthous ulcers ('canker sores') [57, 58]. The leading toothpaste manufacturers still continue to utilize SLS, however, because of its desired foaming ability, acceptable taste and (especially) low cost in relation to other surfactants. Only very few currently marketed toothpastes contain a surfactant other than SLS.

More anecdotal at this moment in time are case reports on mucosal sloughing in relation to the use of antitartar and chemical whitening toothpastes [59]. The high pH of these formulations in combinations with higher flavor contents can ostensibly irritate mucous membranes.

Toothpastes – A Missed Opportunity?

Are fluoride toothpastes more effective than their counterparts 20–30 years ago? What advances have been made in fluoride delivery over the last few decades? Do we fully understand intraoral fluoride delivery and how to optimize it? These are perhaps the most pertinent questions manufacturers and researcher alike should ask themselves. Undoubtedly, our understanding of fluoride delivery has improved considerably since its introduction, but enhancing fluoride substantivity is still the biggest obstacle in reducing the prevalence of dental caries.

Manufacturers, perhaps driven by consumer demand, have gradually moved away from dental caries and introduced several other purposes of toothbrushing over the last few decades – most importantly whitening, but also treatment and prevention of gingivitis, erosion and/or dentin hypersensitivity, breath freshening, etc. Formulations had to be optimized to deliver these benefits (e.g. water content, pH), with manufacturers perhaps sometimes unaware of the effect on fluoride delivery. Understandably, not every new formulation can be tested in a caries clinical trial. But rigorous testing should be conducted to protect the public from products that do not provide a clinically meaningful benefit. Typical examples would be non-fluoride toothpastes marketed with anticaries claims that are not supported by credible scientific evidence or fluoride toothpastes with poor fluoride bioavailability. A joint effort from manufacturers and researchers is therefore required to not only improve fluoride delivery, but also to develop unbiased models that predict the likely clinical outcome [see Tenuta and Cury, this vol.].

References

1 Jardim JJ, Alves LS, Maltz M: The history and global market of oral home-care products. Braz Oral Res 2009; 23(suppl 1):17–22.

2 Horseman RE: The her-story of toothpaste. J Calif Dent Assoc 2006;34: 769–770.

3 http://www.h2g2.com/approved_entry/A2818686; accessed November 2012.

4 http://users.forthnet.gr/ath/abyss/dep1342.htm; accessed November 2012.

5 https://files.nyu.edu/ssg280/public/toothpaste_history.html; accessed November 2012.

6 http://www.huffingtonpost.com/thomas-p-connelly-dds/mouth-health-the-history-_b_702332.html; accessed November 2012.

7 http://www.saveyoursmile.com/toothpaste/toothpaste-a.html; accessed November 2012.

8 http://www.toothpasteworld.com/history.php; accessed November 2012.

9 http://www.buzzle.com/articles/history-of-toothpaste.html; accessed November 2012.

10 http://connecticuthistory.org/aristocratic-dental-cream-gets-squeezed/; accessed November 2012.

11 http://www.fluoride-history.de/p-dentifrice.htm; accessed November 2012.

12 Muhler JC, Radike AW, Nebergall WH, Day HG: The effect of a stannous fluoride-containing dentifrice on caries reduction in children. J Dent Res 1954; 33:606–612.

13 Bibby BG: A test of the effect of fluoride-containing dentifrices on dental caries. J Dent Res 1945;24:297–303.

14 Emslie RD: A history of oral hygiene measures. Comm Dent Oral Epidem 1980;8:225–229.

15 Sjogren K: How to improve oral fluoride retention? Caries Res 2001;35:14–17.

16 Watson CA: Synthetic hydrocolloids and dentifrices. J Soc Cosmet Chem 1970;21: 459–470.

17 Benedek-Spat E: The composition of unstimulated human parotid saliva. Arch Oral Biol 1973;18:39–47.

18 Council Directive 76/768/EEC of 27 July 1976 on the approximation of the laws of the Member States relating to cosmetic products. http://eur-lex.europa.eu/LexUriServ/LexUriServ.do?uri=OJ:L:1976:262:0169:0200:EN:PDF; accessed November 2012.

19 US Food and Drug Administration. CFR – Code of Federal Regulations Title 21 –Food and drugs. Chapter I – Food and Drug Administration Department of Health and Human Services. Subchapter D – Drugs for human use part 355; Anticaries drug products for over-the-counter human use. http://www.accessdata.fda.gov/scripts/cdrh/cfdocs/cfcfr/CFRSearch.cfm?CFRPart=355; accessed November 2012.

20 Peter S, Nayak DG, Philip P, Bijlani NS: Antiplaque and antigingivitis efficacy of toothpastes containing triclosan and fluoride. Int Dent J 2004;54:299–303.

21 Gaffar A, Scherl D, Afflitto J, Coleman EJ: The effect of triclosan on mediators of gingival inflammation. J Clin Periodontol 1995;22:480–484.

22 Young A, Jonski G, Rolla G: Inhibition of orally produced volatile sulfur compounds by zinc, chlorhexidine or cetylpyridinium chloride – effect of concentration. Eur J Oral Sci 2003;111: 400–404.

23 http://www.merriam-webster.com/medlineplus/calculus; accessed November 2012.

24 http://www.merriam-webster.com/dictionary/tartar; accessed November 2012.

25 Simkiss K: Phosphates as crystal poisons of calcification. Biol Rev Cambridge Philosoph Soc 1964;39:487–505.

26 Rykke M, Rolla G, Sonju T: Effect of pyrophosphate on protein adsorption to hydroxyapatite in vitro and on pellicle formation in vivo. Scand J Dent Res 1988;96:517–522.

27 Rykke M, Rolla G: Desorption of acquired enamel pellicle in vivo by pyrophosphate. Scand J Dent Res 1990;98:211–214.

28 White DJ: A new and improved 'dual action' whitening dentifrice technology: Sodium hexametaphosphate. J Clin Dent 2002;13:1–5.

29 Joiner A, Philpotts CJ, Alonso C, Ashcroft AT, Sygrove NJ: A novel optical approach to achieving tooth whitening. J Dent 2008;36:S8–S14.

30 Addy M, Dowell P: Dentine hypersensitivity – a review. Clinical and in vitro evaluation of treatment agents. J Clin Periodontol 1983;10:351–363.

31 Poulsen S, Errobe M, Lescay MY, Glenny AM: Potassium containing toothpastes for dentine hypersensitivity. Cochrane Database Syst Rev 2006;CD001476.

32 Blitzer B: A consideration of the possible causes of dental hypersensitivity: treatment by a strontium-ion dentifrice. Periodontics 1967;5:318–321.

33 Miller JT, Shannon IL, Kilgore WG, Bookman JE: Use of a water-free stannous fluoride-containing gel in the control of dental hypersensitivity. J Periodontol 1969;40:490–491.

34 Du Min Q, Bian Z, Jiang H, Greenspan DC, Burwell AK, Zhong J, et al: Clinical evaluation of a dentifrice containing calcium sodium phosphosilicate (novamin) for the treatment of dentin hypersensitivity. Am J Dent 2008;21: 210–214.

35 Fu YY, Li X, Que KH, Wang MH, Hu DY, Mateo LR, et al: Instant dentin hypersensitivity relief of a new desensitizing dentifrice containing 8.0% arginine, a high cleaning calcium carbonate system and 1450 ppm fluoride: a 3-day clinical study in Chengdu, China. Am J Dent 2010;23: 20A–27A.

36 Barlow AP, Sufi F, Mason SC: Evaluation of different fluoridated dentifrice formulations using an in situ erosion remineralization model. J Clin Dent 2009;20:192–198.

37 Hara AT, Kelly SA, Gonzalez-Cabezas C, Eckert GJ, Barlow AP, Mason SC, et al: Influence of fluoride availability of dentifrices on eroded enamel remineralization in situ. Caries Res 2009;43:57–63.

38 Ganss C, Klimek J, Brune V, Schurmann A: Effects of two fluoridation measures on erosion progression in human enamel and dentine in situ. Caries Res 2004;38:561–566.

39 Young A, Thrane PS, Saxegaard E, Jonski G, Rolla G: Effect of stannous fluoride toothpaste on erosion-like lesions: an in vivo study. Eur J Oral Sci 2006;114:180–183.

40 Hooper SM, Newcombe RG, Faller R, Eversole S, Addy M, West NX: The protective effects of toothpaste against erosion by orange juice: studies in situ and in vitro. J Dent 2007;35:476–481.

41 Duke SA, Rees DA, Forward GC: Increased plaque calcium and phosphorus concentrations after using a calcium carbonate toothpaste containing calcium glycerophosphate and sodium monofluorophosphate. Pilot study. Caries Res 1979;13:57–59.

42 Petersson LG, Birkhed D, Gleerup A, Johansson M, Jonsson G: Caries-preventive effect of dentifrices containing various types and concentrations of fluorides and sugar alcohols. Caries Res 1991;25:74–79.

43 Takatsuka T, Exterkate RAM, ten Cate JM: Effects of Isomalt on enamel de- and remineralization, a combined in vitro pH-cycling model and in situ study. Clin Oral Invest 2008;12:173–177.

44 Kani T, Kani M, Isozaki A, Shintani H, Ohashi T, Tokumoto T: Effect to apatite-containing dentifrices on dental caries in school children. J Dent Health 1989;39:104–109.

45 O'Mullane DM, Kavanagh D, Ellwood RP, Chesters RK, Schafer F, Huntington E, et al: A three-year clinical trial of a combination of trimetaphosphate and sodium fluoride in silica toothpastes. J Dent Res 1997;76:1776–1781.

46 Papas A, Russell D, Singh M, Kent R, Triol C, Winston A: Caries clinical trial of a remineralising toothpaste in radiation patients. Gerodontology 2008;25:76–88.

47 Reynolds EC: Anticariogenic casein phosphopeptides. Protein Peptide Lett 1999;6:295–303.

48 Joiner A: Whitening toothpastes: a review of the literature. J Dent 2010;38:E17–E24.

49 Mehling A, Kleber M, Hensen H: Comparative studies on the ocular and dermal irritation potential of surfactants. Food Chem Tox 2007;45:747–758.

50 Christov NC, Denkov ND, Kralchevsky PA, Ananthapadmanabhan KP, Lips A: Synergistic sphere-to-rod micelle transition in mixed solutions of sodium dodecyl sulfate and cocoamidopropyl betaine. Langmuir 2004;20:565–571.

51 http://encyclopedia2.thefreedictionary.com/Syneresis+(chemistry).

52 Whitford GM: Fluoride in dental products – safety considerations. J Dent Res 1987;66:1056–1060.

53 Burt BA: The changing patterns of systemic fluoride intake. J Dent Res 1992;71:1228–1237.

54 American Academy of Pediatrics: Committee on nutrition, fluoride supplementation. Pediatrics 1986;77:758–761.

55 Institute of Medicine: Dietary Reference Intakes for Calcium, Phosphorus, Magnesium, Vitamin D, and Fluoride. Washington, The National Academies Press, 1997. http://www.nap.edu/openbook.php?record_id=5776; accessed November 2012.

56 Wong MCM, Clarkson J, Glenny AM, Lo ECM, Marinho VCC, Tsang BWK, et al: Cochrane Reviews on the Benefits/Risks of Fluoride Toothpastes. J Dent Res 2011;90:573–579.

57 Chahine L, Sempson N, Wagoner C: The effect of sodium lauryl sulfate on recurrent aphthous ulcers: a clinical study. Compend Cont Edu Dent 1997;18:1238–1240.

58 Shim YJ, Choi JH, Ahn HJ, Kwon JS: Effect of sodium lauryl sulfate on recurrent aphthous stomatitis: a randomized controlled clinical trial. Oral Dis 2012;18:655–660.

59 Kowitz G, Jacobson J, Meng Z, Lucatorto F: The effects of tartar-control toothpaste on the oral soft-tissues. Oral Surg Oral Med Oral Path Oral Radiol Endodont 1990;70:529–536.

Frank Lippert
Department of Preventive and Community Dentistry
Oral Health Research Institute, Indiana University School of Dentistry
415 Lansing Street, Indianapolis, IN 46202 (USA)
E-Mail flippert@iu.edu

van Loveren C (ed): Toothpastes. Monogr Oral Sci. Basel, Karger, 2013, vol 23, pp 15–26
DOI: 10.1159/000350458

Fluorides and Non-Fluoride Remineralization Systems

Bennett T. Amaechi[a] · Cor van Loveren[b]

[a]Department of Comprehensive Dentistry, University of Texas Health Science Center at San Antonio, San Antonio, Tex.,
USA; [b]Department of Preventive Dentistry, Academic Center for Dentistry Amsterdam, University of Amsterdam and
VU University Amsterdam, Amsterdam, The Netherlands

Abstract

Caries develops when the equilibrium between de- and remineralization is unbalanced favoring demineralization. De- and remineralization occur depending on the degree of saturation of the interstitial fluids with respect to the tooth mineral. This equilibrium is positively influenced when fluoride, calcium and phosphate ions are added favoring remineralization. In addition, when fluoride is present, it will be incorporated into the newly formed mineral which is then less soluble. Toothpastes may contain fluoride and calcium ions separately or together in various compounds (remineralization systems) and may therefore reduce demineralization and promote remineralization. Formulating all these compounds in one paste may be challenging due to possible premature calcium-fluoride interactions and the low solubility of CaF_2. There is a large amount of clinical evidence supporting the potent caries preventive effect of fluoride toothpastes indisputably. The amount of clinical evidence of the effectiveness of the other remineralization systems is far less convincing. Evidence is lacking for head to head comparisons of the various remineralization systems.

Copyright © 2013 S. Karger AG, Basel

Fluoride is currently recognized as the main active ingredient in the oral hygiene arsenal responsible for the significant decline in caries prevalence that has been observed worldwide [1]. Ideally, fluoride should be present in the oral cavity 24 h a day. The best way to achieve this should rely as little as possible on the individual's compliance and should be affordable. Toothpaste is most likely to be the best choice for administering fluoride. In many studies, the efficacy of different fluoridated dentifrices has been proven. In addition, toothbrushing combines the application of fluoride with the removal of dental plaque, which not only contributes to caries prevention but also to the prevention of periodontal diseases. Toothpastes can contain fluoride in various chemical forms mainly as sodium fluoride (NaF), sodium monofluorophosphate (Na_2FPO_3), amine fluoride ($C_{27}H_{60}F_2N_2O_3$), stannous fluoride (SnF_2) or combinations of these. An overview of all fluorides permissible is given in the chapter by Lippert [2].

In the 1980s, the concept that fluoride controls caries lesion development primarily through its

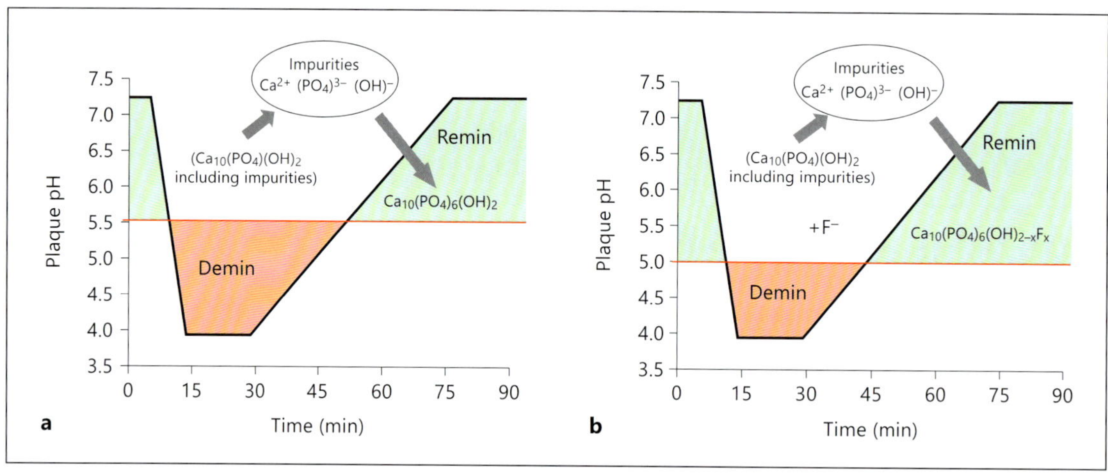

Fig. 1. Caries attack in the absence of fluoride (**a**) and in the presence of fluoride (**b**). In the presence of fluoride, the risk period (red area) is smaller than in the absence of fluoride as a result of a lower critical pH (pH 5.0 vs. 5.5). During remineralization, fluoridated hydroxyapatite is formed which is less soluble than the hydroxyapatite formed in the absence of fluoride.

topical effect on de- and remineralization taking place at the interface between tooth surface and the oral fluids was established [3–5]. During tooth development, insufficient amounts of fluoride are incorporated to give lasting protection after eruption [5, 6].

Caries and Mechanisms of Fluoride Control

Enamel, dentine and root cement consist of an inorganic component (approximately 86, 55 and 45 vol%, respectively), an organic component (approximately 4, 25 and 30 vol%, respectively) and water. The inorganic component is hydroxyapatite, $Ca_{10}(PO_4)_6(OH)_2$. During tooth formation, impurities may be incorporated in the tooth mineral, making the mineral either less or more soluble. Impurities like Mg^{2+}, Na^+, $(CO_3)^{2-}$ or $(HPO_4)^{2-}$ will make the mineral more soluble, and crystals containing these impurities will dissolve preferentially [7]. During de- and remineralization, the impurities will be washed out.

Since the oral fluid, dental plaque and the interstitial fluid of the mineral contain calcium and phosphate ions, it depends on the pH whether the environment of the tooth is saturated, under- or super-saturated with respect to the mineral. When the environment is undersaturated, demineralization will occur, and when the environment is supersaturated, remineralization will take place. When the pH in overlaying dental plaque drops below 5.5, which is called the critical pH, dissolution of enamel starts. This value varies with individual patients. When the pH rises again, over 5.5, remineralization will occur, but impurities that made the mineral more soluble, will not be built in (fig. 1a). As long as remineralization can keep up with the demineralization, cycles of de- and re mineralization will result in a mineral of better quality. This is part of the posteruptive maturation of the mineral. When remineralization cannot keep up with demineralization, i.e. when remineralization is not given sufficient time, caries lesions will develop.

In the presence of fluoride, hydroxyapatite will behave as fluorapatite, which dissolves in the oral environment only as the pH drops below approximately 5.0–4.5 (fig. 1b). This means that the critical pH for demineralization shifts by approximately 0.5–1.0 units to a more acidic critical pH value. When the pH returns to less acidic values above this 'new' critical pH, fluoride will be built into the lattice of the mineral making it less soluble. The promotion of remineralization is a result of the fact that fluoride fits better into the hydroxyapatite lattice than the OH^- ions that it preferentially replaces.

Dentine is more vulnerable to acid dissolution than enamel due to its composition and open structure. The mineral crystals are smaller than those in enamel, which means that the crystal surface area is increased and therefore the crystals are more easily attacked. Dentine also has a much larger organic component (25%) embedded in the mineral compared with enamel (4% organic component). Once the mineral is gone, the organic material is exposed to the oral environment and will be broken down by salivary and bacterial proteolytic enzymes. All these factors together make dentine more vulnerable to caries attack. Dentine demineralizes faster and remineralizes more slowly than enamel under the same experimental conditions [8]. More concentrated fluoride is needed to inhibit demineralization and to enhance remineralization. Dentine seems to benefit from a higher daily frequency of exposure to fluoride [9] and to the combination of fluoride methods [10].

In case of an 'erosive' attack at the mineral, the pH will drop far below the critical pH for even fluorapatite, which explains that the role of fluoride in the protection against erosion is only minor [11].

To interfere with the demineralization and remineralization processes, fluoride must be constantly present in the vicinity of these processes. The closest vicinity is being incorporated in the structure of the crystals, absorbed to the crystal surface and present in the interstitial fluid of the mineral. At some distance, fluoride may be present absorbed to the mineral surface, as a CaF_2 or a CaF_2-like deposit on the mineral surface, free or bound in dental plaque, in saliva or in other so called oral reservoirs, such as the soft tissues [12]. As mentioned by Duckworth, there is no strong evidence for the formation of CaF_2-like material in the mouth following use of conventional F toothpaste [12]. As pointed out above, when fluoride has absorbed to the crystal surface, the crystal behaves like fluorapatite. Furthermore, it may attract calcium to partially demineralized crystals. Fluoride in the interstitial fluid determines the amount of fluoride that absorbs to the crystals and thereby the 'fluorapatite behavior' of the crystals. The concentrations needed in the interstitial fluid for fluoride to be effective are in the sub-ppm range; as little as 0.02 mg/l are already effective [4, 13]. Each depot is, however, important for the effectiveness of fluoride as more distinct depots may deliver fluoride to the closer vicinities of the caries process. The chapters of Duckworth [12] and Tenuta and Cury [14] discuss these issues in more depth.

Fluoride is also known to inhibit the metabolism of oral microorganisms and to affect plaque composition. The concentrations needed for these effects are much higher, and approx. 100× the concentrations needed for the effects on the dynamics of the de- and remineralization processes. Therefore, the interference with the demineralization process and the promotion of remineralization are regarded as the predominant ways by which fluoride exerts its cariostatic and anticaries effects.

Fluoride Toothpaste

Fluoride toothpastes should deliver free or soluble fluoride. Toothpastes can contain fluoride in various chemical forms mainly as NaF, Na_2FPO_3, $C_{27}H_{60}F_2N_2O_3$, SnF_2 or combinations of these. The first formulations of fluoride toothpastes failed to show a significant effect due to the incompatibility of the fluoride compounds and the abrasive system. This problem is solved by either using sodium monofluorophosphate, which is compatible with calcium-containing abrasives, or by using abrasives not providing calcium ions. Sodium monofluorophosphate requires enzymatic hydrolysis to release free fluoride. The relative effectiveness of the various fluoride salts has been the topic of much debate [15, 16], but a systematic review concluded that they were equally effective [17]. This review compared 22 trials with toothpastes containing Na_2FPO_3, 10 trials with NaF toothpastes, 19 with SnF_2 pastes and 5 trials with amine fluoride. The authors emphasized that there is very little to no information from head to head comparisons. It has to be remarked that the studies were conducted with toothpaste of manufacturers who are willing to invest in research and of which it can be assumed that the whole production process is aimed at the highest performance of the pastes. There are toothpaste companies that have lower control of the production process which might result in less well-formulated and less effective products. Recently, a number of articles have been published showing that there are toothpastes on the market in which not all fluoride is available [18, 19]. In these pastes, fluoride may bind to the calcium-containing abrasives after slow hydrolysis of PO_3F^{2-}.

The associate ions will not actively interfere with the working mechanism of fluoride. However, they may facilitate fluoride to reach and adhere to the mineral surface because of an interaction with the surface (SnF_2 and $NaPO_3F$) or decreasing surface tension (amine). With SnF_2, a relatively insoluble stannous trifluorophosphate ($Sn_3F_3PO_4$) layer may be formed, and PO_3F^{2-} may be adsorbed to the mineral surface as associate ion, exchange with orthophosphate or with HPO_4^{2-} in calcium-deficient mineral. In addition, stannous and amine are known to be effective in promoting lower plaque formation and acid pro-

duction either alone or in combination [20–22]. The early SnF_2 formulations were unstable since in aqueous solutions SnF_2 is readily hydrolyzed to form insoluble precipitates of Sn^{4+} (stannic-ion) for instance as stannic fluoride which is ineffective as a dental prophylactic. Also stannic sulfides may be formed with sulfhydryl groups from denatured pellicle which gives a yellow-golden stain [23]. The formation of stannous hydroxyphosphate gives the product a bitter taste. Recent formulations are able to stabilize SnF_2 either by the addition of gluconate or amines keeping the formulations active. Some discoloration may still occur but can be prevented by the abrasives or whitening agents in the pastes.

Desirable Concentration
The clinical efficacy of fluoride toothpaste has been estimated at approximately 24% [17, 24]. Marinho et al. [17] found that the effect of fluoride toothpaste increased with higher baseline levels of D(M)FS, higher fluoride concentration, higher frequency of use and supervised brushing, but was not influenced by exposure to water fluoridation. The exact nature of the dose-response of fluoride in toothpaste however still needs further investigation. There are very few head-to-head comparisons, and therefore Walsh et al. [25] undertook a network meta-analysis utilizing both direct and indirect comparison from randomized controlled trials (table 1). The dose-response relationship is further hampered by the availability of free fluoride in the toothpastes which may depend on the total formulation and on the presence of additional remineralizing systems. These make it impossible to predict whether one toothpaste is better than the other. It was shown that the clinical efficacy of a 500-ppm fluoride toothpaste was similar to a 1,100-ppm toothpaste when used by caries-inactive children, but when the low fluoride toothpaste was used by caries-active children it seemed less effective than the 1,100-ppm formulation [26]. Stookey et al. [27] was not able to show a differ-

Table 1. Direct and network comparison of the clinical effectiveness of toothpastes (pooled DMFS PF) with different fluoride concentrations

Comparison	Direct comparison		Network meta-analysis	
	DMFS PF	95% CI	DMFS PF	95% CI
Placebo vs.				
250 ppm	8.9	−1.6 to 19.4	9.1	−3.7 to 22.0
440–550 ppm	7.9	−6.1 to 21.9	15.4	−1.9 to 32.5
1,000–1,250 ppm	22.2	18.7 to 25.7	23.0	19.4 to 26.6
1,450/1,500 ppm	22	15.3 to 28.9	29.3	21.2 to 37.5
1,700–2,200 ppm			34	16.5 to 50.8
2,400–2,800 ppm	36.6	17.5 to 55.6	35.5	27.2 to 43.6
440–550 ppm vs.				
1,000–1,250 ppm	0.5	−15.0 to 16.0	7.7	−9.5 to 24.8
1,450–1,500 ppm			14.0	−4.8 to 32.7
1,700–2,200 ppm			18.0	−5.5 to 41.8
2,400–2,800 ppm	12.7	−1.7 to 27.0	20.2	2.3 to 38.0
1,000–1,250 ppm vs.				
1,450–1,500 ppm	9.6	2.5 to 16.7	6.3	−1.5 to 14.3
1,700–2,200 ppm	9.4	2.1 to 16.8	10.7	−6.1 to 27.6
2,400–2,800 ppm	12.2	6.0 to 18.4	12.5	4.5 to 20.5
1,450–1,500 ppm vs.				
1,700–2,200 ppm			4.4	−13.2 to 21.9
2,400–2,800 ppm			6.2	−4.6 to 16.8
1,700–2,200 ppm vs.				
2,400–2,800 ppm			1.81	−16.2 to 19.8

ence between a 500-ppm NaF and 1,100-ppm toothpaste in a 2-year clinical trial with caries-active teenagers (9–12 years). The chapter of Tenuta and Cury [14] will further elaborate on surrogate outcomes to measure effectiveness of toothpastes.

The use of topical fluorides in young children is usually associated with the inadvertent ingestion and systematic absorption of fluoride increasing the risk of fluorosis. Although the mild forms of dental fluorosis do not pose a public health problem, more severe forms will be of esthetic concern, especially when the upper anterior teeth are involved. It is therefore important to achieve an appropriate balance between the beneficial and harmful effects of topical fluoride

therapies [28]. To cope with this problem, national guidelines follow a strategy of prescribing toddler toothpaste with 500 ppm F until ages 5–7 or a strategy based on a pea size amount of toothpaste of up to 1,100 ppm F for children aged 2 through 5 years and a 'smear' for children less than 2 years of age. Ecological observations in European countries adopting one of these strategies do not show dramatic differences in caries prevalence in children.

A recent meta-analysis assessed the effects of fluoride toothpastes on the prevention of dental caries in the primary dentition of preschool children [29]. Seven clinical trials were included in this meta-analysis, and most of them compared F toothpastes associated with oral health education

Table 2. Preventive fraction DMFS for low-fluoride and standard fluoride toothpastes

Reference	Year	F %, ppm	PF	95% CI	Weight %
Low-fluoride toothpaste					
Andruškeviciene et al. [30]	2008	500	54	44 to 64	62
Whittle et al. [31]	2008	440	17	−26 to 45	38
Total			40	5 to 74	100
Standard fluoride toothpastes					
Schwarz et al. [32]	1998	1,000	43	19 to 60	19
You et al. [33]	2002	1,100	16	0.12 to 29	24
Rong et al. [34]	2003	1,000	31	9 to 48	20
Jackson et al. [35]	2005	1,450	12	−34 to 44	8
Fan et al. [36]	2008	1,500	42	−29 to 53	28
Total			31	18 to 43	100

against no intervention. When standard F toothpastes (1,000–1,500 ppm) were compared to placebo or no intervention, significant caries reduction at surface level was found (prevented fraction, PF = 31%; 95% CI 18–43; 2,644 participants in 5 studies; table 2). Low-F toothpastes (440–500 ppm) were effective only at surface level (PF = 40%; 95% CI 5–75; 561 participants in 2 studies; table 2).

Recently, 2,800- and 5,000-ppm fluoride toothpastes have been launched as prescription fluoride toothpastes recommended to be used once daily for adults. These are not recommended for children. The benefits of 2,800 ppm have been demonstrated in various clinical trials [27, 37, 38], and the additional caries-preventive effect has to be estimated at around 15% (table 1) [25]. Nordström and Birkhed [39] showed that volunteers aged 14–16 years with DMFS ≥5 using 5,000-ppm F toothpaste had significantly lower caries progression compared to those using 1,450-ppm F toothpaste with a prevented fraction of 40%, with those with poorer compliance showing a slightly higher prevented fraction (42%). Ekstrand et al. [40] showed a 5,000-ppm toothpaste to be more effective in controlling root caries in homebound 75+ year olds than a 1,450-ppm toothpaste in an 8-month experiment. In a 3-month experiment, it was concluded that the dentifrice containing 5,000 ppm F⁻ was significantly better at remineralizing primary root caries lesions than the one containing 1,100 ppm F⁻ [41]. Further studies on the use of these toothpastes on prescription are needed.

Non-Fluoride Remineralization Systems

The action of fluoride in remineralization has to be seen as the 'gold standard' against which other remineralization systems have to compete against, either alone or in combination with fluoride. Ideal remineralization material should diffuse or deliver calcium and phosphate into the (sub)surface lesion or boost the remineralization properties of saliva and oral reservoirs without increasing the risk of calculus formation.

Amorphous Calcium Phosphate

Some commercially available toothpastes are based on unstabilized amorphous calcium phosphate (ACP), where a calcium salt and a phosphate salt are delivered separately intraorally via a dual-chamber device or delivered in a product with a low water activity [42, 43]. As the salts mix with saliva, they dissolve, releasing calcium and phosphate ions. The mixing of calcium ions with phosphate ions results in the immediate precipitation of ACP or, in the presence of fluoride ions, amorphous calcium fluoride phosphate (ACFP). According to Cochrane et al. [43], in the intraoral environment, these phases (ACP and ACFP) are potentially very unstable and may rapidly transform into a more thermodynamically stable, crystalline phase such as hydroxyapatite and fluorhydroxyapatite; thus, it has lower substantivity. However, before phase transformation, calcium and phosphate ions should be transiently bioavailable to promote enamel subsurface lesion remineralization [43]. Clinical studies demonstrated ACFP-forming toothpaste to be superior to fluoride alone in lowering root caries increment, while both are equally effective in lowering coronal caries increment [44]. Although not supported by any clinical evidence, it has been marketed as reducing hypersensitivity, restoring enamel luster, and reducing microleakage related to decay. Its high solubility and low substantivity may necessitate frequent application of the products. However, there is concern on promotion of dental calculus formation with long-term use; therefore, long-term randomized controlled caries clinical trials of the unstabilized ACP/ACFP technologies are needed to demonstrate efficacy in preventing coronal caries and lack of dental calculus promotion with long-term use.

Casein Derivatives
ACP is a reactive and soluble calcium phosphate compound that releases calcium and phosphate ions to convert to apatite and to remineralize the tooth surface when it comes in contact with saliva. Forming on the tooth coronal enamel and within the root dentinal tubules, ACP $[Ca_3(PO_4)_2-nH_2O]$ provides a reservoir of calcium and phosphate ions [45]. Fluoride can be incorporated to provide ACFP with similar characteristics. Casein phosphopeptide (CPP) is a milk-derived phosphoprotein that stabilizes high concentrations of calcium and phosphate ions in a metastable solution supersaturated with respect to the calcium phosphate solid phases at acidic and basic pH as well as in the presence of fluoride ions, forming nanoclusters of CPP-stabilized ACP (CPP-ACP) or CPP-stabilized ACFP (CPP-ACFP) nanocomplexes [43, 46, 47]. CPP-ACP and CPP-ACFP complexes have been shown to provide bioavailable calcium and phosphate ions at the tooth surface, thus inhibiting demineralization and favoring remineralization [48–51]. According to Cochrane et al. [43], CPP-ACP and CPP-ACFP enter the porosities of an enamel subsurface lesion and diffuse down concentration gradients into the body of the subsurface lesion. Once present in the enamel subsurface lesion, these nanocomplexes would release the weakly bound calcium and phosphate ions, which would then deposit into crystal voids. In the presence of fluoride, the mineral formed in the enamel lesion is consistent with fluorapatite or fluorhydroxyapatite [47]. The CPP-ACP nanocomplexes have also been demonstrated to bind onto the tooth surface and into supragingival plaque to significantly increase the level of bioavailable calcium and phosphate ions [52]. Thus, these complexes can function as a remineralization and caries prevention agent by creating a state of supersaturation of calcium and phosphate ions in the oral biofilm, modifying the dynamics of the demineralization-remineralization events when cariogenic challenge occurs [43]. In addition, enzymic breakdown of the CPP has been shown to produce a plaque pH rise through the production of ammonia, and hence contributing to the inhibition of demineralization and promotion of remineralization [53]. The CPP-ACP and the fluoride-containing CPP-ACFP have been incorporated into commercial sugar-free chewing gums, dental cream [43], and toothpaste [54]. However, Azarpazhooh and Limeback [55]

found insufficient clinical trial evidence (in quantity, quality or both) to make a recommendation regarding the long-term effectiveness of CPP-ACP and CPP-ACFP in reducing or eliminating dental caries, white-spot lesions or dentin hypersensitivity.

Tricalcium Phosphate
The application of β-tricalcium phosphate (TCP) in toothpaste and other remineralizing systems such as varnishes and mouthrinses was implemented by combining fluoride and functionalized TCP [56, 57]. Functionalized TCP is a tailored, low-dose calcium phosphate system that is incorporated into a single-phase aqueous or non-aqueous topical fluoride formulation such as dentifrice, gel, rinse or varnish [56, 58]. Supplementation with TCP is therefore designed to enhance fluoride-based nucleation 'seeding' activity, with subsequent remineralization driven by dietary and salivary calcium and phosphate. Ongoing research suggests the calcium oxide polyhedra, which become functionalized with specific organic molecules (e.g. fumaric acid or sodium lauryl sulfate) during the high-energy milling synthesis, appears to coordinate with fluoride to improve the quality of bond formation with loosely bound or broken orthophosphate groups within the enamel lattice [58–61]. Functionalization of TCP serves two major roles: first, it provides a barrier that prevents premature TCP-fluoride interactions, and second, it provides targeted delivery of TCP when applied to the teeth [60]. Although this is a relatively new approach, evidence for the benefits of TCP is mounting. Placebo-controlled clinical studies have demonstrated that relative to fluoride alone, the combination of fluoride plus functionalized TCP can improve remineralization by building stronger, more acid-resistant mineral in both white-spot lesions as well as eroded enamel [57, 62–65]. TCP has been combined with 5,000 ppm F (America), 950 ppm (Asia) and 850 ppm F (Australia) in toothpaste.

NovaMin® (Calcium Sodium Phosphosilicate Bioactive Glass)
NovaMin-containing toothpaste was originally tailored for treatment of hypersensitivity through physical occlusion of exposed dentinal tubules [66]. The potential of this toothpaste to prevent demineralization and/or aid in remineralization of tooth surfaces has been demonstrated in in vitro studies [67]. The mode of action of this material is based on the chemical reactivity with aqueous solutions. When introduced into the oral environment, the material releases sodium, calcium and phosphate which then interact with the oral fluids and result in the formation of a crystalline hydroxycarbonate apatite layer that is structurally and chemically similar to natural tooth mineral [67]. The calcium and phosphate ions are protected by glass, and the glass particles need to be trapped for the calcium and phosphate to be localized. While NovaMin alone and in combination with fluoride can enhance the remineralization of enamel and dentin lesions, as well as prevent demineralization from acid challenges, the combination of therapeutic levels of fluoride with NovaMin increases the remineralization of caries lesions more than either of them used alone [67]. However, the efficacy of NovaMin, both alone and in combination with fluoride, in enhancing remineralization and preventing demineralization still needs to be proved in randomized clinical trials.

Nanohydroxyapatite
Toothpaste based on nano-hydroxyapatite (nHA) has been commercially available in Japan since the 1980s, and was approved as an anticaries agent in 1993 based on randomized anticaries field trials in Japanese school children [68]. An increasing number of reports have shown that nHA has the potential to remineralize caries lesions following addition to toothpastes and mouthrinses [69–71]. Combination of nHA and fluoride enhanced the effectiveness of both nHAP and fluoride [70]. The remineralization

effect increased with increasing nHA concentrations up to 10%, after which the effect plateaued; hence, 10% nHA appeared to be the optimal concentration for remineralization of early enamel lesions with regular daily usage [71]. Nanohydroxyapatite is both bioactive and biocompatible. In toothpaste, it will lower the bioavailable F concentration, with NaF being slightly more of a concern than sodium monofluorophosphate. nHA functions by directly filling up micropores on demineralized tooth surfaces. When it penetrates the enamel pores, it also acts as a template in the remineralization process by continuously attracting large amounts of calcium and phosphate ions from the remineralization solution to the enamel tissue, thus promoting crystal integrity and growth.

Arginine Bicarbonate

Arginine bicarbonate is an amino acid complex with particles of calcium carbonate. Toothpaste containing arginine complex has been commercially available for caries control and hypersensitivity treatment. The arginine complex is responsible for adhering calcium carbonate particles to the mineral surface. When calcium carbonate dissolves slowly, the released calcium is available to remineralize the mineral while the release of carbonate may give a slight local pH rise. In dental plaque and saliva, the fermentation of arginine will also raise the pH [72, 73]. Arginine complex technology is also applied for treatment of hypersensitivity by physical occlusion of dentinal tubules. Arginine bicarbonate can be formulated with sodium monofluorophosphate.

Dicalcium Phosphate Dihydrate ($CaHPO_4 \cdot 2H_2O$; Brushite)

Dicalcium phosphate dihydrate is a precursor for apatite that readily turns into fluorapatite in the presence of fluoride [74]. Wefel and Harless [75] showed in vitro that even a 1-ppm fluoride solution could successfully and rapidly initiate remineralization of lesions after three 2-min pretreatment rinses with a DCPD-forming solution. Dicalcium phosphate dihydrate can be formulated with sodium monofluorophosphate or in a dual chamber system with NaF. Experiments with a dual-chamber dentifrice showed increased levels of free calcium ions in plaque fluid, and these remain elevated for up to 12–18 h after brushing, which fosters improved remineralization when in combination with fluoride [76]. Clinical experiments showed an increased level of anticaries efficacy of a dual-chambered dentifrice tube, with 0.234% NaF in a silica base and dicalcium phosphate dihydrate, compared with a dentifrice containing 0.243% NaF in a silica base [77, 78].

Conclusion

Since the introduction of effective fluoride toothpastes, caries prevalence has declined significantly. Since then, advances in technologies have improved the quality of the pastes not only by increasing the availability of fluoride but also by combining fluoride with calcium- and phosphate-based remineralization systems. Different formulations might vary the effectiveness between products, but it is impossible to compare all pastes head by head and therefore to select the best. Even the dose-response correlation is not so clear cut as might be expected. Careful use of the products might compensate for slight differences in the effectiveness. The best moment to brush the teeth is when there is time to do it carefully. As saliva flow decreases during sleep, which slows down the rate at which fluoride will be washed away, a brushing exercise just before going to bed is expected to be very beneficial. No food, drink or medical syrups should be taken after the last brushing.

References

1 Bratthall D, Hänsel-Petersson G, Sundberg H: Reasons for the caries decline: what do the experts believe? Eur J Oral Sci 1996;104:416–422, discussion 423–425, 430–432.

2 Lippert F: An introduction to toothpaste – Its purpose, history and ingredients; in van Loveren C (ed): Toothpastes. Monogr Oral Sci. Basel, Karger, 2013, vol 23, pp 1–14.

3 Ten Cate JM: In vitro studies on the effects of fluoride on de- and remineralization. J Dent Res 1990;69:614–619, discussion 634–636.

4 Featherstone JD, Glena R, Shariati M, Shields CP: Dependence of in vitro demineralization of apatite and remineralization of dental enamel on fluoride concentration. J Dent Res 1990;69:620–625, discussion 634–636.

5 Fejerskov O: Changing paradigms in concepts on dental caries: consequences for oral health care. Caries Res 200;38:182–191.

6 Weatherell JA, Deutsch D, Robinson C, Hallsworth AS: Fluoride concentrations in developing enamel. Nature 1975;256:230–232.

7 Robinson C: Fluoride and the caries lesion: interactions and mechanism of action. Eur Arch Paediatr Dent 2009;10:136–140.

8 Ten Cate JM, Buijs MJ, Damen JJ: pH-cycling of enamel and dentin lesions in the presence of low concentrations of fluoride. Eur J Oral Sci 1995;103:362–367.

9 Laheij AM, van Strijp AJ, van Loveren C: In situ remineralisation of enamel and dentin after the use of an amine fluoride mouthrinse in addition to twice daily brushings with amine fluoride toothpaste. Caries Res 2010;44:260–266.

10 Vale GC, Tabchoury CP, Del Bel Cury AA, Tenuta LM, ten Cate JM, Cury JA: APF and dentifrice effect on root dentin demineralization and biofilm. J Dent Res 2011;90:77–81.

11 Ganss C, Schulze K, Schlueter N: Toothpaste and erosion; in van Loveren C (ed): Toothpastes. Monogr Oral Sci. Basel, Karger, 2013, vol 23, pp 88–95.

12 Duckworth RM: Pharmacokinetics in the oral cavity: Fluoride and other active ingredients; in van Loveren C (ed): Toothpastes. Monogr Oral Sci. Basel, Karger, 2013, vol 23, pp 121–135.

13 Ten Cate JM, Featherstone JD: Mechanistic aspects of the interactions between fluoride and dental enamel. Crit Rev Oral Biol Med 1991;2:283–296.

14 Tenuta LMA, Cury JA: Laboratory and human studies to estimate anticaries efficacy of fluoride toothpastes; in van Loveren C (ed): Toothpastes. Monogr Oral Sci. Basel, Karger, 2013, vol 23, pp 104–120.

15 Stookey GK, DePaola PF, Featherstone JD, Fejerskov O, Möller IJ, Rotberg S, Stephen KW, Wefel JS: A critical review of the relative anticaries efficacy of sodium fluoride and sodium monofluorophosphate dentifrices. Caries Res1993;27:337–360.

16 Garcia-Godoy F: Clinical significance of the conclusions from the International Scientific Assembly on the Comparative Anticaries Efficacy of Sodium Fluoride and Sodium Monofluorophosphate Dentifrices. Am J Dent 1993;6:S4.

17 Marinho VC, Higgins JP, Sheiham A, Logan S: Fluoride toothpastes for preventing dental caries in children and adolescents. Cochrane Database Syst Rev 2003;CD002278.

18 van Loveren C, Moorer WR, Buijs MJ, van Palenstein Helderman WH: Total and free fluoride in toothpastes from some non-established market economy countries. Caries Res 2005;39:224–230.

19 Benzian H, Holmgren C, Buijs M, van Loveren C, van der Weijden F, van Palenstein Helderman W: Total and free available fluoride in toothpastes in Brunei, Cambodia, Laos, the Netherlands and Suriname. Int Dent J 2012;62:213–221.

20 Madléna M, Dombi C, Gintner Z, Bánóczy J: Effect of amine fluoride/stannous fluoride toothpaste and mouthrinse on dental plaque accumulation and gingival health. Oral Dis 2004;10:294–297.

21 Gerardu VA, van Loveren C, Heijnsbroek M, Buijs MJ, van der Weijden GA, ten Cate JM: Effects of various rinsing protocols after the use of amine fluoride/stannous fluoride toothpaste on the acid production of dental plaque and tongue flora. Caries Res 2006;40:245–250.

22 Paraskevas S, van der Weijden GA: A review of the effects of stannous fluoride on gingivitis. J Clin Periodontol 2006;33:1–13.

23 Ellingsen JE, Eriksen HM, Rölla G: Extrinsic dental stain caused by stannous fluoride. Scand J Dent Res 1982;90:9–13.

24 Twetman S: Caries prevention with fluoride toothpaste in children: an update. Eur Arch Paediatr Dent 2009;10:162–167.

25 Walsh T, Worthington HV, Glenny AM, Appelbe P, Marinho VC, Shi X: Fluoride toothpastes of different concentrations for preventing dental caries in children and adolescents. Cochrane Database Syst Rev 2010;CD007868.

26 Lima TJ, Ribeiro CC, Tenuta LM, Cury JA: Low-fluoride dentifrice and caries lesion control in children with different caries experience: a randomized clinical trial. Caries Res 2008;42:46–50.

27 Stookey GK, Mau MS, Isaacs RL, Gonzalez-Gierbolini C, Bartizek RD, Biesbrock AR: The relative anticaries effectiveness of three fluoride-containing dentifrices in Puerto Rico. Caries Res 2004;38:542–550.

28 Do LG, Spencer AJ: Risk-benefit balance in the use of fluoride among young children. J Dent Res 2007;86:723–728.

29 Dos Santos AP, Nadanovsky P, de Oliveira BH: A systematic review and meta-analysis of the effects of fluoride toothpastes on the prevention of dental caries in the primary dentition of preschool children. Community Dent Oral Epidemiol DOI: 10.1111/j.1600-0528.2012.00708.x.

30 Andruskeviciene V, Milciuviene S, Bendoraitiene E, Saldunaite K, Vasiliauskiene I, Slabsinskiene E, Narbutaite J: Oral health status and effectiveness of caries prevention programme in kindergartens in Kaunas city (Lithuania). Oral Health Prev Dent 2008;6:343–348.

31 Whittle JG, Whitehead HF, Bishop CM: A randomised control trial of oral health education provided by a health visitor to parents of pre-school children. Community Dent Health 2008;25:28–32.

32 Schwarz E, Lo EC, Wong MC: Prevention of early childhood caries – results of a fluoride toothpaste demonstration trial on Chinese preschool children after three years. J Public Health Dent 1998;58:12–18.

33 You BJ, Jian WW, Sheng RW, Jun Q, Wa WC, Bartizek RD, Biesbrock AR: Caries prevention in Chinese children with sodium fluoride dentifrice delivered through a kindergarten-based oral health program in China. J Clin Dent 2002;13:179–184.

34 Rong WS, Bian JY, Wang WJ, Wang JD: Effectiveness of an oral health education and caries prevention program in kindergartens in China. Community Dent Oral Epidemiol 2003;31:412–416.

35 Jackson RJ, Newman HN, Smart GJ, Stokes E, Hogan JI, Brown C, Seres J: The effects of a supervised toothbrushing programme on the caries increment of primary school children, initially aged 5–6 years. Caries Res 2005;39: 108–115.

36 Fan X, Li X, Wan H, Hu D, Zhang YP, Volpe AR, DeVizio W: Clinical investigation of the anticaries efficacy of a 1.14% sodium monofluorophosphate (SMFP) calcium carbonate-based dentifrice: a two-year caries clinical trial on children in China. J Clin Dent 2008;19:134–137.

37 Biesbrock AR, Gerlach RW, Bollmer BW, Faller RV, Jacobs SA, Bartizek RD: Relative anti-caries efficacy of 1,100, 1,700, 2,200, and 2,800 ppm fluoride ion in a sodium fluoride dentifrice over 1 year. Community Dent Oral Epidemiol 2001;29:382–389.

38 Bartizek RD, Gerlach RW, Faller RV, Jacobs SA, Bollmer BW, Biesbrock AR: Reduction in dental caries with four concentrations of sodium fluoride in a dentifrice: a meta-analysis evaluation. J Clin Dent 2001;12:57–62.

39 Nordström A, Birkhed D: Preventive effect of high-fluoride dentifrice (5,000 ppm) in caries-active adolescents: a 2-year clinical trial. Caries Res 2010;44: 323–331.

40 Ekstrand K, Martignon S, Holm-Pedersen P: Development and evaluation of two root caries controlling programmes for home-based frail people older than 75 years. Gerodontology 2008;25:67–75.

41 Baysan A, Lynch E, Ellwood R, Davies R, Petersson L, Borsboom P: Reversal of primary root caries using dentifrices containing 5,000 and 1,100 ppm fluoride. Caries Res 2001;35:41–46.

42 Tung MS, Eichmiller FC: Amorphous calcium phosphates for tooth mineralization. Compend Contin Educ Dent 2004;25(suppl 1):S9–S13.

43 Cochrane NJ, Cai F, Huq NL, Burrow MF, Reynolds EC: New approaches to enhanced remineralization of tooth enamel. J Dent Res 2010;89:1187–1197.

44 Papas A, Russell D, Singh M, Kent R, Triol C, Winston A: Caries clinical trial of a remineralising toothpaste in radiation patients. Gerodontology 2008;25: 76–88.

45 Chow LC, Takagi S, Vogel GL: Amorphous calcium phosphate: the contention of bone. J Dent Res 1998;77:6, author reply 7.

46 Cross KJ, Huq NL, Palamara JE, Perich JW, Reynolds EC: Physicochemical characterization of casein phosphopeptide-amorphous calcium phosphate nanocomplexes. J Biol Chem 2005;280: 15362–15369.

47 Cochrane NJ, Saranathan S, Cai F, Cross KJ, Reynolds EC: Enamel subsurface lesion remineralisation with casein phosphopeptide stabilised solutions of calcium, phosphate and fluoride. Caries Res 2008;42:88–97.

48 Slade GD, Caplan DJ: Impact of analytic conventions on outcome measures in two longitudinal studies of dental caries. Community Dent Oral Epidemiol 2000; 28:202–210.

49 Cai F, Shen P, Morgan MV, Reynolds EC: Remineralization of enamel subsurface lesions in situ by sugar-free lozenges containing casein phosphopeptide-amorphous calcium phosphate. Aust Dent J 2003;48:240–243.

50 Oshiro M, Yamaguchi K, Takamizawa T, Inage H, Watanabe T, Irokawa A, Ando S, Miyazaki M: Effect of CPP-ACP paste on tooth mineralization: an FE-SEM study. J Oral Sci 2007;49:115–120.

51 Yamaguchi K, Miyazaki M, Takamizawa T, Inage H, Kurokawa H: Ultrasonic determination of the effect of casein phosphopeptide-amorphous calcium phosphate paste on the demineralization of bovine dentin. Caries Res 2007;41: 204–207.

52 Reynolds EC, Cai F, Shen P, Walker GD: Retention in plaque and remineralization of enamel lesions by various forms of calcium in a mouthrinse or sugar-free chewing gum. J Dent Res 2003;82:206–211.

53 Reynolds EC, Riley PF: Protein dissimilation by human salivary-sediment bacteria. J Dent Res 1989;68:124–129.

54 Reynolds EC, Cai F, Cochrane NJ, Shen P, Walker GD, Morgan MV, Reynolds C: Fluoride and casein phosphopeptide-amorphous calcium phosphate. J Dent Res 2008;87:344–348.

55 Azarpazhooh A, Limeback H: Clinical efficacy of casein derivates: a systematic review of literature. J. Am Dent Assoc 2008;139:915–924.

56 Pfarrer AM, Karlinsey RL: Challenges of implementing new remineralization technologies. Adv Dent Res 2009;21: 79–82.

57 Karlinsey RL, Pfarrer AM: Fluoride plus functionalized β-TCP: a promising combination for robust remineralization. Adv Dent Res 2012;24:48–52.

58 Karlinsey RL, Mackey AC: Solid-state preparation and dental application of an organically-modified calcium phosphate. J Mater Sci 2009;44:346–349.

59 Karlinsey RL, Mackey AC, Walker ER, Frederick KE: Spectroscopic evaluation of native, milled, and functionalized β-TCP seeding into dental enamel lesions. J Mater Sci 2009;44:5013–5016.

60 Karlinsey RL, Mackey AC, Walker ER, Frederick KE: Preparation, characterization, and in vitro efficacy of an acid-modified β-TCP material for dental hard-tissue remineralization. Acta Biomater 2010;6:969–978.

61 Karlinsey RL, Mackey AC, Walker ER, Frederick KE: Surfactant-modified β-TCP: structure, properties, and in vitro remineralization of subsurface enamel lesions. J Mater Sci Mater Med 2010;21:2009–2020.

62 Amaechi BT, Ramalingam K, Mensinksai PK, Narjibfard K, Mackey AC, Karlinsey RL: Remineralization of eroded enamel by a NaF rinse containing a novel calcium phosphate agent in an in situ model: a pilot study. Clin Cosmet Invest Dent 2010;2:93–100.

63 Mensinkai PK, Ccahuana-Vasquez RA, Chedjieu I, Amaechi BT, Mackey AC, Walker TJ, Blanken DD, Karlinsey RL: In situ remineralization of white-spot enamel lesions by 500 and 1,100 ppm F dentifrices. Clin Oral Investig 2012;16:1007–1014.

64 Amaechi BT, Ramalingam K, Mensinkai PK, Chedjieu I: In situ remineralization of early caries by a new high-fluoride dentifrice. Gen Dent 2012;60:e186–e192.

65 Mathews MS, Amaechi BT, Ramalingam K, Ccahuana-Vasquez RA, Chedjieu IP, Mackey AC, Karlinsey RL: In situ remineralisation of eroded enamel lesions by NaF rinses. Arch Oral Biol 2012;57:525–530.

66 Du Min Q, Bian Z, Jiang H, Greenspan DC, Burwell AK, Zhong J, Tai BJ: Clinical evaluation of a dentifrice containing calcium sodium phosphosilicate (NovaMin) for the treatment of dentin hypersensitivity. Am J Dent 2008;21: 210–214.

67 Burwell AK, Litkowski LJ, Greenspan DC: Calcium sodium phosphosilicate (NovaMin®): remineralization potential. Adv Dent Res 2009;21:35–39.

68 Kani K, Kani M, Isozaki A, Shintani H, Ohashi T, Tokumoto T: Effect of apatite-containing dentifrices on dental caries in school children. J Dent Health 1989; 19:104–109.

69 Lu KL, Zhang JX, Meng XC, Li XY: Remineralization effect of the nano-HA toothpaste on artificial caries. Key Eng Mater 2007;330–332:267–270.

70 Kim MY, Kwon HK, Choi CH, Kim BI: Combined effects of nano-hydroxyapatite and NaF on remineralization of early caries lesion. Key Eng Mater 2007; 330–332:1347–1350.

71 Huang SB, Gao SS, Yu HY: Effect of nano-hydroxyapatite concentration on remineralization of initial enamel lesion. Biomed Mater 2009;4:034104.

72 Kleinberg I: Effect of varying sediment and glucose concentrations on the pH and acid production in human salivary sediment mixtures. Arch Oral Biol 1967; 12:1457–1473.

73 Lamberts BL, Pederson ED, Shklair IL: Salivary pH-rise activities in caries-free and caries-active naval recruits. Arch Oral Biol 1983;28:605–608.

74 Chow LC, Guo MK, Hsieh CC, Hong YC: Apatitic fluoride increase in enamel from a topical treatment involving intermediate $CaHPO_4 \cdot 2H_2O$ formation, an in vivo study. Caries Res 1981;15:369–376.

75 Wefel JS, Harless JD: The use of saturated DCPD in remineralization of artificial caries lesions in vitro. J Dent Res 1987; 66:1640–1643.

76 Sullivan RJ, Masters J, Cantore R, Roberson A, Petrou I, Stranick M, Goldman H, Guggenheim B, Gaffar A: Development of an enhanced anticaries efficacy dual component dentifrice containing sodium fluoride and dicalcium phosphate dihydrate. Am J Dent 2001;14:3A–11A.

77 Silva MF, Melo EV, Stewart B, De Vizio W, Sintes JL, Petrone ME, Volpe AR, Zhang Y, McCool JJ, Proskin HM: The enhanced anticaries efficacy of a sodium fluoride and dicalcium phosphate dihydrate dentifrice in a dual-chambered tube. A 2-year caries clinical study on children in Brazil. Am J Dent 2001;14: 19A–23A.

78 Boneta AE, Neesmith A, Mankodi S, Berkowitz HJ, Sánchez L, Mostler K, Stewart B, Sintes J, De Vizio W, Petrone ME, Volpe AR, Zhang YP, McCool JJ, Bustillo E, Proskin HM: The enhanced anticaries efficacy of a sodium fluoride and dicalcium phosphate dihydrate dentifrice in a dual-chambered tube. A 2-year caries clinical study on children in the United States of America. Am J Dent 2001; 14:13A–17A.

Bennett T. Amaechi, BDS, MS, PhD
Department of Comprehensive Dentistry
University of Texas Health Science Center at San Antonio
7703 Floyd Curl Drive, San Antonio, TX 78229-3900 (USA)
E-Mail amaechi@uthscsa.edu

van Loveren C (ed): Toothpastes. Monogr Oral Sci. Basel, Karger, 2013, vol 23, pp 27–44
DOI: 10.1159/000350465

Antiplaque and Antigingivitis Toothpastes

Mariano Sanz · Jorge Serrano · Margarita Iniesta · Isabel Santa Cruz · David Herrera

Etiology and Therapy of Periodontal Diseases Research Group, Faculty of Odontology, University Complutense, Madrid, Spain

Abstract

Dentifrices are a general term used to describe preparations that are used together with a toothbrush with the purpose to clean and/or polish the teeth. Active toothpastes were first formulated in the 1950s and included ingredients such as urea, enzymes, ammonium phosphate, sodium lauryl sarcosinate and stannous fluoride. Later, therapeutic agents were included. Today's toothpastes have two objectives: to help the toothbrush in cleaning the tooth surface and to provide a therapeutic effect. The therapeutic effect may have an antiplaque or anti-inflammatory basis when the nature of the agents is antimicrobial. Plaque inhibitory and antiplaque activity of toothpastes used for chemical plaque control is evaluated in distinct consecutive stages, the last being home use randomized clinical trials of at least 6 months' duration. In this chapter, the scientific evidence supporting the use of the most common antiplaque agents, included in toothpaste formulations, is reviewed, with a special emphasis on 6-month clinical trials, and systematic reviews with meta-analyses of the mentioned studies. Among the active agents, the following have been included in toothpastes: enzymes, amine alcohols, herbal or natural products, triclosan, bisbiguanides (chlorhexidine), quaternary ammonium compounds (cetylpyridinium chloride) and different metal salts (zinc salts, stannous fluoride, stannous fluoride with amine fluoride). Dentifrices are the ideal vehicles for any active ingredient used as an oral health preventive measure since they are used in combination with toothbrushing, which is the most frequently employed oral hygiene method. The most important indications of dentifrices with active ingredients are associated with long-term use to prevent bacterial biofilm formation, mostly in gingivitis patients or in patients on supportive periodontal therapy.

Dentifrices are a general term used to describe preparations that are used together with a toothbrush with the purpose to clean and/or polish the teeth. Dentifrices can be prepared as powders, gels or toothpastes depending on the water content. Toothpastes usually, but not necessarily, have high water content, while powders have almost none. In gels, most of the water content is replaced by a humectant. In the present chapter, the terms dentifrice and toothpaste are used indistinctively.

Human beings were always conscious of the importance of using toothpaste as part of oral hygiene practices. In fact, the first known tooth cream was reported in Egypt, back in 3000–5000

BC. Archaeological research has also suggested that Greek and Roman civilizations used a powder from crushed bones from different animals as a dentifrice. Around 500 BC, Chinese added flavorings to the powders, such as ginseng and other herbs. The modern era of therapeutically active toothpastes, however, did not start until the 1950s, when the first chemically active ingredients were added, such as urea, enzymes, ammonium phosphate, sodium lauryl sarcosinate and stannous fluoride.

Overall, modern toothpastes have both cosmetic and therapeutic objectives: to help the toothbrush in cleaning the tooth surface and provide a fresh breath (the cosmetic effect) and to provide a therapeutic effect, mainly through anticaries, antihalitosis, antiplaque or anti-inflammatory effects.

Composition of Toothpastes

Toothpastes are formulated by combining multiple ingredients, and special attention must be paid to avoid the possible interactions that may occur among them. Among the ingredients that are usually part of a dentifrice formulation, the most important are listed in table 1 [see the chapter by Lippert for more details, see page 1–14]. In addition, different active agents, being antimicrobial in nature, have been included in toothpastes to provide a therapeutic effect aiming to help in controlling plaque and gingivitis. The adjunctive use of these toothpastes may increase the efficacy of toothbrushing alone since the mechanical action of the toothbrush will reduce the amount of biofilm and disrupt its structure, thus facilitating the pharmacological mechanism of action of the toothpaste formulation [1]. Among the active agents, the following have been included in toothpastes: enzymes, amine alcohols, natural products, triclosan, bisbiguanides (chlorhexidine, CHX), quaternary ammonium compounds (cetylpyridinium chloride, CPC) and different metal salts (zinc salts, stannous fluoride, stannous fluoride with amine fluoride, AmF).

The present review will also consider gels, if they are used together with toothbrushing, as part of plaque control. Since gels do not include abrasives or detergents, they are easier to formulate, but their pharmacokinetics are less predictable. In addition, both dentifrices and gels lack the ability to access difficult to reach areas, such as the tonsils, the dorsum of the tongue, etc.

Mechanisms of Action and Classification of the Active Ingredients

Oral hygiene products used for chemical plaque control have been categorized according to their mechanism of action [2] as: (a) antimicrobial agents, when demonstrating a bacteriostatic or bactericidal effect in vitro; (b) plaque-reducing/inhibitory agents, when demonstrating an in vivo significant quantitative or qualitative effect on plaque levels, which may not have a significant effect on gingivitis and/or caries; (c) antiplaque agents, when demonstrating an in vivo significant effect on plaque levels sufficient to achieve a significant benefit in terms of gingivitis and/or caries control; (d) antigingivitis agents, when demonstrating an in vivo significant reduction in gingival inflammation without, necessarily, reducing dental plaque levels.

The previous definitions are widely accepted in Europe, but in North America the term antiplaque refers more often to agents capable of significantly reducing plaque levels and antigingivitis to agents capable of significantly reducing gingivitis levels.

Antiplaque activity may be achieved by different mechanisms of action: (a) by preventing bacterial adhesion; (b) by limiting bacterial growth and/or coaggregation; (c) by disrupting an already established biofilm; (d) by altering the composition and/or pathogenicity of the biofilm (see fig. 1). Its efficacy should be demonstrated in well-designed clinical trials through quantitative (re-

Table 1. Toothpaste ingredients, adapted from Davies et al. [168]

Abrasives	Surfactants	Humectants
Alumina	Amine fluorides	Glycerol
Aluminium trihydrate	Dioctyl sodium	PEG 8 (polyoxyethylene
Bentonite	sulfosuccinate	glycol esters)
Calcium carbonate	Sodium lauryl sulfate	Pentatol
Calcium pyrophosphate	Sodium N lauryl sarcosinate	PPG (polypropylene
Dicalcium phosphate	Sodium stearyl fumarate	glycol ethers)
Kaolin	Sodium stearyl lactate	Sorbitol
Methacrylate	Sodium lauryl sulfoacetate	Water
Perlite (a natural volcanic glass)		Xylitol
Polyethylene		
Pumice		
Silica		
Sodium bicarbonate		
Sodium metaphosphate		

Thickeners	Flavors	Preservatives
Carbopols	Aniseed	Alcohols
Carboxymethyl cellulose	Clove oil	Benzoic acid
Carrageenan	Eucalyptus	Ethyl parabens
Hydroxyethyl cellulose	Fennel	Formaldehyde
Plant extracts (alginate, guar gum, gum arabic)	Menthol	Methylparabens
Silica thickeners	Peppermint	Phenolics (methyl, ethyl, propyl)
Sodium alginate	Spearmint	Polyaminopropyl biguanide
Sodium aluminum silicates Viscarine	Vanilla	
Xanthan gum	Wintergreen	

Colors	Film agents	Sweeteners
Chlorophyll	Cyclomethicone	Acesulfame
Titanium dioxide	Dimethicone	Aspartame
	Polydimethylsiloxane	Saccharine
	Siliglycol	Sorbitol

duction of the number of microorganisms) and/or qualitative (altering the vitality of the biofilm) effects [1].

Evaluation of the Plaque Inhibitory and Antiplaque Activity of Toothpastes

In order to demonstrate the plaque inhibitory and antiplaque activity of toothpastes used for chemical plaque control, different consecutive stages of evaluation have been proposed, the last being the home use randomized clinical trial of at least 6-months' duration [3].

In vitro Studies

Toothpaste formulations including active agents combine different ingredients that may interact among themselves and lose their activity. It is therefore important to test the in vitro bioavailability of the active agents, as well as their adsorption to different surfaces. In vitro studies evaluating product

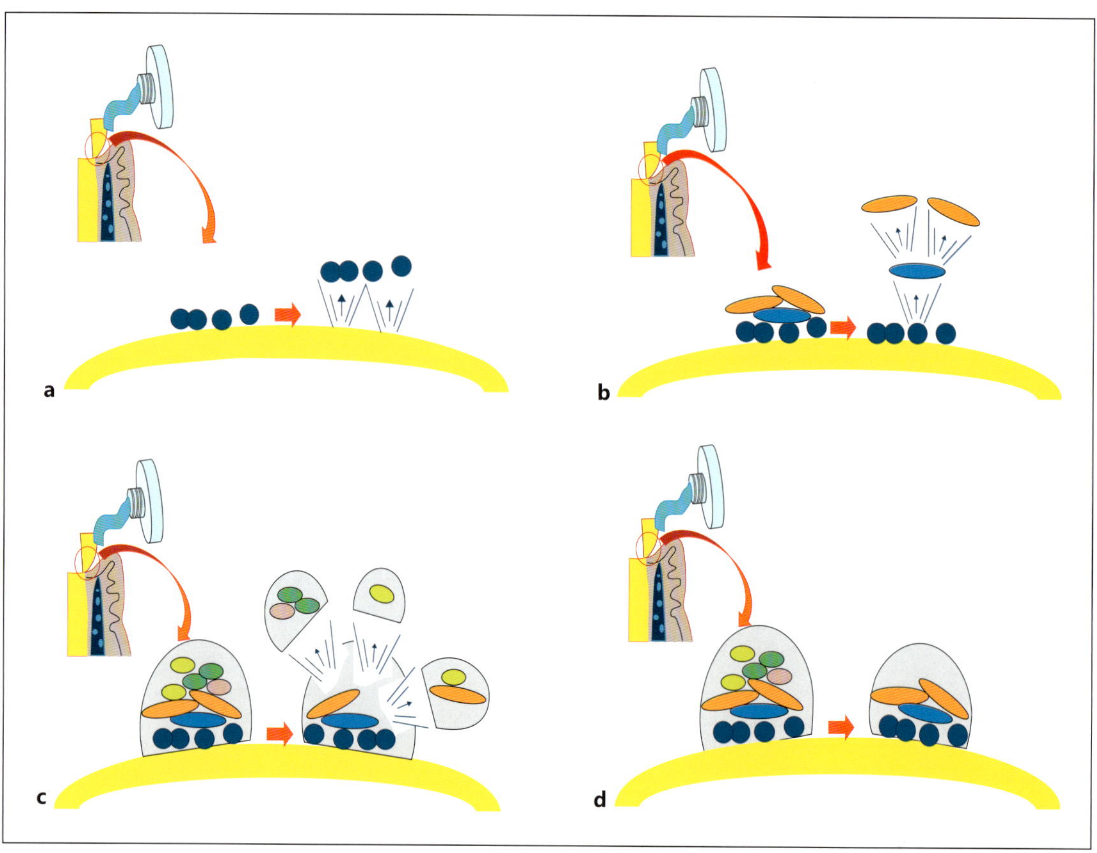

Fig. 1. Mechanisms of action of dentifrices. **a** Prevention of bacterial adhesion. **b** Interference with bacterial growth and/or coaggregation. **c** Elimination of an already established biofilm. **d** Alteration of the pathogenicity of the biofilm.

uptake are usually performed using different chemical methodologies, such as spectrophotometry.

For evaluating the toothpaste antimicrobial activity, different microbiological in vitro assays have been developed. They usually measure the minimum inhibitory concentrations and the minimum bactericidal concentrations against a battery of the most common oral bacterial species. This information is usually of limited value, since when using the toothpaste in vivo, there are many different factors that affect its antibacterial activity and spectrum of action. Moreover, this antibacterial activity is usually tested with isolated bacteria as planktonic cells, while in the oral environment bacteria are organized in complex biofilms. Recently, in vitro biofilm models have been developed for testing oral health products with antimicrobial activity, thus better simulating the real-life conditions [4–6].

In vivo Study Models
Similar to in vitro models, the product uptake is evaluated in depot studies that assess the retention of the agent in the subject's mouth after a single use of the toothpaste. This is usually performed by measuring the agent level in saliva or in dental plaque. These results, however, do not provide information on the activity of the

product [7–12; see the chapter by Duckworth, this vol.].

There are standardized in vivo models to evaluate the antiplaque activity of oral health products used for chemical plaque control. Although most of these models have been developed for assessing mouthrinse formulations, toothpastes have also been studied by applying them in trays or by transforming the toothpaste in an aqueous solution or in slurry.

- In vivo antimicrobial studies are usually designed as crossover trials (with at least a placebo and, preferably, also a positive control, normally a CHX mouthrinse, in which the amount of bacteria in saliva is measured before and after a single use of a tested formulation.
- Plaque regrowth studies are also usually designed as crossover trials (with at least a placebo and preferably also a positive control), in which plaque regrowth after a professional prophylaxis is measured for a short period of time (normally 3–4 days), and only the use of the tested toothpaste is allowed as oral hygiene method (no toothbrushing). In these studies, the plaque inhibitory capacity of the toothpaste is tested [13–17].
- Experimental gingivitis studies have the same design as plaque regrowth studies but usually utilize longer evaluation times (typically 12–28 days) and assess clinically relevant outcome variables (plaque and gingivitis indices) [18, 19]. Experimental gingivitis studies can be also designed as parallel studies since during this evaluation time, no mechanical hygiene is allowed.
- In vivo biofilm study models assess the efficacy of the toothpaste formulations in different surfaces, such as enamel, dentine or other materials, which are included in devices inserted in the subject's mouth during different evaluation periods. Once retrieved, the biofilm organized on these surfaces is analyzed and measured [20, 21].

Home Use Clinical Trials
It is a general consensus that the plaque inhibitory and antiplaque activity of oral health products needs to be demonstrated in long-term (at least 6 months), home use, randomized clinical trials. These studies not only demonstrate the efficacy of the product, but also its safety, by evidencing the lack of relevant side effects. In these studies, the use of the tested formulations should be adjunctive to mechanical plaque control (toothbrushing). These home use clinical trials should have certain characteristics to provide accepted results [22]:

a Experimental design. They should be adequately controlled (negative and/or positive controls) and blinded (double blind, including patients and examiner).
b Duration. They should be designed with a minimum of 6 months to allow for an adequate evaluation of their long-term efficacy, being able to compensate for the likely Hawthorne effect [23] and to monitor the absence of relevant adverse events.
c Microbiological evaluation. They should include the adequate microbiological methods to assess the product's antimicrobial activity as well as the absence of microbiological adverse effects, such as the overgrowth of pathogenic, opportunist or resistant strains.

Concerning validity of clinical outcome measures, plaque and gingival indices are the primary outcome variables in home use studies. They are usually assessed with well-validated indices (although most of them rely on a subjective evaluation), although a previous training of the examiners is mandatory with adequate intra- and inter-examiner calibration trials.

Oral health products, when demonstrating significant efficacy in terms of plaque and gingivitis reductions in, at least, two 6-month independent clinical trials, have received a 'seal of approval' by relevant agencies, such as the American Dental Association and the Food and Drug Administration.

In the following section, the scientific evidence supporting the use of the most common agents included in toothpaste formulations is reviewed,

Table 2. Summary of meta-analyses of 6-month home use randomized clinical trials in terms of plaque levels

Active agent (vehicle)	First author and year	n	WMD	p value	95% CI	Heterogeneity		
						p value	I^2, %	method
Triclosan and copolymer (dentifrice)	Gunsolley, 2006	17	0.82	<0.0001	NA	high	>75[a]	random
	Hioe, 2005	9	0.48	<0.0001	0.24–0.73	<0.00001	97.2	random
	Davies, 2004	11	0.48	<0.00001	0.32–0.64	<0.00001	95.7	random
Triclosan and zinc citrate (dentifrice)	Hioe, 2005	6	0.07	<0.00001	0.05–0.10	0.53	0	random
	Gunsolley, 2006	NA	NA	NA	NA		NA	NA
Stannous fluoride (dentifrice)	Gunsolley, 2006	5	0.17	significant	NA	low	<25[a]	NA
	Paraskevas, 2006	4	0.31	0.01	0.07–0.54	<0.0001	91.7	random

n = Number of studies included in the meta-analyses; WMD = weighted mean difference between test and placebo groups; CI = confidence interval; NA = not available.
[a] Estimated.

Table 3. Summary of meta-analyses of 6-month home use randomized clinical trials in terms of gingivitis levels

Active agent (vehicle)	First author and year	n	WMD	p value	95% CI	Heterogeneity		
						p value	I^2, %	method
Triclosan and copolymer (dentifrice)	Gunsolley, 2006	16	0.86	<0.001	NA	<0.001		
	Hioe, 2005	8	0.24	<0.0001	0.13–0.35	<0.00001	98.3	random
	Davies, 2004	14	0.26	<0.00001	0.18–0.34	<0.00001	96.5	random
								NA
Triclosan and zinc citrate (dentifrice)	Hioe, 2005	4	10.8%[a]	<0.00001	8.93–12.69	0.48	0	random
	Gunsolley, 2006	1	NA	NA	NA		NA	NA
Stannous fluoride (dentifrice)	Gunsolley, 2006	6	0.44	<0.001	NA	0.010	91.1	NA
	Paraskevas, 2006	6	0.15	<0.00001	0.11–0.20	<0.00001		random

[a] Effect on bleeding.

with special emphasis on 6-month, home use, clinical trials and on systematic reviews with meta-analyses of 6-month studies (see tables 2, 3).

Enzymes

Specific agents include glucose oxidase and amyloglucosidase. Their mechanisms of action rely on the catalyzation of thiocyanate into hypothiocyanite through the salivary lactoperoxidase system. Clinical studies with gingivitis patients have shown contradictory results, and no long-term (6-month) studies are available [24–27].

Amine Alcohols

Specific agents include delmopinol and octapinol. Their mechanism of action is through the inhibition and disruption of the biofilm extracellular matrix, and therefore they are not antimicrobial agents since they disrupt an already established biofilm. They also inhibit glycan synthesis by *Streptococcus mutans* [28, 29] and thus reduce bacteria acid production [30]. Delmopinol has been marketed as toothpaste in concentrations of 0.2%, in combination with 0.11% fluoride as sodium fluoride (NaF). It has been clinically evaluated just as a mouthrinse at concentrations of 0.1 and 0.2% [16, 31–34] but not as toothpaste.

Metal Salts: Zinc Salts
Specific agents include zinc lactate, zinc citrate, zinc sulphate or zinc chloride. Zinc salts have shown antibacterial action due to their ability to inhibit bacterial adhesion, metabolic activity and growth. Zinc products have been evaluated for plaque control, but also focused on halitosis control [35–39; see the chapter by Dadamio et al., this vol.], tartar control [40, 41; see the chapter by van Loveren and Duckworth, this vol.], or healing properties in presence of ulcers [42]. Some products have demonstrated some efficacy on plaque [43] and gingivitis [44, 45]: a 12-week study reported a 20.7% reduction in plaque and 38.1% in gingivitis, of a 0.1% o-cymen-5-ol and 0.6% zinc chloride dentifrice, when compared to a control dentifrice (p < 0.0001) [44]; however, only one 6-month trial is available [45], demonstrating reductions of 25.3% in plaque and 18.8% in gingivitis, when compared to the placebo.

In summary, when they are used as single ingredients, they have limited effects on plaque; but they may also be used in combination with other active agents (triclosan, CPC, CHX), which may improve substantivity and efficacy.

Metal Salts: Stannous Fluoride
Stannous fluoride has been included in dentifrices and gels since 1940s. The mechanism of action of the stannous ion is through adherence to the bacterial surface, inhibition of bacterial colonization, penetration into the bacteria cytoplasm and interference with the bacterial metabolism [46].

The combination of stannous and fluoride, chemically SnF_2, is difficult to formulate in oral hygiene products due to the lack of stability of this formulation in presence of water [47]. Several formulations have been tested, but the two most commonly evaluated are the combination of stannous fluoride and AmF (addressed in the following section), and 0.454% stabilized stannous fluoride combined or not with sodium hexametaphosphate (SHMP). Several 6-month studies have been published, evaluating gel or dentifrice products, more frequently with the 0.454% SnF_2 formulation [48–52], but also with SnF_2 plus SHMP [53–55] and older formulations [56, 57]. There are two published systematic reviews evaluating their efficacy in randomized clinical trials. In one of them, the 0.454% SnF_2 formulation provided significant benefits in terms of gingivitis (weighted mean difference, WMD, 0.441, p < 0.001, but with significant heterogeneity, p = 0.010) [58]. In the other systematic review [59], data pooling was performed at the final study visit, assuming that no differences were found at baseline, and there was limited availability of data, which prevented the meta-analysis. In addition, the results combined different SnF_2 formulations, including the combination with AmF. The results demonstrated significant differences, favoring the test group, in terms of gingival index (WMD –0.15), modified gingival index (WMD –0.21) and plaque index (WMD –0.31), also demonstrating a significant heterogeneity. Gels formulated with 0.4% stannous fluoride have also been evaluated, reporting reductions in gingival inflammation and in bleeding on probing [56, 60]. The observed additional reductions in bleeding and gingival inflammation amounted for 67% and 50%, respectively, as compared to the control, after 3 months [60].

Metal Salts: Stannous Fluoride with Amine Fluoride
AmF was developed in the 1950s at the University of Zurich. Its formulation in combination

with stannous fluoride (AmF/SnF_2) has demonstrated an increased bactericidal activity when compared with AmF alone. Its antimicrobial mechanism of action is through antiglycolytic activities. The activity of AmF/SnF_2 formulated as dentifrice lasts during 8 h after its use [61], although clinical trials have not demonstrated a significant benefit when used as dentifrice alone [62–65]. When used in combination with a mouthrinse, significant effects over plaque, but not over gingivitis [65], have been shown: plaque reductions versus baseline were 16%, ($p < 0.001$).

Natural Products

Specific agents include sanguinarine extract and other herbal ingredients (chamomile, echinacea, sage, myrrh, rhatany, peppermint oil). Sanguinarine is an alkaloid obtained from the plant *Sanguinaria canadensis* which has demonstrated low bactericidal capacity in an in vitro biofilm model [4], while its clinical evaluation has reported contradictory results [66–68]. At least five home use, 6-month, oral hygiene trials were performed in the 1980s and early 1990s, assessing sanguinarine extract with zinc chloride, used as dentifrice [69, 70] or used in combination with mouthrinse [71–73]. This combination reported significant reductions in terms of plaque and gingivitis: plaque reductions versus placebo ranged between 30% [71] and 13% [73]; for gingivitis, the respective range was 39–16%.

Triclosan

Triclosan [5-chloro-2-(2, 4 dichlorophenoxy) phenol] is a non-ionic bisphenolic, broad-spectrum antibacterial agent [74]. Triclosan has been widely formulated in dentifrices usually in combination with polyvinyl-methyl ether maleic acid copolymer, zinc citrate or pyrophosphate, in order to improve the substantivity and/or the antimicrobial activity. With these formulations, it can be detected for up to 8 h in dental plaque [75]. Triclosan has also demonstrated anti-inflammatory effects [76–78] through the inhibition of the cyclooxygenase and lipoxygenase pathways, by reducing the synthesis of prostaglandins and leukotrienes.

Three triclosan dentifrice formulations (triclosan with copolymer, triclosan with zinc citrate, triclosan with pyrophosphate) have been tested in 6-month, home use, randomized clinical trials. A dentifrice containing triclosan and zinc citrate was extensively evaluated in the 1990s [79–85]. The results of two systematic reviews provide conflicting results. In one, a limited meta-analysis demonstrated a small but significant effect on plaque (WMD –0.07, $p < 0.00001$) and a more important effect on gingival bleeding reduction (WMD –10.81%, $p < 0.00001$) [86]. Conversely, no significant differences were observed in the other systematic review evaluating changes between baseline and end of study [58]. A dentifrice with triclosan and copolymer has also been extensively evaluated in 6-month clinical trials [50, 79, 82, 87–99]. In a limited meta-analysis over final visit values, a significant effect was observed on plaque using the Turesky modification of the plaque index (WMD –0.48, $p < 0.0001$) and on gingivitis using the Talbott modification of the gingival index (WMD –0.24, $p < 0.0001$). In both cases, significant heterogeneity was shown [86]. In another meta-analysis, evaluating changes between baseline and final visit, a significant effect in plaque was observed (WMD 0.823), with significant differences in 14 out of the 18 included arms; a significant effect was also observed for gingivitis (WMD 0.858). In both cases, a significant heterogeneity was reported [58]. A dentifrice containing triclosan and pyrophosphate have been evaluated less frequently [79, 80, 99, 100], and the results are conflicting, also demonstrating a significant heterogeneity [58].

Bisbiguanides: Chlorhexidine

CHX is an active agent against Gram-positive and Gram-negative bacteria, yeasts and viruses, including the human immunodeficiency and hepatitis B viruses [101]. Its mechanism of action is bacteriostatic at low concentrations, by increasing the bacterial plasmatic membrane permeability [102, 103]. At higher concentrations, it is bactericidal by inducing intracytoplasmic precipitation and cellular death [104, 105]. When tested against biofilms, CHX has demonstrated its capacity to penetrate and to actively alter the biofilm formation and cause bacterial death [4, 106]. In addition to its antimicrobial effect, CHX interferes with bacterial adhesion [104, 107–110], interacts with salivary glycoproteins and also reduces the activity of bacterial enzymes involved in glycan production (glycosyl transferase C) [111].

The CHX molecule is highly cationic and binds reversibly to oral tissues [8, 9], evidencing a slow release that allows for sustained antimicrobial effects for up to 12 h [112]. Due to its cationic characteristic, this molecule is difficult to formulate in dentifrices due to the risk of inactivation with other anionic ingredients. There are, however, two published 6-month studies evaluating CHX-containing dentifrices: dentifrices with 1% CHX [113] and with 0.4% CHX in combination with zinc [114] demonstrated significant benefits in terms of plaque and gingival inflammation. The use of a 1% CHX dentifrice produced 19% of additional reduction in terms of plaque and 7% in terms of gingival inflammation, as compared to the control [113]. A 0.4% CHX dentifrice with zinc resulted in reductions of 27% and 12%, respectively, as compared with the control [114].

CHX gels for use with a toothbrush or applied in trays are available at different concentrations, (0.1, 0.12, 0.2, 0.5 and 1%), although the amount of CHX delivered when used with a toothbrush is not predictable [115]. When applied in a dental tray, a reduction in the levels of plaque and inflammation has been reported [116–118], although the acceptance by patients and therapists (used in disabled patients) was not good [119]. CHX gels may also be used for other purposes, such as prevention of alveolitis after tooth extraction [120, 121]. Its use has also been suggested as part of the full-mouth disinfection protocols, including tongue brushing with 1% CHX gel for 1 min and subgingival irrigation of pockets with 1% CHX gel [122, 123]. More recently, it has been evaluated in peri-implant mucositis therapy [124], although with limited effects.

Quaternary Ammonium Compounds
Specific agents include benzylconium chloride and CPC. Their mechanisms of action rely on the hydrophilic part of the CPC molecule that interacts with the bacterial cell membrane, leading to its disruption, alteration of the bacterial cell metabolism growth inhibition and finally cell death [125, 126]. CPC is a monocationic agent due the positive charge of the mentioned active hydrophilic part. This characteristic allows rapid adsorption of this molecule to oral surfaces [127] with a substantivity of approximately 3–5 h [128], although it also rapidly loses its activity or becomes neutralized [127]. Its formulation is also complex since it is easily inactivated by other ingredients, which makes the study of its bioavailability important. There are no 6-month clinical trials assessing the efficacy of CPC-containing toothpastes.

Safety and Adverse Effects

One of the limitations of the use of toothpastes with active ingredients is the risk of adverse effects and possible interactions with other ingredients.

- Enzymes. No relevant adverse effects have been described.
- Amine alcohols. The most relevant side effects described are tooth staining and possible occurrence of a transient sensation of numbing and burning of the mucosa and/or the tongue.

- Zinc salts. At low concentrations, no adverse effects have been reported.
- Stannous fluoride and stannous fluoride with AmF. Their main limiting factor may be tooth staining [65, 129, 130]. This limiting factor is not associated with formulations including SHMP.
- Natural products. The use of sanguinarine has been associated with oral leukoplakia [131].
- Triclosan. There are no relevant side effects, but the formation of a carcinogenic product (chloroform) was demonstrated in an in vitro study, when combining triclosan with the free chlorine present in water [132]. In addition, a possible environmental hazard has been suggested since triclosan is detected in the food chain. No convincing evidence is available to support the mentioned risks.
- CHX. Several adverse events have been reported with the use of this molecule, including: hypersensitivity reaction after oral use [133], neurosensory deafness when the product is placed in the middle ear [134], taste alterations and presence of a bitter taste [135, 136], uni-or bilateral parotid tumefaction [137, 138], staining, either of teeth, mucosa, tongue dorsum or restorations [137], mucosal erosion [139], or even alterations in the wound healing process (suggested from in vitro studies). In vivo studies, however, have not found interference with the healing process, but on the contrary, a better resolution of the inflammation was reported [140]. Heating during long periods of time can induce the formation of 4-chloroaninine, which has been shown to be cancerogenic and mutagenic. No adverse microbiological changes, including the overgrowth of opportunistic strains, are induced after long-term use [112, 141, 142].
- Quaternary ammonium compounds. The reported adverse effects are similar, although less frequent than with CHX formulations, and include tooth and tongue staining, transient gingival irritation and aphthous ulcers in some individuals [143]. In addition, no significant changes in the oral microbiota or overgrowth of opportunistic species have been observed [144].

Interactions between Toothpaste Ingredients

The complexity of toothpaste formulations may lead to the interference among ingredients, resulting in a limited activity. The best known example is CHX. CHX digluconate forms low solubility salts with anions, such as phosphate, sulphate or chloride; therefore, anionic detergents may reduce CHX activity when formulated in a toothpaste [24]. CHX may interfere with abrasives, and it is incompatible with sodium monofluorophosphate and other fluorides due to the formation of non-soluble salts (in vitro) [145]. Anionic thickeners, such as carboxymethyl cellulose, should not be used in a formulation with CHX, requiring non-ionic thickeners, such as cellulose ethers.

Among the other active agents, CPC is a monocationic molecule, which may also be inhibited by different toothpaste ingredients, especially detergents [146].

Indications of Toothpastes with Plaque Inhibitory and/or Antiplaque Activity

Dentifrices are the ideal vehicles for any active ingredient used as an oral health preventive measure, since they are used in combination with toothbrushing, which is the most frequently employed oral hygiene method. However, there are also a number of disadvantages, such as the difficulties in their formulation due to the likely interactions between the active agents and the other dentifrice ingredients. Their pharmacokinetics are less predictable than those of mouthrinses, and they will not reach to areas of difficult access, such as the tonsils or the dorsum of the tongue. Furthermore, in some specific situations, such as when used after surgical interventions or in disabled patients, their use together with toothbrushing might not be possible since patients may be instructed not to brush or they may not be able to brush.

Toothpastes with active ingredients, therefore, should not be recommended in single-use applications (e.g. preoperative use) or in situations where mechanical plaque control is suboptimal or impossible. The most important indication is their long-term use to prevent biofilm formation, mostly in gingivitis patients or in patients on supportive periodontal therapy.

There are specific recommendations for special patient categories:

- In patients with fixed or removable orthodontic appliances. A common strategy to improve mechanical plaque removal in these patients is the addition, as part of the oral hygiene regimen, of a chemotherapeutic antimicrobial agent. Amine/stannous fluoride [147] or sanguinarine [71] in the form of mouthrinses combined with toothpastes or gels, have been evaluated in clinical studies. Most of these clinical studies have reported significant benefits in the adjunctive use of these products, although the magnitude of the reported benefits might not have a clear clinical relevance.
- In periodontitis patients. Together with an adequate professional supportive periodontal therapy program, chemical agents may be recommended to improve biofilm control and to decrease the risk of disease progression. A careful consideration of the risk-benefit ratio should be made since these patients will be in supportive therapy for life. A dentifrice with triclosan and copolymer evaluated for 2 years demonstrated a significant reduction in the presence of deep pockets and sites with clinical attachment and bone loss [148–150].

- In patients with dental implants. The use of different agents (CHX, triclosan, stannous fluoride) may help to control biofilms and decrease the risk of peri-implant diseases [151–153]. In a randomized trial, triclosan/copolymer significantly improved clinical and microbiological variables, as compared with a fluoride dentifrice, after 6 months [153].
- In the general population. Its main use should be the treatment of gingivitis by reaching a balance between the biofilm and the host response, thus maintaining a gingival health status. Dentifrices containing triclosan and copolymer [58, 86] as well as stannous fluoride [58, 130] have demonstrated antiplaque efficacy in 6-month clinical trials. The available data from the systematic reviews show the clinical benefit of its daily use when compared with the provision of oral hygiene instructions. In spite of these benefits, the daily usage of antiseptic products in the general population is still a subject of controversy since optimal results may be also achieved without the adjunctive antiseptic [58].

Other indications of the long-term use of toothpastes with antimicrobial ingredients may be the prevention of the other oral conditions.

- In caries prevention. Dentifrices with triclosan and copolymer or a zinc salt have demonstrated anticaries activity [154] even in long-term studies [155]. In high-risk patients, amine and stannous fluoride may also be recommended based on the proven remineralization and anticaries action [156, 157].
- In the prevention of recurrent aphthous ulcers. CHX usage may reduce incidence, duration and severity, including ulcers in patients with fixed orthodontic appliances [158]. Triclosan formulation may also decrease the incidence of oral ulcers [159].
- In halitosis therapy and secondary prevention. Different chemical agents and formulations have been evaluated, with two main aims: antibacterial and interference with volatilization of odoriferous compounds. Among the most eval-

uated agents, the following may be highlighted: triclosan with zinc or copolymer [160–163], or CHX, especially if combined with zinc salts and CPC in a mouthrinse formulation [164–166]. In order to be effective, these agents need to be used in conjunction with adequate oral hygiene and tongue scrapping or brushing [167; see the chapter by Dadamio et al., this vol.].

Conclusions

Dentifrices are normally used in combination with toothbrushing, providing a cosmetic (cleaning, fresh breath) and often also a therapeutic (caries, periodontal diseases, halitosis control) benefit.

Different ingredients have been included as active components in dentifrice formulations depending on the therapeutic claim. When the objective is the control of plaque and gingivitis, enzymes, amine alcohols, herbal extracts, triclosan, bisbiguanides, quaternary ammonium compounds and metal salts, have been utilized. Depending on their activity, they can be categorized as antimicrobial, plaque inhibitory, antiplaque or antigingivitis. Antiplaque agents are those able to significantly affect plaque and gingivitis, and they should be preferred in the treatment of gingivitis and the prevention of periodontal diseases. The efficacy of these products should be demonstrated in well-designed, 6-month, home use, randomized clinical trials.

Dentifrices based on zinc salts have shown only limited effects on plaque. However, they may improve the substantivity and efficacy of other active agents when formulated together.

Stabilized stannous fluoride formulations, especially if combined with SHMP, have shown reductions in both plaque and gingivitis. Stannous fluoride in combination with AmF may reduce plaque levels, but only if combined with a mouthrinse with the same active ingredients.

A dentifrice with sanguinarine extract has demonstrated conflicting results, but its clinical use is not recommended due to its association with leukoplakia.

Triclosan-based products have an effect on plaque and inflammation, but the results when comparing different studies and formulations have shown high heterogeneity. The best results have been demonstrated in a formulation with a proprietary copolymer that enhances substantivity.

CHX-based (0.1% or 0.4% with zinc) dentifrices have produced significant reductions in plaque and gingivitis, but are usually associated with adverse effects, especially tooth staining. They may also be used for other indications such as alveolitis after tooth extraction, full-mouth disinfection protocols or peri-implant disease therapy.

Dentifrices represent the ideal vehicle for the application of active agents in the prevention (and therapy) of the most prevalent oral diseases, caries and periodontal diseases, since they are used in combination with toothbrushing, perhaps the most compliant behavior of modern human beings. Dentifrices, however, can be produced with complex formulations that may interfere with the activity of the therapeutic agents, and therefore the efficacy of any newly marketed dentifrice should be tested in well-designed randomized clinical trials. Formulations with triclosan (especially with copolymer), stannous fluoride (with SHMP) and CHX have demonstrated significant antiplaque efficacy. These products are clearly indicated in high-risk patient groups such as periodontitis patients, subjects with dental implants or patients with fixed orthodontic appliances. The daily usage of these antiseptic products in the general population is still a subject of controversy since optimal results may also be achieved without the adjunctive active ingredient.

References

1 Commission FDI: Mouthrinses and periodontal disease. Int Dent J 2002;52:346–352.

2 Lang NP, Newman HN: Consensus report of sesion II; in Lang Np, Karring T, Lindhe J (eds): Proceedings of the 2nd European Workshop on Periodontology, Chemicals in Periodontics. London, Quintessence, 1997, pp 192–195.

3 Addy M, Moran JM: Clinical indications for the use of chemical adjuncts to plaque control: chlorhexidine formulations. Periodontol 2000 1997;15:52–54.

4 Shapiro S, Giertsen E, Guggenheim B: An in vitro oral biofilm model for comparing the efficacy of antimicrobial mouthrinses. Caries Res 2002;36:93–100.

5 Socransky SS, Haffajee AD: Dental biofilms: difficult therapeutic targets. Periodontol 2000 2002;28:12–55.

6 Xu KD, McFeters GA, Stewart PS: Biofilm resistance to antimicrobial agents. Microbiology 2000;146:547–549.

7 Bonesvoll P: Retention and plaque-inhibiting effect in man of chlorhexidine after multiple mouth rinses and retention and release of chlorhexidine after toothbrushing with a chlorhexidine gel. Arch Oral Biol 1978;23:295–300.

8 Bonesvoll P, Lokken P, Rolla G: Influence of concentration, time, temperature and pH on the retention of chlorhexidine in the human oral cavity after mouth rinses. Arch Oral Biol 1974;19:1025–1029.

9 Bonesvoll P, Lokken P, Rolla G, Paus PN: Retention of chlorhexidine in the human oral cavity after mouth rinses. Arch Oral Biol 1974;19:209–212.

10 Gjermo P, Bonesvoll P, Hjeljord LG, Rolla G: Influence of variation of pH of chlorhexidine mouth rinses on oral retention and plague-inhibiting effect. Caries Res 1975;9:74–82.

11 Gjermo P, Bonesvoll P, Rolla G: Relationship between plaque-inhibiting effect and retention of chlorhexidine in the human oral cavity. Arch Oral Biol 1974;19:1031–1034.

12 Rolla G, Loe H, Schiott CR: Retention of chlorhexidine in the human oral cavity. Arch Oral Biol 1971;16:1109–1116.

13 Addy M, Willis L, Moran J: Effect of toothpaste rinses compared with chlorhexidine on plaque formation during a 4-day period. J Clin Periodontol 1983;10:89–99.

14 Arweiler NB, Henning G, Reich E, Netuschil L: Effect of an amine-fluoride-triclosan mouthrinse on plaque regrowth and biofilm vitality. J Clin Periodontol 2002;29:358–363.

15 Harrap GJ: Assessment of the effect of dentifrices on the growth of dental plaque. J Clin Periodontol 1974;1:166–174.

16 Moran J, Addy M, Wade WG, Maynard JH: A comparison of delmopinol and chlorhexidine on plaque regrowth over a 4-day period and salivary bacterial counts. J Clin Periodontol 1992;19:749–753.

17 Pizzo G, La CM, Licata ME, Pizzo I, D'Angelo M: The effects of an essential oil and an amine fluoride/stannous fluoride mouthrinse on supragingival plaque regrowth. J Periodontol 2008;79:1177–1183.

18 Löe H: Experimental gingivitis in man. J Periodontol 1965;36:177–187.

19 Löe H, Schiott CR: The effect of mouthrinses and topical application of chlorhexidine on the development of dental plaque and gingivitis in man. J Periodontal Res 1970;5:79–83.

20 Pan P, Barnett ML, Coelho J, Brogdon C, Finnegan MB: Determination of the in situ bactericidal activity of an essential oil mouthrinse using a vital stain method. J Clin Periodontol 2000;27:256–261.

21 Sreenivasan PK, Mattai J, Nabi N, Xu T, Gaffar A: A simple approach to examine early oral microbial biofilm formation and the effects of treatments. Oral Microbiol Immunol 2004;19:297–302.

22 American Dental Association: Guidelines for acceptance of chemotherapeutic products for the control of supragingival dental plaque and gingivitis. Council of Dental Therapeutics. J Am Dent Assoc 1986;112:529–532.

23 Overholser CD Jr: Longitudinal clinical studies with antimicrobial mouthrinses. J Clin Periodontol 1988;15:517–519.

24 Addy M: Chlorhexidine compared with other locally delivered antimicrobials. A short review. J Clin Periodontol 1986;13:957–964.

25 Hatti S, Ravindra S, Satpathy A, Kulkarni RD, Parande MV: Biofilm inhibition and antimicrobial activity of a dentifrice containing salivary substitutes. Int J Dent Hyg 2007;5:218–224.

26 Kirstila V, Lenander-Lumikari M, Tenovuo J: Effects of a lactoperoxidase-system-containing toothpaste on dental plaque and whole saliva in vivo. Acta Odontol Scand 1994;52:346–353.

27 Moran J, Addy M, Newcombe R: Comparison of the effect of toothpastes containing enzymes or antimicrobial compounds with a conventional fluoride toothpaste on the development of plaque and gingivitis. J Clin Periodontol 1989;16:295–299.

28 Elworthy AJ, Edgar R, Moran J, Addy M, Movert R, Kelty E, et al: A 6-month home-usage trial of 0.1% and 0.2% delmopinol mouthwashes (II). Effects on the plaque microflora. J Clin Periodontol 1995;22:527–532.

29 Rundegren J, Simonsson T, Petersson LG, Hansson E: Effect of delmopinol on the cohesion of glucan-containing plaque formed by *Streptococcus mutans* in a flow cell system. J Dent Res 1992;71:1792–1796.

30 Simonsson T, Hvid EB, Rundegren J, Edwardsson S: Effect of delmopinol on in vitro dental plaque formation, bacterial production and the number of microorganisms in human saliva. Oral Microbiol Immunol 1991;6:305–309.

31 Abbott DM, Gunsolley JC, Koertge TE, Payne EL: The relative efficacy of 0.1% and 0.2% delmopinol mouthrinses in inhibiting the development of supragingival dental plaque and gingivitis in man. J Periodontol 1994;65:437–441.

32 Claydon N, Hunter L, Moran J, Wade WG, Kelty E, Movert R, et al: A 6-month home-usage trial of 0.1% and 0.2% delmopinol mouthwashes (I). Effects on plaque, gingivitis, supragingival calculus and tooth staining. J Clin Periodontol 1996;23:220–228.

33 Collaert B, Attstrim R, De Bruyn H, Movert R: The effect of delmopinol rinsing on dental plaque formation and gingivitis healing. J Clin Periodontol 1992;19:274–280.

34 Zee KY, Rundegren J, Attstrîm R: Effect of delmopinol hydrochloride mouthrinse on plaque formation and gingivitis in 'rapid' and 'slow' plaque formers. J Clin Periodontol 1997;24:486–491.

35 Navada R, Kumari H, Le S, Zhang J: Oral malodor reduction from a zinc-containing toothpaste. J Clin Dent 2008;19:69–73.

36 Newby CS, Rowland JL, Lynch RJ, Bradshaw DJ, Whitworth D, Bosma ML: Benefits of a silica-based fluoride toothpaste containing o-cymen-5-ol, zinc chloride and sodium fluoride. Int Dent J 2011;61(suppl 3):74–80.

37 Newby EE, Hickling JM, Hughes FJ, Proskin HM, Bosma MP: Control of oral malodour by dentifrices measured by gas chromatography. Arch Oral Biol 2008;53(suppl 1):S19–S25.

38 Young A, Jonski G: Effect of a single brushing with two Zn-containing toothpastes on VSC in morning breath: a 12 h, randomized, double-blind, crossover clinical study. J Breath Res 2011;5: 046012.

39 Young A, Jonski G, Rolla G: Inhibition of orally produced volatile sulfur compounds by zinc, chlorhexidine or cetylpyridinium chloride – effect of concentration. Eur J Oral Sci 2003;111:400–404.

40 Lobene RR, Soparkar PM, Newman MB, Kohut BE: Reduced formation of supragingival calculus with use of fluoride-zinc chloride dentifrice. J Am Dent Assoc 1987;114:350–352.

41 Sowinski J, Petrone DM, Battista G, Simone AJ, Crawford R, Patel S, et al: Clinical efficacy of a dentifrice containing zinc citrate: a 12-week calculus clinical study in adults. Compend Contin Educ Dent 1998;19(suppl 2):16–19.

42 Pories WJ, Henzel JH, Rob CG, Strain WH: Acceleration of wound healing in man with zinc sulphate given by mouth. Lancet 1967;1:121–124.

43 Gunbay S, Bicakci N, Guneri T, Kirilmaz L: The effect of zinc chloride dentifrices on plaque growth and oral zinc levels. Quintessence Int 1992;23:619–624.

44 Kakar A, Newby EE, Ghosh S, Butler A, Bosma ML: A randomised clinical trial to assess maintenance of gingival health by a novel gel to foam dentifrice containing 0.1%w/w o-cymen-5-ol, 0.6%w/w zinc chloride. Int Dent J 2011; 61(suppl 3):21–27.

45 Williams C, McBride S, Mostler K, Petrone DM, Simone AJ, Crawford R, et al: Efficacy of a dentifrice containing zinc citrate for the control of plaque and gingivitis: a 6-month clinical study in adults. Compend Contin Educ Dent 1998;19(suppl 2):4–15.

46 Tinanoff N: Review of the antimicrobial action of stannous fluoride. J Clin Dent 1990;2:22–27.

47 Miller JT, Shannon IL, Kilgore WG, Bookman JE: Use of a water-free stannous fluoride-containing gel in the control of dental hypersensitivity. J Periodontol 1969;40:490–491.

48 Beiswanger BB, Doyle PM, Jackson R, Mallatt ME, Mau M, Bollmer BW, et al: The clinical effect of dentifrices containing stabilised stannous fluoride on plaque formation and gingivitis – a six-month study with ad libitum brushing. J Clin Dent 1995;6: 46–53.

49 Mankodi S, Petrone DM, Battista G, Petrone ME, Chaknis P, DeVizio W, et al: Clinical efficacy of an optimized stannous fluoride dentifrice. 2. A 6-month plaque/gingivitis clinical study, northeast USA. Compend Contin Educ Dent 1997;18:10–15.

50 McClanahan SF, Beiswanger BB, Bartizek RD, Lanzalaco AC, Bacca L, White DJ: A comparison of stabilized stannous fluoride dentifrice and triclosan/copolymer dentifrice for efficacy in the reduction of gingivitis and gingival bleeding: six-month clinical results. J Clin Dent 1997;8: 39–45.

51 Perlich MA, Bacca LA, Bollmer BW, Lanzalaco AC: The clinical effect of a stabilized stannous fluoride dentifrice on plaque formation, gingivitis and gingival bleeding: a six-month study. J Clin Dent 1995;6:54–58.

52 Williams C, McBride S, Bolden TE, Mostler K, Petrone DM, Petrone ME, et al: Clinical efficacy of an optimized stannous fluoride dentifrice. 3. A 6-month plaque/gingivitis clinical study, southeast USA. Compend Contin Educ Dent 1997;18:16–20.

53 Boneta AE, Aguilar MM, Romeu FL, Stewart B, DeVizio W, Proskin HM: Comparative investigation of the efficacy of triclosan/copolymer/sodium fluoride and stannous fluoride/sodium hexametaphosphate/zinc lactate dentifrices for the control of established supragingival plaque and gingivitis in a six-month clinical study. J Clin Dent 2010;21:117–123.

54 Mallatt M, Mankodi S, Bauroth K, Bsoul SA, Bartizek RD, He T: A controlled 6-month clinical trial to study the effects of a stannous fluoride dentifrice on gingivitis. J Clin Periodontol 2007;34: 762–767.

55 Mankodi S, Bartizek RD, Winston JL, Biesbrock AR, McClanahan SF, He T: Anti-gingivitis efficacy of a stabilized 0.454% stannous fluoride/sodium hexametaphosphate dentifrice. J Clin Periodontol 2005;32:75–80.

56 Boyd RL, Chun YS: Eighteen-month evaluation of the effects of a 0.4% stannous fluoride gel on gingivitis in orthodontic patients. Am J Orthod Dentofacial Orthop 1994;105:35–41.

57 Wolff LF, Pihlstrom BL, Bakdash MB, Aeppli DM, Bandt CL: Effect of toothbrushing with 0.4% stannous fluoride and 0.22% sodium fluoride gel on gingivitis for 18 months. J Am Dent Assoc 1989;119:283–289.

58 Gunsolley JC: A meta-analysis of six-month studies of antiplaque and antigingivitis agents. J Am Dent Assoc 2006; 137:1649–1657.

59 Paraskevas S, van der Weijden GA: A review of the effects of stannous fluoride on gingivitis. J Clin Periodontol 2006;33: 1–13.

60 Tinanoff N, Manwell MA, Zameck RL, Grasso JE: Clinical and microbiological effects of daily brushing with either NaF or SnF$_2$ gels in subjects with fixed or removable dental prostheses. J Clin Periodontol 1989;16:284–290.

61 Weiland B, Netuschil L, Hoffmann T, Lorenz K: Substantivity of amine fluoride/stannous fluoride following different modes of application: a randomized, investigator-blind, placebo-controlled trial. Acta Odontol Scand 2008;66:307–313.

62 Sgan-Cohen HD, Gat E, Schwartz Z: The effectiveness of an amine fluoride/stannous fluoride dentifrice on the gingival health of teenagers: results after six months. Int Dent J 1996;46:340–345.

63 Shapira L, Shapira M, Tandlich M, Gedalia I: Effect of amine fluoride-stannous fluoride containing toothpaste (Meridol) on plaque and gingivitis in adults: a six-month clinical study. J Int Acad Periodontol 1999;1:117–120.

64 Mengel R, Wissing E, Schmitz-Habben A, Flores-de-Jacoby L: Comparative study of plaque and gingivitis prevention by AmF/SnF$_2$ and NaF. A clinical and microbiological 9-month study. J Clin Periodontol 1996;23:372–378.

65 Paraskevas S, Versteeg PA, Timmerman MF, Van der Velden U, van der Weijden GA: The effect of a dentifrice and mouth rinse combination containing amine fluoride/stannous fluoride on plaque and gingivitis: a 6-month field study. J Clin Periodontol 2005;32:757–764.

66 Moran J: A clinical trial to assess the efficacy of sanguinarine-zinc mouthrinse (Veadent) compared with chlorhexidine mouthrinse (Corsodyl). J Clin Periodontol 1988;15:612–616.

67 Quirynen M, Marechal M, van Steenberghe D: Comparative antiplaque activity of sanguinarine and chlorhexidine in man. J Clin Periodontol 1990;17:223–227.

68 Scherer W, Gultz J, Lee SS, Kaim JM: The ability of an herbal mouthrinse to reduce gingival bleeding. J Clin Dent 1998;9:97–100.

69 Lobene RR, Soparkar PM, Newman MB: The effects of a sanguinaria dentifrice on plaque and gingivitis. Compend Contin Educ Dent 1986;(suppl 7):S185–S188.

70 Mauriello SM, Bader JD: Six-month effects of a sanguinarine dentifrice on plaque and gingivitis. J Periodontol 1988;59:238–243.

71 Hannah JJ, Johnson JD, Kuftinec MM: Long-term clinical evaluation of toothpaste and oral rinse containing sanguinaria extract in controlling plaque, gingival inflammation, and sulcular bleeding during orthodontic treatment. Am J Orthod Dentofacial Orthop 1989; 96:199–207.

72 Harper DS, Mueller LJ, Fine JB, Gordon JM, Laster LL: Clinical efficacy of a dentifrice and oral rinse containing sanguinaria extract and zinc chloride during 6 months of use. J Periodontol 1990;61: 352–358.

73 Kopczyk RA, Abrams H, Brown AT, Matheny JL, Kaplan AL: Clinical and microbiological effects of a sanguinaria-containing mouthrinse and dentifrice with and without fluoride during 6 months of use. J Periodontol 1991;62: 617–622.

74 Ciancio SG: Antiseptics and antibiotics as chemotherapeutic agents for periodontitis management. Compendium 2000;21:59–78.

75 Gilbert RJ, Williams PE: The oral retention and antiplaque efficacy of triclosan in human volunteers. Br J Clin Pharmacol 1987;23:579–583.

76 Barkvoll P, Rolla G: Triclosan protects the skin against dermatitis caused by sodium lauryl sulphate exposure. J Clin Periodontol 1994;21:717–719.

77 Gaffar A, Scherl D, Afflitto J, Coleman EJ: The effect of triclosan on mediators of gingival inflammation. J Clin Periodontol 1995;22:480–484.

78 Kjaerheim V, Skaare A, Barkvoll P: Antiplaque, antibacterial and anti- inflammatory properties of triclosan mouthrinse in combination with zinc citrate or polyvinylmethylether maleic acid (PVA-MA) copolymer. Eur J Oral Sci 1996;104: 529–534.

79 Palomo F, Wantland L, Sanchez A, Volpe AR, McCool J, DeVizio W: The effect of three commercially available dentifrices containing triclosan on supragingival plaque formation and gingivitis: a six month clinical study. Int Dent J 1994;44(suppl 1):75–81.

80 Renvert S, Birkhed D: Comparison between 3 triclosan dentifrices on plaque, gingivitis and salivary microflora. J Clin Periodontol 1995;22:63–70.

81 Stephen KW, Saxton CA, Jones CL, Ritchie JA, Morrison T: Control of gingivitis and calculus by a dentifrice containing a zinc salt and triclosan. J Periodontol 1990;61:674–679.

82 Svatun B, Sadxton CA, Huntington E, Cummins D: The effects of three silica dentifrices containing Triclosan on supragingival plaque and calculus formation and on gingivitis. Int Dent J 1993; 43(suppl 1):441–452.

83 Svatun B, Saxton CA, Huntington E, Cummins D: The effects of a silica dentifrice containing Triclosan and zinc citrate on supragingival plaque and calculus formation and the control of gingivitis. Int Dent J 1993;43(suppl 1):431–439.

84 Svatun B, Saxton CA, Rolla G: Six-month study of the effect of a dentifrice containing zinc citrate and triclosan on plaque, gingival health, and calculus. Scand J Dent Res 1990;98:301–304.

85 Svatun B, Saxton CA, Rolla G, van der Ouderaa FJ: One-year study of the efficacy of a dentifrice containing zinc citrate and triclosan to maintain gingival health. Scand J Dent Res 1989;97:242–246.

86 Hioe KP, van der Weijden GA: The effectiveness of self-performed mechanical plaque control with triclosan containing dentifrices. Int J Dent Hyg 2005; 3:192–204.

87 Allen DR, Battista GW, Petrone DM, Petrone ME, Chaknis P, DeVizio W, et al: The clinical efficacy of Colgate Total Plus Whitening Toothpaste containing a special grade of silica and Colgate Total Fresh Stripe Toothpaste in the control of plaque and gingivitis: a six-month clinical study. J Clin Dent 2002;13:59–64.

88 Bolden TE, Zambon JJ, Sowinski J, Ayad F, McCool JJ, Volpe AR, et al: The clinical effect of a dentifrice containing triclosan and a copolymer in a sodium fluoride/silica base on plaque formation and gingivitis: a six-month clinical study. J Clin Dent 1992;3:125–131.

89 Charles CH, Sharma NC, Galustians HJ, Qaqish J, McGuire JA, Vincent JW: Comparative efficacy of an antiseptic mouthrinse and an antiplaque/antigingivitis dentifrice. A six-month clinical trial. J Am Dent Assoc 2001;132:670–675.

90 Cubells AB, Dalmau LB, Petrone ME, Chaknis P, Volpe AR: The effect of a Triclosan/copolymer/fluoride dentifrice on plaque formation and gingivitis: a six-month clinical study. J Clin Dent 1991;2:63–69.

91 Deasy MJ, Singh SM, Rustogi KN, Petrone DM, Battista G, Petrone ME, et al: Effect of a dentifrice containing triclosan and a copolymer on plaque formation and gingivitis. Clin Prev Dent 1991;13:12–19.

92 Denepitiya JL, Fine D, Singh S, DeVizio W, Volpe AR, Person P: Effect upon plaque formation and gingivitis of a triclosan/copolymer/fluoride dentifrice: a 6-month clinical study. Am J Dent 1992; 5:307–311.

93 Garcia-Godoy F, DeVizio W, Volpe AR, Ferlauto RJ, Miller JM: Effect of a triclosan/copolymer/fluoride dentifrice on plaque formation and gingivitis: a 7-month clinical study. Am J Dent 1990;3:15–26.

94 Hu D, Zhang J, Wan H, Zhang Y, Volpe AR, Petrone ME: Efficacy of a triclosan/copolymer dentifrice in the control of plaque and gingivitis: a six-month study in China. Hua XiKou QiangYiXueZa Zhi 1997;15:333–335.

95 Kanchanakamol U, Umpriwan R, Jotikasthira N, Srisilapanan P, Tuongratanaphan S, Sholitkul W, et al: Reduction of plaque formation and gingivitis by a dentifrice containing triclosan and copolymer. J Periodontol 1995;66:109–112.

96 Lindhe J, Rosling B, Socransky SS, Volpe AR: The effect of a triclosan-containing dentifrice on established plaque and gingivitis. J Clin Periodontol 1993;20: 327–334.

97 Mankodi S, Walker C, Conforti N, DeVizio W, McCool JJ, Volpe AR: Clinical effect of a triclosan-containing dentifrice on plaque and gingivitis: a six-month study. Clin Prev Dent 1992;14:4–10.

98 Triratana T, Kraivaphan P, Amornchat C, Rustogi KN, Petrone MP, Volpe AR: Effect of a triclosan-copolymer pre-brush mouthrinse on established plaque formation and gingivitis: a six month clinical study in Thailand. J Clin Dent 1995;6:142–147.

99 Winston JL, Bartizek RD, McClanahan SF, Mau MS, Beiswanger BB: A clinical methods study of the effects of triclosan dentifrices on gingivitis over six months. J Clin Dent 2002;13:240–248.

100 Grossman E, Hou L, Bollmer BW, Court LK, McClary JM, Bennett S, et al: Triclosan/pyrophosphate dentifrice: dental plaque and gingivitis effects in a 6-month randomized controlled clinical study. J Clin Dent 2002; 13:149–157.

101 Wade WG, Addy M: In vitro activity of a chlorhexidine-containing mouthwash against subgingival bacteria. J Periodontol 1989;60:521–525.

102 Hugo WB, Longworth AR: Some aspects of the mode of action of chlorhexidine. J Pharm Pharmacol 1964;16:655–662.

103 Hugo WB, Longworth AR: Cytological aspects of the mode of action of chlorhexidine diacetate. J Pharm Pharmacol 1965;17:28–32.

104 Fine DH: Mouthrinses as adjuncts for plaque and gingivitis management. A status report for the American Journal of Dentistry. Am J Dent 1988;1:259–263.

105 Hugo WB, Longworth AR: The effect of chlorhexidine on the electrophoretic mobility, cytoplasmic constituents, dehydrogenase activity and cell walls of *Escherichia coli* and *Staphylococcus aureus*. J Pharm Pharmacol 1966; 18:569–578.

106 Arweiler NB, Netuschil L, Reich E: Alcohol-free mouthrinse solutions to reduce supragingival plaque regrowth and vitality. A controlled clinical study. J Clin Periodontol 2001;28:168–174.

107 Jenkins S, Addy M, Newcombe RG: Comparison of two commercially available chlorhexidine mouthrinses. II. Effects on plaque reformation, gingivitis and tooth staining. Clin Prev Dent 1989;11:12–16.

108 Jenkins S, Addy M, Wade WG: The mechanism of action of chlorhexidine. A study of plaque growth on enamel inserts in vivo. J Clin Periodontol 1988; 15:415–424.

109 Rolla G, Melsen B: On the mechanism of the plaque inhibition by chlorhexidine. J Dent Res 1975;54:57–62.

110 Wolff LF: Chemotherapeutic agents in the prevention and treatment of periodontal disease. Northwest Dent 1985; 64:15–24.

111 Vacca-Smith AM, Bowen WH: Effects of some antiplaque agents on the activity of glycosyltransferases of *Streptococcus mutans* adsorbed onto saliva-coated hydroxyapatite and in solution. Biofilms 1996;1:1360–1365.

112 Schiott CR, Loe H, Jensen SB, Kilian M, Davies RM, Glavind K: The effect of chlorhexidine mouthrinses on the human oral flora. J Periodontal Res 1970; 5:84–89.

113 Yates R, Jenkins S, Newcombe RG, Wade WG, Moran J, Addy M: A 6-month home usage trial of a 1% chlorhexidine toothpaste (1). Effects on plaque, gingivitis, calculus and toothstaining. J Clin Periodontol 1993;20:130–138.

114 Sanz M, Vallcorba N, Fabregues S, Muller I, Herkstroter F: The effect of a dentifrice containing chlorhexidine and zinc on plaque, gingivitis, calculus and tooth staining. J Clin Periodontol 1994;21:431–437.

115 Saxen L, Niemi ML, Ainamo J: Intra-oral spread of the antimicrobial effect of a chlorhexidine gel. Scand J Dent Res 1976;84:304–307.

116 Francis JR, Hunter B, Addy M: A comparison of three delivery methods of chlorhexidine in handicapped children. I. Effects on plaque, gingivitis, and toothstaining. J Periodontol 1987; 58:451–455.

117 Pannuti CM, Saraiva MC, Ferraro A, Falsi D, Cai S, Lotufo RF: Efficacy of a 0.5% chlorhexidine gel on the control of gingivitis in Brazilian mentally handicapped patients. J Clin Periodontol 2003;30:573–576.

118 Slot DE, Rosema NA, Hennequin-Hoenderdos NL, Versteeg PA, Van DV, van der Weijden GA: The effect of 1% chlorhexidine gel and 0.12% dentifrice gel on plaque accumulation: a 3-day non-brushing model. Int J Dent Hyg 2010;8:294–300.

119 Francis JR, Addy M, Hunter B: A comparison of three delivery methods of chlorhexidine in handicapped children. II. Parent and house-parent preferences. J Periodontol 1987;58:456–459.

120 Hita-Iglesias P, Torres-Lagares D, Flores-Ruiz R, Magallanes-Abad N, Basallote-Gonzalez M, Gutierrez-Perez JL: Effectiveness of chlorhexidine gel versus chlorhexidine rinse in reducing alveolar osteitis in mandibular third molar surgery. J Oral Maxillofac Surg 2008;66:441–445.

121 Minguez-Serra MP, Salort-Llorca C, Silvestre-Donat FJ: Chlorhexidine in the prevention of dry socket: effectiveness of different dosage forms and regimens. Med Oral Patol Oral Cir Bucal 2009;14:e445–e449.

122 Bollen CM, Mongardini C, Papaioannou W, van SD, Quirynen M: The effect of a one-stage full-mouth disinfection on different intra-oral niches. Clinical and microbiological observations. J Clin Periodontol 1998;25:56–66.

123 Bollen CM, Vandekerckhove BN, Papaioannou W, Van EJ, Quirynen M: Full- versus partial-mouth disinfection in the treatment of periodontal infections. A pilot study: long-term microbiological observations. J Clin Periodontol 1996;23: 960–970.

124 Heitz-Mayfield LJ, Salvi GE, Botticelli D, Mombelli A, Faddy M, Lang NP: Anti-infective treatment of peri-implant mucositis: a randomised controlled clinical trial. Clin Oral Implants Res 2011;22:237–241.

125 Merianos JJ: Quaternary ammonium antimicrobial compounds; in Block SS (ed): Disinfection, Sterilization and Preservation. Philadelphia, Lea & Febiger, 1991, pp 225–255.

126 Smith RN, Anderson RN, Kolenbrander PE: Inhibition of intergeneric coaggregation among oral bacteria by cetylpyridinium chloride, chlorhexidine digluconate and octenidine dihydrochloride. J Periodontal Res 1991;26: 422–428.

127 Bonesvoll P, Gjermo P: A comparision between chlorhexidine and some quaternary ammonium compounds with regard to retention, salivary concentration and plaque-inhibiting effect in the human mouth after mouth rinses. Arch Oral Biol 1978;23:289–294.

128 Roberts WR, Addy M: Comparison of the in vivo and in vitro antibacterial properties of antiseptic mouthrinses containing chlorhexidine, alexidine, cetyl pyridinium chloride and hexetidine. Relevance to mode of action. J Clin Periodontol 1981;8: 295–310.

129 Brecx MC, Macdonald LL, Legary K, Cheang M, Forgay MG: Long-term effects of Meridol and chlorhexidine mouthrinses on plaque, gingivitis, staining, and bacterial vitality. J Dent Res 1993;72:1194–1197.

130 Paraskevas S, Timmerman MF, Van der Velden U, van der Weijden GA: Additional effect of dentifrices on the instant efficacy of toothbrushing. J Periodontol 2006;77:1522–1527.

131 Mascarenhas AK, Allen CM, Moeschberger ML: The association between Viadent use and oral leukoplakia – results of a matched case-control study. J Public Health Dent 2002;62: 158–162.

132 Rule KL, Ebbett VR, Vikesland PJ: Formation of chloroform and chlorinated organics by free-chlorine-mediated oxidation of triclosan. Environ Sci Technol 2005;39:3176–3185.

133 Beaudouin E, Kanny G, Morisset M, Renaudin JM, Mertes M, Laxenaire MC, et al: Immediate hypersensitivity to chlorhexidine: literature review. Allerg Immunol (Paris) 2004;36:123–126.

134 Aursnes J: Ototoxic effect of iodine disinfectants. Acta Otolaryngol 1982; 93:219–226.

135 Breslin PA, Tharp CD: Reduction of saltiness and bitterness after a chlorhexidine rinse. Chem Senses 2001;26: 105–116.

136 Marinone MG, Savoldi E: Chlorhexidine and taste. Influence of mouthwashes concentration and of rinsing time. Minerva Stomatol 2000;49:221–226.

137 Flotra L, Gjermo P, Rolla G, Waerhaug J: Side effects of chlorhexidine mouth washes. Scand J Dent Res 1971;79: 119–125.

138 van der Weijden GA, Ten Heggeler JM, Slot DE, Rosema NA, Van der Velden U: Parotid gland swelling following mouthrinse use. Int J Dent Hyg 2010;8: 276–279.

139 Almqvist H, Luthman J: Gingival and mucosal reactions after intensive chlorhexidine gel treatment with or without oral hygiene measures. Scand J Dent Res 1988;96:557–560.

140 Sanz M, Newman MG, Anderson L, Matoska W, Otomo-Corgel J, Saltini C: Clinical enhancement of postperiodontal surgical therapy by a 0.12% chlorhexidine gluconate mouthrinse. J Periodontol 1989;60: 570–576.

141 Schiott CR, Briner WW, Kirkland JJ, Loe H: Two years oral use of chlorhexidine in man. III. Changes in sensitivity of the salivary flora. J Periodontal Res 1976;11:153–157.

142 Schiott CR, Briner WW, Loe H: Two year oral use of chlorhexidine in man. II. The effect on the salivary bacterial flora. J Periodontal Res 1976;11:145–152.

143 Lobene RR, Kashket S, Soparkar PM: The effect of cetylpyridinium chloride on human plaque bacteria and gingivitis. Pharmacol Therapeut Dent 1979;4: 33–47.

144 Ciancio SG, Mather ML, Bunnell HL: Clinical evaluation of a quaternary ammonium-containing mouthrinse. J Periodontol 1975;46:397–401.

145 Barkvoll P, Rolla G, Bellagamba S: Interaction between chlorhexidine digluconate and sodium monofluorophosphate in vitro. Scand J Dent Res 1988; 96:30–33.

146 Sheen S, Owens J, Addy M: The effect of toothpaste on the propensity of chlorhexidine and cetyl pyridinium chloride to produce staining in vitro: a possible predictor of inactivation. J Clin Periodontol 2001;28: 46–51.

147 Ogaard B, Alm AA, Larsson E, Adolfsson U: A prospective, randomized clinical study on the effects of an amine fluoride/stannous fluoride toothpaste/mouthrinse on plaque, gingivitis and initial caries lesion development in orthodontic patients. Eur J Orthod 2006;28:8–12.

148 Bruhn G, Netuschil L, Richter S, Brecx MC, Hoffmann T: Effect of a toothpaste containing triclosan on dental plaque, gingivitis, and bleeding on probing – an investigation in periodontitis patients over 28 weeks. Clin Oral Investig 2002;6: 124–127.

149 Rosling B, Dahlen G, Volpe AR, Furuichi Y, Ramberg P, Lindhe J: Effect of triclosan on the subgingival microbiota of periodontitis-susceptible subjects. J Clin Periodontol 1997;24:881–887.

150 Rosling B, Wannfors B, Volpe AR, Furuichi Y, Ramberg P, Lindhe J: The use of a triclosan/copolymer dentifrice may retard the progression of periodontitis. J Clin Periodontol 1997;24: 873–880.

151 Ciancio SG, Lauciello F, Shibly O, Vitello M, Mather M: The effect of an antiseptic mouthrinse on implant maintenance: plaque and peri-implant gingival tissues. J Periodontol 1995;66: 962–965.

152 Di Carlo F, Quaranta A, Di AL, Ronconi LF, Quaranta M, Piattelli A: Influence of amine fluoride/stannous fluoride mouthwashes with and without chlorhexidine on secretion of proinflammatory molecules by peri-implant crevicular fluid cells. Minerva Stomatol 2008;57:215–221, 221–225.

153 Sreenivasan PK, Vered Y, Zini A, Mann J, Kolog H, Steinberg D, et al: A 6-month study of the effects of 0.3% triclosan/copolymer dentifrice on dental implants. J Clin Periodontol 2011; 38:33–42.

154 Panagakos FS, Volpe AR, Petrone ME, DeVizio W, Davies RM, Proskin HM: Advanced oral antibacterial/anti-inflammatory technology: a comprehensive review of the clinical benefits of a triclosan/copolymer/fluoride dentifrice. J Clin Dent 2005;16(suppl): S1–S19.

155 Mann J, Vered Y, Babayof I, Sintes J, Petrone ME, Volpe AR, et al: The comparative anticaries efficacy of a dentifrice containing 0.3% triclosan and 2.0% copolymer in a 0.243% sodium fluoride/silica base and a dentifrice containing 0.243% sodium fluoride/silica base: a two-year coronal caries clinical trial on adults in Israel. J Clin Dent 2001;12:71–76.

156 Paraskevas S, Danser MM, Timmerman MF, van der Velden U, Van der Weijden GA: Amine fluoride/stannous fluoride and incidence of root caries in periodontal maintenance patients. A 2 year evaluation. J Clin Periodontol 2004;31:965–971.

157 Tinanoff N, Hock J, Camosci D, Hellden L: Effect of stannous fluoride mouthrinse on dental plaque formation. J Clin Periodontol 1980;7:232–241.

158 Shaw WC, Addy M, Griffiths S, Price C: Chlorhexidine and traumatic ulcers in orthodontic patients. Eur J Orthod 1984;6:137–140.

159 Skaare A, Herlofson BB, Barkvoll P: Mouthrinses containing triclosan reduce the incidence of recurrent aphthous ulcers. J Clin Periodontol 1996;23:778–781.

160 Hu D, Zhang YP, Petrone M, Volpe AR, DeVizio W, Giniger M: Clinical effectiveness of a triclosan/copolymer/sodium fluoride dentifrice in controlling oral malodor: a 3-week clinical trial. Oral Dis 2005;11(suppl 1):51–53.

161 Niles HP, Hunter CM, Vazquez J, Williams MI, Cummins D: Clinical comparison of Colgate Total Advanced Fresh vs a commercially available fluoride breath-freshening toothpaste in reducing breath odor overnight: a multiple-use study. Compend Contin Educ Dent 2003;24(suppl 9):29–33.

162 Sharma NC, Galustians HJ, Qaquish J, Galustians A, Rustogi KN, Petrone ME, et al: The clinical effectiveness of a dentifrice containing triclosan and a copolymer for controlling breath odor measured organoleptically twelve hours after toothbrushing. J Clin Dent 1999;10:131–134.

163 van Steenberghe D: Breath malodor. Curr Opin Periodontol 1997;4:137–143.

164 Roldán S, Herrera D, Santacruz I, O'Connor A, Gonzalez I, Sanz M: Comparative effects of different chlorhexidine mouth-rinse formulations on volatile sulphur compounds and salivary bacterial counts. J Clin Periodontol 2004;31:1128–1134.

165 Roldán S, Winkel EG, Herrera D, Sanz M, van Winkelhoff AJ: The effects of a new mouthrinse containing chlorhexidine, cetylpyridinium chloride and zinc lactate on the microflora of oral halitosis patients: a dual-centre, double-blind placebo-controlled study. J Clin Periodontol 2003;30:427–434.

166 Winkel EG, Roldán S, van Winkelhoff AJ, Herrera D, Sanz M: Clinical effects of a new mouthrinse containing chlorhexidine, cetylpyridinium chloride and zinc-lactate on oral halitosis. A dual-center, double-blind placebo-controlled study. J Clin Periodontol 2003;30:300–306.

167 Roldán S, Herrera D, Sanz M: Biofilms and the tongue: therapeutical approaches for the control of halitosis. Clin Oral Investig 2003;7:189–197.

168 Davies R, Scully C, Preston AJ: Dentifrices – an update. Med Oral Patol Oral Cir Bucal 2010;15:e976–e982.

Mariano Sanz
Facultad de Odontología
Plaza Ramón y Cajal s/n (Ciudad Universitaria)
ES–28040 Madrid (Spain)
E-Mail marianosanz@odon.ucm.es

van Loveren C (ed): Toothpastes. Monogr Oral Sci. Basel, Karger, 2013, vol 23, pp 45–60
DOI: 10.1159/000350472

The Role of Toothpastes in Oral Malodor Management

Jesica Dadamio · Isabelle Laleman · Marc Quirynen

Department of Periodontology, Catholic University of Leuven, Leuven, Belgium

Abstract

One out of four people suffers from persistent bad breath. In most of the cases, the cause can be found in the mouth, with the presence of tongue coating as the leading factor, followed by gingivitis and periodontitis, and it is referred to as oral malodor. Because oral malodor is the result of the degradation of organic substrates by anaerobic bacteria of the oral cavity, the management is mostly done by masking the odorous compounds or eliminating the cause (bacteria and their substrates) either mechanically or chemically. Toothpaste formulations have been modified to carry antimicrobial and oxidizing agents with an impact on the process of oral malodor formation. We performed extensive literature search regarding the effect of dedicated toothpastes in the management of oral malodor. The main characteristics of the in vitro and in vivo investigations and their most relevant findings are presented for discussion. Even though the amount of publications regarding this topic is far smaller than for others such as caries, plaque control and whitening, antibacterial ingredients such as triclosan and metal ions like stannous and zinc appear to be effective in the control of oral malodor. On the other hand, data supporting the use of hydrogen peroxide, baking soda, essential oils and flavors in the management of oral malodor are rather few and inconclusive.

Introduction

Definition, Epidemiology and Causes of Oral Malodor

Halitosis, breath malodor and bad breath are common terms used to define an unpleasant odor emanating from the oral cavity. This chronic condition should not be confused with transient situations caused by some food consumption (garlic, spices), or with the morning bad breath experienced upon awakening that will disappear after breakfast or oral hygiene [1]. Most cases of bad breath are caused by oral conditions, and only then does the term 'oral malodor' apply [2].

People suffering from bad breath often remain completely unaware of their own oral emission [3, 4], whereas others without halitosis are convinced that they suffer from it. These situations are referred in the literature as 'bad breath paradox' and 'imaginary halitosis', respectively. Self-perception of breath malodor is notoriously unreliable [5].

Even though bad breath is a common complaint among the general population and can lead to personal discomfort and social embarrassment, its incidence remains poorly documented. Three large-scale studies [6–8] and some smaller investigations [9–11] have been conducted to establish the incidence of this condition. Independently of the method used to assess oral malodor and of the study population, their results pointed out that about 1 out of 4 people suffers from persistent bad breath. Accordingly, in 2003 a report of the American Dental Association estimated a bad breath prevalence of 25% [12].

Although the existence of bad breath has been described thousands of years ago, Greek and Roman writers wrote about it, the topic still remains as one of the biggest taboos in the modern society. In the largest series published until now, more than 90% of 2,000 patients attending a bad breath clinic [13] had complaints for more than 1 year, reaching even up to 15 years in 16% of the cases. Most of them searched for help at several other places, and less than 30% of the subjects were referred to the bad breath clinic by a health care professional (general practitioner, dentist or medical/oral specialist). This indicates that the lack of knowledge around this topic is not restricted to the general population but also to medical services.

As mentioned before, the cause of the bad breath mostly can be found in the oral cavity. This was the case for 75.8% of the 2,000 above-mentioned patients [13]; with tongue coating being the predominant cause either alone (43.3%) or in combination with gingivitis and periodontitis (18.2%). The presence of tongue coating has been related to several factors of which the level of oral hygiene appears to be the most important [14].

In less than 3% of the patients, bad breath had an extraoral origin, with a wide variety of pathologies, but predominantly associated to gastrointestinal disorders (table 1). Other non-oral causes of halitosis are less frequent and include disturbances of the upper and lower respiratory tract, some systemic diseases, metabolic disorders and carcinomas [15, 16].

A special situation arises when an obvious breath malodor cannot be perceived by others but the patient is convinced that he or she suffers from it. This 'imaginary halitosis', also called pseudo-halitosis, represents between 15 and 25% of the patients attending bad breath clinics [13, 17]. If after treatment of either genuine halitosis or diagnosis of pseudo-halitosis, the patient still believes that bad breath is present, we speak of 'halitopho-

Table 1. Etiology of halitosis in 2,000 patients attending a halitosis clinic

Cause	Percent
Oral	
Tongue coating	43.4
Gingivitis	3.8
Periodontitis	7.4
Combination of tongue coating with gingivitis or periodontitis	18.2
Xerostomia	2.5
Teeth related	0.4
Candida	0.2
	75.8
Ear/nose/throat (ENT)	
Tonsillitis	0.7
Rhinitis	0.6
Sinusitis	0.2
Nose obstruction	0.4
	1.9
Extra-oral	
GI	1.3
Trimethylaminuria	0.1
Other diseases	0.3
Medication	0.1
Hormonal	0.1
Diet	0.5
	2.3
Combination	
ENT/oral cause	2.1
GI/oral cause	1.7
	3.8
Pseudo-halitosis	15.7
Unknown	0.8

GI = Gastrointestinal. Adapted with permission from Quirynen et al. [13].

bia' [2] – a condition with a strong psychological component that implies a real challenge for bad breath clinics.

Oral malodor is the result of the degradation of organic substrates by anaerobic bacteria. During the process of bacterial putrefaction, different components such as peptides present in saliva, food debris, gingival crevicular fluid, interdental plaque, shed epithelial cells, postnasal drip and blood are hydrolyzed to sulfide- and non-sulfide-containing amino acids. The proteolytic degradation of sulfide containing amino acids (cysteine, cystine and methionine) by Gram-negative bacteria produce sulphur-containing gases like hydrogen sulfide (H_2S) and methyl mercaptan (CH_3SH) [18]. Other compounds such as indole and skatole, the amines putrescine and cadaverine and the carboxylic acids acetic, butyric and propionic acid are also formed by proteolytic degradation of non-sulfide-containing amino acids by oral microorganisms. Indole and skatole are mainly formed by bacterial degradation of tryptophan [19]. Lysine and ornithine are the most important substrates for the production of cadaverine and putrescine [20]. Organic acids (i.e. acetic, butyric and isovaleric) are also found as fermentation products of oral bacteria.

Some of these final products of bacterial activity – as the sulphur ones – are very volatile and contribute largely to the breath odor [21], others like biogenic amines are in a non-volatile status at the normal pH of the oral cavity and may only contribute under specific conditions (e.g. oral dryness) [22]. These compounds, however, can be detected in saliva, and their presence has shown to correlate with the presence of oral malodor [23–25].

The oral cavity is colonized by over 500 bacterial species, many of which can degrade proteins, peptides and amino acids. At least 82 species can produce H_2S from cysteine and another 25 are able to generate CH_3SH from methionine. They include *Treponema denticola, Por-*

phyromonas gingivallis, Prevotella intermedia and *Eubacterium* species [26]. In vitro studies have demonstrated the ability of Gram-negative anaerobic bacteria of the oral cavity to produce volatile sulphur compounds (VSCs) from serum and other sources of proteins [27–30]. Recently, the presence of *Solobacterium moorei*, a Gram-positive bacterium, has been linked to oral malodor [31, 32].

Diagnostic Strategies

Current methods for diagnosis of oral malodor are based either on the subjective detection of the presence of an unpleasant smell (organoleptic or hedonic procedure) and/or the objective measurement of VSCs.

The organoleptic rating or scoring (OLS), considered as the 'gold standard method', is done by simply sniffing the breath air by a trained and calibrated judge. The air is rated on its intensity and unpleasantness. Different scales and definitions have been proposed: a 9-point hedonic rating (HR) scale [33], a 6-point intensity scale [34] and a 4-point scale based on the distance at which the odor can be perceived [35]. The intensity scale proposed by Rosenberg and McCulloch [34], with OLS of 0 representing absence of odor, 1 given for barely noticeable, 2 for slight, 3 for moderate, 4 for strong, and 5 for severe malodor, is the most commonly used. The main drawbacks of this technique are its intrinsic subjectivity, the necessity of calibration and training of the odor judges [36, 37] and the embarrassment for the patient when undergoing the examination. Because the smell that characterizes bad breath arises from the combination of several malodor compounds, the human nose is, until now, the only 'sensor' able to recognize oral malodor as entity [38].

Gas chromatography is probably the most objective and reproducible method for the measurement of the VSCs [39]. Unfortunately, it is not suitable for routine analysis since it is expensive, not portable and needs trained personnel. In order to overcome these practical drawbacks, several portable devices have been developed. Two of the most commonly used devices are the Halimeter[®] (Interscan Coorporation, Chatsworth, US) and the OralChroma™ (Abilit Corporation, Kanagawa, Japan). Based on an enclosed liquid electrochemical cell, the Halimeter provides a digital readout of the VSC concentration in air aspirated from the oral cavity. It cannot discriminate between the different sulphur gases and shows different sensitivity for each of them [40]. The OralChroma is designed as a simple GC system with a highly sensitive metal oxide semiconductor gas sensor as detector. It is able to detect separately the three main sulphur compounds, even though the peak integration is not always perfect and needs to be corrected manually [41]. Measurements with both devices have shown to correlate well with the OLS [42, 43]. Because of their high specificity, they can be used to prove the absence of malodor in case of imaginary halitosis/pseudo-halitosis [44].

Oral Malodor Management

In an effort to prevent or at least alleviate oral malodor, several treatment strategies have been developed. Because the offensive smell arises from the metabolic degradation of available substrates by certain microorganisms, it seems logic that this condition can be ameliorated by (a) masking the unpleasant smell, (b) reducing substrate availability, (c) reducing bacterial load or (d) converting volatile malodor compounds to non-volatiles forms [45].

Mints, chewing gums and sprays are used to mask the malodor [46–48]. Since they do not deal with the etiology of the malodor, they are only effective for very short periods of time.

Eliminating the cause of the malodor can be done mechanically or chemically. Given that tongue coating is the major etiological factor for oral malodor [13, 49] cleaning the tongue on a regular basis is recommended [50]. The tongue can be cleaned with a normal toothbrush, but preferably with a tongue scraper [51]. The cleaning of the tongue seems to reduce the substrate for putrefaction, rather than the bacterial load. It also improves the taste sensation [52]. Toothpastes and mouth rinses are the most common products used to deliver active chemical ingredients such as antibacterial and oxidizing agents into the oral cavity.

Toothpastes in the Management of Oral Malodor

Fluoride toothpastes are used to clean teeth, control plaque and prevent caries. Additional ingredients can be incorporated to provide supplementary benefits like controlling or preventing oral malodor. This chapter aimed to review the relevant investigations regarding the effect of toothpastes on parameters associated with oral malodor.

Two independent reviewers (J.D. and I.L.) screened relevant medical databases (PubMed and Embase) up to June 2012. Twenty-seven articles reporting results of in vivo studies and 5 other in vitro and ex vivo reports were retrieved. Hydrogen peroxide and baking soda; metal ions (e.g. stannous and zinc); antibacterial compounds, and a variety of flavors, essential oils and even detergents have been proposed to have an added value in the management of oral malodor.

The majority (65%) of the in vivo studies used a crossover design. The number of volunteers varied between 10 and 96 subjects. Only healthy volunteers were recruited. Not all the studies included a certain level of VSC, objectionable OLS or unpleasant HR as inclusion criterion. Instead, volunteers were asked to refrain from oral hygiene and eating or drinking the morning of the examination in order to mimic morning bad breath.

Except for one study where the toothpaste was used as slurry [53], all subjects used the pastes only for manual tooth brushing on their customary

Table 2. Summary of in vivo studies assessing effectiveness of toothpastes with different active components in controlling oral malodor

First author, year	Active component	Design (inclusion criterion)	Subjects	Use	Time	Reduction in oral malodor indicator
Grigor, 1992	H_2O_2	crossover (none)	10	once	IA	59%[#] in thiols in saliva
Niles, 1995	BS	n.r.	16	once	3	43.8%[#] in VSC (GC)
Brunette, 1998	BS	crossover (VSC >2 ng/10 ml)	11	once	IA; 1 ,2 ,3 h	>50% in VSC (GC)
	BS	crossover (OLS ≥4)	39 / 38	once	1, 2, 3 h	>73, >48, >28% in OLS of breath / 53, 41, 31% in OLS of breath
Bradshaw, 2005	flavor	crossover (none)	24	once	2 h	>70%[*, #] in OLS breath
Peruzzo, 2008	flavor	crossover (none)	50	3 × day/1 month	ON	24%[§] in VSC (Halimeter) / 33%[*, §] in OLS of breath
Peruzzo, 2008	SLS	crossover (none)	25	3 × day/1 month	ON	38%[#] in VSC (Halimeter) / 33%[#] in OLS of breath
Newby, 2008	SLS	crossover (VSC >300 ppb)	20	once	IA; 1, 2, 3, 7 h	up to 80%[*, §] in VSC levels (GC)
Bosman, 2008	SLS	crossover (none)	34	once	IA	1.3 log[§] anaerobic bacteria and BPB removed
Olshan, 2000	EO	intersubject (HR >4)	40 / 45	once	0.5, 1, 2, 3, 4 h	up to 40%[*, #] in HR of breath / up to 37%[*, #] in HR of breath

Time signifies measurement time after last product use. IA = Immediately after; ON = overnight; BS = baking soda; EO = essential oils; GC = gas chromatography; BPB = black pigmented bacteria; n.r. = not reported. Studies performed with VSC levels or OLS as inclusion criteria (morning bad breath model) are shown in *italics*. * Significant with respect to baseline; [#] significant with respect to placebo; [§] significant with respect to other treatment.

manner; tongues were not brushed or scraped. Only 5 studies included supervised brushing. A single use or a twice-a-day brushing during a week was the most common schedule. Longer intervals were less frequent and did not exceed a month. Small, and therefore probably negligible, differences in the standardization of the amount of toothpaste and time of brushing were also observed. The effect of the pastes in breath malodor indicators was evaluated at time intervals oscillating between immediately after use to overnight (12 h).

Tables 2–5 contain all the relevant information from the in vivo studies regarding the different active components. This information together with the findings of the in vitro and ex vivo studies is discussed in more detail below. Data regarding the use of hydrogen peroxide, baking soda, flavors, essential oils and detergents are summarized in table 2. Evidence supporting the use of metal ions in the formulations is presented in tables 3 and 4. Table 5 summarizes the available information for the use of triclosan alone and with extra active components.

Hydrogen Peroxide

The ability of oxidizing agents to delay the degradation of thiol precursors in saliva has been suggested a while ago in the context of a research

Table 3. Summary of in vivo studies assessing effectiveness of toothpaste formulations with SnF_2 in controlling oral malodor

First author, year	Active component	Design (inclusion criterion)	Subjects	Use	Time	Reduction in oral malodor indicator
Gerlach, 1998	SnF_2	intersubject (OLS >4)	96	2×/day, 5 days	3, 8 h after first use	8[#], 14%[#] in VSC levels (Halimeter) 38[#], 13% in OLS of breath
					3, 8 h after last use	14[#], 16%[#] in VSC levels (Halimeter) 37[#], 19%[#] in OLS of breath
Quirynen, 2002	SnF_2	crossover (none)	16	2×/day, 1 week	ON after 3 days and 1 week	>40%* in OLS of breath 21% in OLS of tongue
Chen, 2010	SnF_2	crossover (VSC >120 ppb)	33	3×/day, 1 day	ON, 4 h (28 h)	47[#], 69%[#] in VSC levels (Halimeter)
Feng, 2010	SnF_2	metanalysis (VSC >120 ppb)	100	2×/day, 1 day	3–4 h, ON, 3–4 h (27–28 h)	52[#], 24[#],59%[#] in VSC levels (Halimeter)

Time signifies measurement time after last product use. Studies performed with VSC levels or OLS as inclusion criteria (morning bad breath model) are shown in *italics*. * Significant with respect to baseline; [#] significant with respect to placebo; [§] significant with respect to other treatment.

Table 4. Summary of in vivo studies assessing effectiveness of toothpastes formulations with zinc ions alone and combined with other active ingredient in controlling oral malodor

First author, year	Active component	Design (inclusion criterion)	Subjects	Use	Time	Reduction in oral malodor indicator
Newby, 2008	Zn^{2+}	crossover (VSC >300 ppb)	16	once	IA, 1 h	82*[,#,§], 44%*[,#,§] in VSC levels (GC)
Navada, 2008	Zn^{2+}	intersubject (VSC >120 ppb, OLS ≥3)	94	2×/day, 1 month	2 h after first/ last use	68*[,#], 42%*[,#] in VSC levels (Halimeter) 28*[,#], 28%*[,#] in OLS of breath
Young, 2011	Zn^{2+}	crossover (none)	28	once	ON	68[#,§], 47%[#,§] in H_2S and CH_3SH (GC)
Payne, 2011	Zn^{2+} and o-cymen-5-ol	crossover (H_2S >300 ppb)	78	2×/day, 1 week	ON, IA, 1, 2, 3 h	33*[,§] to 97%*[,§] in H_2S (GC) 27*[,§] to 77%*[,§] in CH_3SH (GC)

Time signifies measurement time after last product use. Studies performed with VSC levels or OLS as inclusion criteria (morning bad breath model) are shown in *italics*. * Significant with respect to baseline; [#] significant with respect to placebo; [§] significant with respect to other treatment.

Table 5. Summary of in vivo studies assessing effectiveness of triclosan/copolymer-containing toothpastes in controlling oral malodor

First author, year	Active component	Design (inclusion criterion)	Subjects	Use	Time	Oral malodor indicator
Niles, 1999	TCN+PVM/MA	crossover (VSC >20 ng/ml)	20	2×/day, 1 week	7 h, ON	65.3[*, §] and 41.2%[*, §] in VSC levels (GC)
Sharma, 1999	TCN+PVM/MA	intersubject (HR ≥6)	32	once	12 h	28%[*] in HR of breath
Screnivasan, 2003	TCN+PVM/MA	crossover (none)	20	2×/day, 1 week	2, 4 h, ON	62[*], 52[*], 49%[*] in bacterial counts in saliva rinse 79[*], 72[*], 66%[*] in BPB counts in saliva rinse
Hu, 2005	TCN+PVM/MA	intersubject (HR ≥6)	41	2×/day, 3 weeks	1 day; 1, 2, 3 weeks	>50%[*, #] in HR of breath
Niles, 2005	TCN+PVM/MA	crossover (VSC >300 ppb)	34	2×/day, 1 week	1 week	57%[*, #] in VSC levels (GC)
Vazquez, 2005	TCN+PVM/MA	crossover (none)	30	2×/day, 1 week	2, 4 h, ON	82[*], 80[*], 22% in BPB counts in saliva rinse
Fine, 2006	TCN+PVM/MA	crossover (none)	15	2×/day, 1 week	6 h, ON	>88%[*] in bacterial counts in saliva rinse, TC and plaque >81%[*] in BPB counts in in saliva rinse, TC and plaque
Sharma, 2007	TCN+PVM/MA	intersubject (HR ≥6)	39	once	12 h	28%[*, §] in HR of breath
Raven, 1996	TCN+PVM/MA+Zn^{2+}	crossover (none)	16 24	once 2×/day, 3 weeks	IA; 1, 2, 3 h ON after 1 day, 1 and 3 weeks	80[*, #], 74[*, #], 46[*, #], 44[*, #] and 22%[#] in VSC levels (GC) 15, 22 and 37%[*, #] in VSC levels (GC)
Sharma, 2002	TCN+PVM/MA +special silica	intersubject (HR ≥6)	42	once	12 h	23.5%[*] in HR of breath
Hu, 2008	TCN+PVM/MA +special silica	intersubject (HR ≥6)	40	once	ON	33.1%[*, §] in HR of breath 60.8%[*, §] in bacterial counts of plaque

Time signifies measurement time after last product use. TC = Tongue coating; TCN = triclosan. Studies performed with VSC levels or OLS as inclusion criteria (morning bad breath model) are shown in *italics*. [*] Significant with respect to baseline; [#] significant with respect to placebo; [§] significant with respect to other treatment.

combining in vivo and in vitro observations. The in vitro experiment showed the ability of a hydrogen peroxide solution (27.5% w/w) to reduce the concentration of salivary thiols. Additionally, when saliva samples were incubated for 24 h with different amounts of hydrogen peroxide, a reduction up to 75% of thiols compared to baseline could be observed. The in vivo study compared the effect of a paste containing baking soda and H$_2$O$_2$ versus a fluoride control. After 30 min, the test paste caused a decrease in the salivary thiols of 59% compared to the 12.5% of the control one [54]. Even though these first results were promising, no further reports on the use of this oxidizing agent in the management of oral malodor were available. Peroxides are used in bleaching treatments [55] and are also listed as active components of whitening toothpastes [56].

Baking Soda (Sodium Bicarbonate)
Even before the introduction of modern tooth-paste, sodium bicarbonate and salt have been used as dentifrices [57]. A short-term, but significant reduction in VSC levels in the oral cavity (43.8%) was observed when using a sodium bicarbonate/fluoride dentifrice [58]. Brunette et al. [59] investigated the impact of the concentration of baking soda on the ability of reducing mouth odor. Using commercially available dentifrices as well as experimental pastes, Brunette's group demonstrated that formulations containing more than 15% baking soda provided real benefits, reducing the odor to acceptable levels. When zinc ions were added to the formulation, the reduction in the levels of VSC exceeded 50%. Interestingly, each author proposed a different mechanism of action. While Niles and Gaffar [58] attributed the reduction to the conversion to a non-odorous form; Brunette et al. [59] suggested that baking soda exerts an antibacterial activity by disruption of outer membranes. Moreover, a mild abrasive action of the compound contributes to the removal of bacteria from dental surfaces. Later research demonstrating enhanced plaque removal by baking soda dentifrices supported Brunette's theory [60].

Flavors
Flavors are incorporated into oral care products as excipients [56], and they are undoubtedly one of most important attributes influencing consumer acceptance and appreciation. Flavors include a wide range of compounds, and they are believed to deliver breath-freshening benefits via masking. Additionally, some of them are known to have antimicrobial effect [29]. It has been suggested that the presence of flavoring agents could stimulate saliva flow, speeding up the clearance of bacteria and thus altering the sequence of events that leads to oral malodor.

Bradshaw et al. [61] selected flavor ingredients with proven in vitro ability of inhibiting VSC production to be tested in a panel of 24 subjects. The effect of toothpaste formulations containing one of the breath-freshening flavors on the HRs of the participants was evaluated every half an hour for 2 h after brushing. The 'Boudica' flavor showed significant reductions in the breath scores when compared with a standard flavor at all the time points. A formulation with the 'Theseus' flavor was not only better than an unflavored paste but also as good as a paste containing 0.1% triclosan. Similar data were obtained when comparing the breath-freshening flavor 'Herakles' with a standard-flavored product containing 0.2% zinc sulphate. Every compound exceeded 70% reductions in the malodor indicators [61]. The authors attribute the effect of the flavors to their ability to interfere with the VSC production rather than to masking. Later, a flavor-containing dentifrice was compared with a similar unflavored formulation in a crossover study involving 50 healthy volunteers. The participants brushed for a month, 3 times per day with one of the toothpastes. The flavoring agent seemed to reduce morning bad breath by decreasing the formation of VSC by 24% [62].

Sodium Lauryl Sulfate
Anionic detergents such as sodium lauryl sulfate (SLS) are used as surfactants in many toothpaste formulations [56]. It has been suggested that the substantivity of SLS in the oral cavity might influence the antimicrobial activity of a dentifrice [63]. However, even though it is (one compound, SLS) extensively used in oral care products, only little evidence is available regarding the possible effect of SLS against oral malodor. One report compared the effect of toothpaste with and without SLS on morning bad breath of healthy volunteers. After 30 days of use, the formulation containing SLS caused a 38 and 33% reduction in VSC and OLS, respectively [64]. In another study, a 'gel-to-foam' toothpaste containing higher levels of SLS (2% w/w, usual concentrations do not exceed 1.5% w/w) showed a significant reduction in VSC levels. The effect was even better than the one ob-

served with a triclosan-containing dentifrice, probably due an increased removal of debris from the mouth because of the elevated surfactant level [65]. To support this theory, a study has been carried out to assess the ability of the gel-to-foam dentifrice to remove oral debris and bacteria. The gel-to-foam dentifrice showed 1.3 log greater removal of total anaerobes and VSC-producing bacteria than a triclosan-containing toothpaste. A greater distribution of the dentifrice components, maximizing surface cleaning efficacy has been proposed as mechanism of action [66].

Essential Oils

Ethereal or essential oils are used in perfumes, cosmetics, soaps and for flavoring food and drinks. There is only one publication reporting the short-term beneficial effects on oral malodor of toothpastes containing such compounds. The dentifrice was able to reduce up to 40% the hedonic ratings of 40 volunteers. During the first 90 min, the reductions were significantly better than the ones obtained with the control toothpaste. The addition of zinc ions to the formulation extended the benefit up to 120 min [33].

SnF$_2$/Amine Fluoride

Stannous ions, like other metals, are able to capture VSC [67–69]. They exhibit an antibacterial and antiplaque action by reducing the glycolytic activity in microorganisms and delaying bacterial growth [70]. The amine fluoride included in the formulation stabilizes the stannous ion, which is translated into an extended presence of this last one in the oral cavity increasing therefore its effect [71, 72]. Several studies evaluated the favorable effect of this ion in mouthrinses and toothpastes for the prevention of plaque formation and gingivitis [73]. Quirynen et al. [53, 74] evaluated the effect of slurry of SnF$_2$/amine fluoride toothpaste in vivo (2002) and also in an in vitro model (2003). When rinsing with the slurry was the only oral hygiene measure, a slight decrease in OLS of

breath over the time could be recorded. The level of VSC compounds showed minor fluctuations, and changes in the bacterial load of saliva and tongue were negligible. The inferior efficacy of the slurry when compared with a mouthrinse with the same formulation was probably due to the reduced solubility of the paste and to a lower amount of active ingredients [53].

The first evidence of the clinical utility of stannous fluoride dentifrice in the management of oral malodor was highlighted by the research of Gerlach et al. [75]. Following cumulative use, stannous fluoride showed to be superior to both sodium fluoride pyrophosphate and sodium fluoride/triclosan copolymer formulations in reducing both OLS and VSC levels.

Recently, a meta-analysis of 4 randomized controlled clinical trials demonstrated the superior short-term and overnight benefit of a stannous-containing dentifrice versus a control dentifrice [76] on morning bad breath. The reductions in VSC levels averaged 24% overnight while exceeding 50% for the short-term effect. Independent data of one of the randomized controlled clinical trials also included the evaluation of an additional effect by tongue brushing [77]. No differences were observed, and the authors attributed this to a very weak intervention. The tongue was divided into three sections (front, middle and back), and only one stroke per section was applied.

Zinc Ions

Zinc ions bind to sulphur ions in VSCs leading to the formation of poorly soluble zinc sulfides that can be easily removed from the oral cavity [78]. Even though zinc ions have a lower affinity than stannous ions, their capacity to inhibit the VSC is bigger [79]. Significant short-term reductions in the level of VSC in subjects with morning bad breath have been reported in a small study evaluating a toothpaste containing zinc chloride. Two formulations with identical zinc ion concentration but different pH (6.2 vs. 9.2) showed a clearly different benefit in reducing oral malodor. The formulation with the most neutral pH delivered greater benefits with up to 82% of reduction in the VSC levels immediately after use. The authors suggested that the effect of zinc salts is not only dependent on their concentration but also the pH of the formulation [65]. The chemical neutralization of VSC compounds by zinc salts is known to be concentration dependent [80]. In a bigger set of volunteers with objectionable morning breath, the short- (2 h after brushing) and long-term (overnight after 1 month of use) effect of a toothpaste containing zinc sulphate was evaluated [81]. The reductions in the VSC (68 and 42%, respectively) and in the OLS levels (30 and 28%, respectively) were significant compared with baseline and the placebo toothpaste.

Recently, the single effect of toothpastes containing zinc as zinc gluconate or as zinc citrate was evaluated in volunteers with morning bad breath [82]. Both toothpastes reduced for 12 h the oral VSC levels and also the amount of H_2S produced by a cysteine challenge. The toothpaste with zinc citrate (experimental) was more effective (35 and 68% reduction in H_2S and methyl mercaptan, respectively) than a marketed formulation containing zinc gluconate (12 and 47% for the same compounds) probably because of the presence of a copolymer and slightly higher concentration of zinc ions. In dry state and without the presence of a copolymer, zinc citrate has shown to be less effective than zinc acetate or gluconate [69, 80].

Zinc and Other Active Components
3-methyl-4-propan-2-ylphenol or *o-cymen-5-ol* is a substituted phenol used in cosmetic products as a preservative to prolong the shelf-life of formulas. Recently, the first data of toothpaste containing zinc ions and o-cymen-5-ol have been presented. Three in vitro models illustrated that the observed effects on the VSC levels were mostly due to the action of the zinc present in the formulation. However, it has been suggested that o-cymen-5-ol may be able to reduce VCS levels by a direct antimicrobial effect or interference with bacterial activities [83]. When combined with zinc chloride, o-cymen-5-ol resulted in a spectrum of antimicrobial activities greater than for each ingredient alone [84]. The clinical utility of the formulation has been reported in an in vivo study. Subjects with morning bad breath (VSC levels higher than 300 ppb) used the test paste or a sodium fluoride control dentifrice during a week. The levels of VSC were monitored overnight, immediately after and every hour up to 3 h after use. Reductions caused by the paste containing zinc chloride and o-cymen-5-ol ranged from 33 to 97% and 27 to 77% for H_2S and methyl mercaptan, respectively; they were, at all time points, significantly superior to the reference paste [85]. A toothpaste containing zinc lactate and cetylpyridinium chloride is commercially available. Cetylpyridinium chloride is a quaternary ammonium compound with demonstrated effectiveness as an antiplaque agent [86]. There is however no scientific literature available supporting the benefit of this combination in oral malodor management.

Triclosan
2,4,4′-trichloro-2′hydroxydiphenyl ether or triclosan is a broad-spectrum antibacterial agent that has been in use for at least 30 years in personal care products. With the cytoplasmatic membrane of bacteria as primary target, triclosan's action can vary from interrupting essential amino acids uptake to cellular leakage in both Gram-positive and Gram-negative bacteria [87]. Because of its lipophilic nature, triclosan tends to partition into a hydrophobic oil phase and thereby become unavailable for adsorption onto oral surfaces. To overcome this limitation, triclosan can be solubilized in flavoring oils or anionic detergents (sodium dodecyl sulfate, sodium lauroyl sarcosinate, propylene glycol or polyethylene glycol). Copolymers like polyvi-

nylmethyl ether maleic acid (PVM/MA) are added to increase oral retention and decrease the rate of release. This characteristic has been outlined in a small study examining the impact of triclosan-containing toothpaste, with and without solubilizing agents. In a set of volunteers with morning bad breath, a paste containing triclosan and zinc, but without flavor oil, was not able to reduce the breath levels of VSC further than 15 min [87]. The same was observed by Nogueira-Filho [89] when evaluating the effect of triclosan formulations without copolymer but with the addition of zinc. The paste was not able to reduce the increase in VSC during the development of experimental gingivitis. In vivo studies demonstrated that triclosan lost its anti-VSC effect when solubilized in oil, in an uncharged detergent or in a chromophor, whereas it maintained its effect when solubilized in a combination of sodium lauryl sulphate, propylene glycol and water [68].

Several studies have illustrated the effect of formulations based on triclosan and a copolymer in the management of oral malodor. Niles et al. [90] assessed chromatographically the effect of a paste containing triclosan and PVM/MA in volunteers with high VSC levels. After brushing their teeth for a week with the test paste or a placebo (fluoride) paste, an 'all day' (7 h) and 'overnight' reduction in the levels of VSC could be demonstrated. For individuals that initially exhibited unpleasant breath (HR >5), 2 studies reported a 28% reduction in the breath scores, 12 h after a single use of the same formulation [91, 92]. Later on, the long-term effect of the formulation was demonstrated in a study involving 40 subjects with unpleasant breath that brushed twice a day for 3 weeks with a triclosan-containing paste. Reductions of more than 50% were observed in the breath scores at the end of every treatment week [93]. In an independent group of volunteers with high VSC levels, a 1-week use of the paste showed to have a similar effect. A 57% reduction over-night was achieved with the test paste while the placebo effect was only 10% [94].

To support the evidence on the reduction in OLS and VSC compounds, the in vitro antimicrobial effect of triclosan has been evaluated. A slurry of a triclosan toothpaste showed to be effective in reducing the number of total bacteria and black pigmented bacteria in a mixture of oral bacteria obtained by a mix of saliva and tongue scrapings [95]. Moreover, significant reduction in bacterial load was observed when plaque and saliva samples were incubated for 30–120 s with triclosan toothpaste [96].

Three crossover studies on healthy volunteers were performed to assess the in vivo antimicrobial effect. All of them evaluated the amount of bacteria recovered from saliva rinses before and after brushing twice a day during a week with a fluoride dentifrice or the test paste containing triclosan. Significant overnight reductions (between 49 and 89%) were observed for the total bacteria as well as for H_2S-producing species [97–99]. Samples of plaque and tongue coating showed even more marked reductions (up to 91.4 and 93.4% for total bacteria and 81.1 and 84.5% for H_2S-producing species, respectively) [99].

Triclosan Combined with other Active Ingredients

The added value of zinc, flavors and special-grade silica to the basic triclosan-containing formulation (0.3% triclosan, 0.243% sodium fluoride and 2% of copolymer) of the above mentioned studies, has been evaluated. Two crossover studies demonstrated the short- and long-term reduction in VSC levels by a triclosan/zinc paste. The short-term reductions fluctuated between 80 and 22% and were significantly different from the placebo paste up to 3 h. The overnight effect was evident after 21 days of regular use of the product. Shorter interval evaluations (1 and 7 days) did not reach significance [100]. Moreover, a formulation containing triclosan with the addition of zinc was able to reduce the increase in VSC occurring during the development of experimental gingivitis [83].

The antimicrobial efficacy and the ability of reducing VSC formation of a triclosan-containing dentifrice, with and without flavor, were assessed using an in vitro breath VSC model. Both formulations showed to have similar effects and were significantly better than a control fluorinated dentifrice [101].

Optimized formulations containing silica have shown to be as effective as the basic formulation in reducing morning bad breath [102]. A 33.1% reduction in OLS and 60.8% in the bacterial counts of plaque have been reported after single use of a toothpaste containing special grade silica [103].

Discussion

To our surprise, the amount of literature supporting the use of dedicated toothpastes in the treatment of oral malodor was far smaller than on other topics such as caries, plaque control and tooth whitening. Only 27 scientific articles reported results of in vivo studies, and few other in vitro and ex vivo reports provided supporting evidence. Formulations with eight different active compounds claimed to have an effect on the management of oral malodor. The diversity of active ingredients and the rather small number of publications made that with the exception of triclosan the number of publications per formulation was low.

When evaluating the results of the in vivo studies, some considerations should be made. The VSC level and/or the OLS of the breath were the most common indicators used to assess the effect of the toothpastes. A minority of studies evaluated the impact on the microbiology of the oral cavity. In spite of the relevant role of the tongue coating in the etiology of oral malodor [13] and the direct correlation between the presence of tongue coating and the level of oral hygiene [14], none of the articles reported the impact of tooth brushing on the amount of coating of the volunteers.

It is also important to note that most of the studies have been carried out on volunteers with morning bad breath and not in real malodor patients. Morning bad breath is frequently used as model in research regarding oral malodor. Although useful, the information obtained with this model should be carefully interpreted. Furthermore, while for some studies the level of malodor was not even an inclusion criterion, for others where the criterion was defined the threshold differed enormously (i.e. 120 vs. 300 ppb VSC). The studies included therefore volunteers with different degrees of malodor.

Even though statistically significant reductions in the malodor indicators have been demonstrated, the 'real' effect of the pastes remains unclear. Breath evaluations in which the unpleasant smell was no longer detected (e.g. OLS <2; HR <6), or where the VSC level was below the 'threshold of objectionableness' (MM <0.5 ng/10ml; H_2S <1.5 ng/10 ml) [104] have not been reported.

Finally, most of the research has been carried out or sponsored by the manufacturer. The risk of publication bias (only positive results) should be at least considered.

Regardless of the limitations pointed out previously, some general conclusions can be made. For toothpastes containing hydrogen peroxide, baking soda, essential oils and flavors as active components, only few studies are available, and they only showed a short-term effect on oral malodor indicators. Data supporting their beneficial effect on oral malodor are therefore scarce and inconclusive. A little more is known in the case of formulations containing metal ions. Studies supporting the short-term as well as the overnight decrease in oral malodor indicators caused by both stannous and zinc ions can be found in the literature. The biggest amount of evidence was found for triclosan.

Several publications have demonstrated the short-term and the overnight effect of triclosan on oral malodor due to its antibacterial and antiplaque activity.

Conclusions

Considering the central role of tongue coating in the development of halitosis [13] and the fact that the level of oral hygiene appears to be the main influencing factor [14], tooth brushing appears to be crucial in the management of oral malodor. From a theoretical point of view, one could assume that brushing should be able to prevent the formation of the coating, and dedicated toothpastes should have an extra added value on this effect. Once the coating is present, brushing may need to be reinforced with mechanical cleaning of the tongue (brushing or scraping). Unfortunately, none of the studies reviewed here has assessed properly this issue, and therefore scientific evidence supporting these assumptions is still needed.

In spite of these limitations, antibacterial agents such as triclosan and metal ions such as stannous and zinc appear to be effective in the control of oral malodor. For other ingredients like hydrogen peroxide, baking soda, essential oils and flavors, data supporting their beneficial effect on oral malodor are rather few and inconclusive.

References

1 Van Steenberghe D, Quirynen M: Breath Malodor. Clinical Periodontology and Implant Dentistry, Oxford, Blackwell Munksgaard, 2003, pp 512–518.

2 Yaegaki K, Coil JM: Examination, classification, and treatment of halitosis; clinical perspectives. J Can Dent Assoc 2000; 66:257–261.

3 Spouge J: Halitosis: a review of its causes and treatment. Dent Practit 1964;14: 307–317.

4 Rosenberg M, Kozlovsky A, Gelernter I, Cherniak O, Gabbay J, Baht R, Eli I: Self-estimation of oral malodor. J Dent Res 1995;74:1577–1582.

5 Eli I, Baht R, Koriat H, Rosenberg M: Self-perception of breath odor. J Am Dent Assoc 2001;132:621–626.

6 Miyazaki H, Sakao S, Katoh Y, Takehara T: Correlation between volatile sulphur compounds and certain oral health measurements in the general population. J Periodontol 1995;66:679–684.

7 Söder B, Johansson B, Söder PO: The relation between foetor ex ore, oral hygiene and periodontal disease. Swed Dent J 2000;24:73–82.

8 Liu XN, Shinada K, Chen XC, Zhang BX, Yaegaki K, Kawaguchi Y: Oral malodor-related parameters in the Chinese general population. J Clin Periodontol 2006; 33:31–36.

9 Nadanovsky P, Carvalho LBM, Ponce de Leon A: Oral malodour and its association with age and sex in a general population in Brazil. Oral Dis 2007;13:105–109.

10 Iwanicka-Grzegorek E, Michalik J, Kepa J, Wierzbicka M, Aleksinski M, Pierzynowska E: Subjective patients' opinion and evaluation of halitosis using halimeter and organoleptic scores. Oral Dis 2005;11(suppl 1):86–88.

11 Knaan T, Cohen D, Rosenberg M: O23 Predicting bad breath in the non-complaining population. Oral Dis 2005;11: 105–106.

12 ADA Council on Scientific Affairs: Oral malodor. J Am Dent Assoc 2003;134: 209–214.

13 Quirynen M, Dadamio J, Van den Velde S, De Smit M, Dekeyser C, Van Tornout M, Vandekerckhove B: Characteristics of 2,000 patients who visited a halitosis clinic. J Clin Periodontol 2009;36:970–975.

14 Van Tornout M, Dadamio J, Coucke W, Quirynen M: Tongue coating: related factors. J Clin Periodontol 2013;40:180–185.

15 Tangerman A: Halitosis in medicine: a review. Int Dent J 2002;52(suppl 3):201–206.

16 Scully C, Greenman J: Halitosis (breath odor). Periodontol 2000 2008;48:66–75.

17 Seemann R, Bizhang M, Djamchidi C, Kage A, Nachnani S: The proportion of pseudo-halitosis patients in a multidisciplinary breath malodour consultation. Int Dent J 2006;56:77–81.

18 Wåler SM: On the transformation of sulfur-containing amino acids and peptides to volatile sulfur compounds (VSC) in the human mouth. Eur J Oral Sci 1997;105:534–537.

19 Jensen MT, Jensen BB: Gas chromatographic determination of indole and 3-methylindole (skatole) in bacterial culture media, intestinal contents and faeces. J Chromatogr B Biomed Appl 1994;655:275–280.

20 Patocka J, Kuehn GD: Natural polyamines and their biological consequence in mammals. Acta Medica (Hradec Kralove) 2000;43:119–124.

21 Van den Velde S, Van Steenberghe D, Van Hee P, Quirynen M: Detection of odorous compounds in breath. J Dent Res 2009;88:285–289.

22 Kleinberg I, Wolff MS, Codipilly DM: Role of saliva in oral dryness, oral feel and oral malodour. Int Dent J 2002; 52(suppl 3):236–240.

23 Goldberg S, Kozlovsky A, Gordon D, Gelernter I, Sintov A, Rosenberg M: Cadaverine as a putative component of oral malodor. J Dent Res 1994;73:1168–1172.

24 Kleinberg I, Codipilly M: The Biological Basis of Oral Malodor Formation. Bad Breath, Research Perspectives. Tel-Aviv, Ramot Publishing, 1995, pp 13–39.

25 Dadamio J, Van Tornout M, Vancauwenberghe F, Federico R, Dekeyser C, Quirynen M: Clinical utility of a novel colorimetric chair side test for oral malodour. J Clin Periodontol 2012;39:645–650.

26 Loesche WJ, Kazor C: Microbiology and treatment of halitosis. Periodontol 2000 2002;28:256–279.

27 Persson S, Claesson R, Carlsson J: The capacity of subgingival microbiotas to produce volatile sulfur compounds in human serum. Oral Microbiol Immunol 1989;4:169–172.

28 Persson S, Edlund MB, Claesson R, Carlsson J: The formation of hydrogen sulfide and methyl mercaptan by oral bacteria. Oral Microbiol Immunol 1990; 5:195–201.

29 Quirynen M, Van Eldere J, Pauwels M, Bollen CM, Van Steenberghe D: In vitro volatile sulfur compound production of oral bacteria in different culture media. Quintessence Int 1999;30:351–356.

30 Nakano Y, Yoshimura M, Koga T: Methyl mercaptan production by periodontal bacteria. Int Dent J 2002;52(suppl 3): 217–220.

31 Haraszthy VI, Zambon JJ, Sreenivasan PK, Zambon MM, Gerber D, Rego R, Parker C: Identification of oral bacterial species associated with halitosis. J Am Dent Assoc 2007;138:1113–1120.

32 Haraszthy VI, Gerber D, Clark B, Moses P, Parker C, Sreenivasan PK, Zambon JJ: Characterization and prevalence of *Solobacterium moorei* associated with oral halitosis. J Breath Res 2008;2: 017002.

33 Olshan AM, Kohut BE, Vincent JW, Borden LC, Delgado N, Qaqish J, Sharma NC, McGuire JA: Clinical effectiveness of essential oil-containing dentifrices in controlling oral malodor. Am J Dent 2000;13:18C–22C.

34 Rosenberg M, McCulloch CA: Measurement of oral malodor: current methods and future prospects. J Periodontol 1992;63:776–782.

35 Seemann R: Measurement of Halitosis. Halitosis. Patients with Oral Malodor in Daily Dental Practice, Quintessence. Berlin, Filippi A, 2006, pp 39–50.

36 Doty RL, Shaman P, Applebaum SL, Giberson R, Siksorski L, Rosenberg L: Smell identification ability: changes with age. Science 1984;226:1441–1443.

37 Nachnani S, Majerus G, Lenton P, Hodges J, Magallanes E: Effects of training on odor judges scoring intensity. Oral Dis 2005;11(suppl 1):40–44.

38 Hatt H: Molecular and cellular basis of human olfaction. Chem Biodivers 2004; 1:1857–1869.

39 Murata T, Yamaga T, Iida T, Miyazaki H, Yaegaki K: Classification and examination of halitosis. Int Dent J 2002; 52(suppl 3):181–186.

40 Furne J, Majerus G, Lenton P, Springfield J, Levitt DG, Levitt MD: Comparison of volatile sulfur compound concentrations measured with a sulfide detector vs gas chromatography. J Dent Res 2002;81:140–143.

41 Tangerman A, Winkel EG: The portable gas chromatograph OralChroma™: a method of choice to detect oral and extra-oral halitosis. J Breath Res 2008;2: 017010.

42 Rosenberg M, Kulkarni GV, Bosy A, McCulloch CA: Reproducibility and sensitivity of oral malodor measurements with a portable sulphide monitor. J Dent Res 1991;70:1436–1440.

43 Shimura M, Yasuno Y, Iwakura M, Shimada Y, Sakai S, Suzuki K, Sakamoto S: A new monitor with a zinc-oxide thin film semiconductor sensor for the measurement of volatile sulfur compounds in mouth air. J Periodontol 1996;67: 396–402.

44 Vandekerckhove B, Van den Velde S, De Smit M, Dadamio J, Teughels W, Van Tornout M, Quirynen M: Clinical reliability of non-organoleptic oral malodour measurements. J Clin Periodontol 2009;36:964–969.

45 Quirynen M, Zhao H, Van Steenberghe D: Review of the treatment strategies for oral malodour. Clin Oral Investig 2002; 6:1–10.

46 Reingewirtz Y, Girault O, Reingewirtz N, Senger B, Tenenbaum H: Mechanical effects and volatile sulfur compound-reducing effects of chewing gums: comparison between test and base gums and a control group. Quintessence Int 1999; 30:319–323.

47 Suarez FL, Furne JK, Springfield J, Levitt MD: Morning breath odor: influence of treatments on sulfur gases. J Dent Res 2000;79:1773–1777.

48 Yaegaki K, Coil JM, Kamemizu T, Miyazaki H: Tongue brushing and mouth rinsing as basic treatment measures for halitosis. Int Dent J 2002;52(suppl 3):192–196.

49 Bosy A, Kulkarni GV, Rosenberg M, McCulloch CA: Relationship of oral malodor to periodontitis: evidence of independence in discrete subpopulations. J Periodontol 1994;65:37–46.

50 Danser MM, Gómez SM, Van der Weijden GA: Tongue coating and tongue brushing: a literature review. Int J Dent Hyg 2003;1:151–158.

51 Outhouse TL, Al-Alawi R, Fedorowicz Z, Keenan JV: Tongue scraping for treating halitosis. Cochrane Database Syst Rev 2006;CD005519.

52 Quirynen M, Avontroodt P, Soers C, Zhao H, Pauwels M, Van Steenberghe D: Impact of tongue cleansers on microbial load and taste. J Clin Periodontol 2004; 31:506–510.

53 Quirynen M, Avontroodt P, Soers C, Zhao H, Pauwels M, Coucke W, Van Steenberghe D: The efficacy of amine fluoride/stannous fluoride in the suppression of morning breath odour. J Clin Periodontol 2002;29:944–954.

54 Grigor J, Roberts AJ: Reduction in the levels of oral malodor precursors by hydrogen peroxide: in vitro and in vivo assessments. J Clin Dent 1992;3:111–115.

55 Sulieman MAM: An overview of tooth-bleaching techniques: chemistry, safety and efficacy. Periodontol 2000 2008;48: 148–169.

56 Davies R, Scully C, Preston AJ: Dentifrices – an update. Med Oral Patol Oral Cir Bucal 2010;15:e976–e982.

57 Fischman SL: The history of oral hygiene products: how far have we come in 6000 years? Periodontol 2000 1997;15:7–14.

58 Niles HP, Gaffar A: Advances in Mouth Odor Research. Bad Breath: Research Perspectives. Ramat Aviv, Ramot Publishing, 1995, pp 55–69.

59 Brunette DM, Proskin HM, Nelson BJ: The effects of dentifrice systems on oral malodor. J Clin Dent 1998;9:76–82.

60 Putt MS, Milleman KR, Ghassemi A, Vorwerk LM, Hooper WJ, Soparkar PM, Winston AE, Proskin HM: Enhancement of plaque removal efficacy by tooth brushing with baking soda dentifrices: results of five clinical studies. J Clin Dent 2008;19:111–119.

61 Bradshaw DJ, Perring KD, Cawkill PM, Provan AF, McNulty DA, Saint EJ, Richards J, Munroe MJ, Behan JM: Creation of oral care flavours to deliver breath-freshening benefits. Oral Dis 2005; 11(suppl 1):75–79.

62 Peruzzo DC, Salvador SL, Sallum AW, Nogueira-Filho G da R: Flavoring agents present in a dentifrice can modify volatile sulphur compounds (VSCs) formation in morning bad breath. Braz Oral Res 2008;22:252–257.

63 Jenkins S, Addy M, Newcombe R: Triclosan and sodium lauryl sulphate mouthwashes (I). Effects on salivary bacterial counts. J Clin Periodontol 1991;18:140–184.

64 Peruzzo DC, Salvador SL, Sallum AW, Da Nogueira-Filho GR: Effects of sodium lauryl sulphate (SLS), present in dentifrice, on volatile sulphur compound (VSC) formation in morning bad breath. J Int Acad Periodontol 2008;10:130–136.

65 Newby EE, Hickling JM, Hughes FJ, Proskin HM, Bosma MP: Control of oral malodour by dentifrices measured by gas chromatography. Arch Oral Biol 2008;53(suppl 1):S19–S25.

66 Bosma MP, McNab R, Gallagher A, Baxter K, Shanga G, Middleton A: Removal of oral debris and bacteria during supervised tooth brushing. Arch Oral Biol 2008;53(suppl 1):S26–S30.

67 Pauling L: General Chemistry, ed 3. San Francisco, WH Freeman, 1988.

68 Young A, Jonski G, Rölla G, Wåler SM: Effects of metal salts on the oral production of volatile sulfur-containing compounds (VSC). J Clin Periodontol 2001;28:776–781.

69 Rölla G, Jonski G, Young A: The significance of the source of zinc and its anti-VSC effect. Int Dent J 2002;52(suppl 3):233–235.

70 Rølla G, Ellingsen JE: Clinical effects and possible mechanisms of action of stannous fluoride. Int Dent J 1994;44:99–105.

71 Gehring F: Effect of amine fluoride and sodium fluoride on the germs of plaque flora (in German). Dtsch Zahnarztl Z 1983;38(suppl 1):S36–S40.

72 Shani S, Friedman M, Steinberg D: The anticariogenic effect of amine fluorides on *Streptococcus sobrinus* and glucosyltransferase in biofilms. Caries Res 2000;34:260–267.

73 Paraskevas S, Van der Weijden GA: A review of the effects of stannous fluoride on gingivitis. J Clin Periodontol 2006;33:1–13.

74 Quirynen M, Zhao H, Avontroodt P, Soers C, Pauwels M, Coucke W, Van Steenberghe D: A salivary incubation test for evaluation of oral malodor: a pilot study. J Periodontol 2003;74:937–944.

75 Gerlach RW, Hyde JD, Poore CL, Stevens DP, Witt JJ: Breath effects of three marketed dentifrices: a comparative study evaluating single and cumulative use. J Clin Dent 1998;9:83–88.

76 Feng X, Chen X, Cheng R, Sun L, Zhang Y, He T: Breath malodor reduction with use of a stannous-containing sodium fluoride dentifrice: a meta-analysis of four randomized and controlled clinical trials. Am J Dent 2010;23:27B–31B.

77 Chen X, He T, Sun L, Zhang Y, Feng X: A randomized cross-over clinical trial to evaluate the effect of a 0.454% stannous fluoride dentifrice on the reduction of oral malodor. Am J Dent 2010;23:175–178.

78 Tonzetich J: Direct gas chromatographic analysis of sulphur compounds in mouth air in man. Arch Oral Biol 1971;16:587–597.

79 Wåler SM: The effect of some metal ions on volatile sulfur-containing compounds originating from the oral cavity. Acta Odontol Scand 1997;55:261–264.

80 Young A, Jonski G, Rölla G: The oral anti-volatile sulphur compound effects of zinc salts and their stability constants. Eur J Oral Sci 2002;110:31–34.

81 Navada R, Kumari H, Le S, Zhang J: Oral malodor reduction from a zinc-containing toothpaste. J Clin Dent 2008;19:69–73.

82 Young A, Jonski G: Effect of a single brushing with two Zn-containing toothpastes on VSC in morning breath: a 12 h, randomized, double-blind, cross-over clinical study. J Breath Res 2011;5:046012.

83 Burnett GR, Stephen AS, Pizzey RL, Bradshaw DJ: In vitro effects of novel toothpaste actives on components of oral malodour. Int Dent J 2011;61(suppl 3):67–73.

84 Newby CS, Rowland JL, Lynch RJM, Bradshaw DJ, Whitworth D, Bosma ML: Benefits of a silica-based fluoride toothpaste containing o-cymen-5-ol, zinc chloride and sodium fluoride. Int Dent J 2011;61(suppl 3):74–80.

85 Payne D, Gordon JJ, Nisbet S, Karwal R, Bosma ML: A randomised clinical trial to assess control of oral malodour by a novel dentifrice containing 0.1%w/w o-cymen-5-ol, 0.6%w/w zinc chloride. Int Dent J 2011;61(suppl 3):60–66.

86 Haps S, Slot DE, Berchier CE, Van der Weijden GA: The effect of cetylpyridinium chloride-containing mouth rinses as adjuncts to toothbrushing on plaque and parameters of gingival inflammation: a systematic review. Int J Dent Hyg 2008;6:290–303.

87 Volpe AR, Petrone ME, De Vizio W, Davies RM, Proskin HM: A review of plaque, gingivitis, calculus and caries clinical efficacy studies with a fluoride dentifrice containing triclosan and PVM/MA copolymer. J Clin Dent 1996;7(suppl):S1–S14.

88 Hoshi K, Van Steenberghe D: The effect of tongue brushing or toothpaste application on oral malodour reduction; in van Steenberghe D, Rosenberg M (eds): Bad Breath: A Multidisciplinary Approach. Leuven, Leuven University Press, 1996, pp 255–264.

89 Nogueira-Filho GR, Duarte PM, Toledo S, Tabchoury CPM, Cury JA: Effect of triclosan dentifrices on mouth volatile sulphur compounds and dental plaque trypsin-like activity during experimental gingivitis development. J Clin Periodontol 2002;29:1059–1064.

90 Niles HP, Vazquez J, Rustogi KN, Williams M, Gaffar A, Proskin HM: The clinical effectiveness of a dentifrice containing triclosan and a copolymer for providing long-term control of breath odor measured chromatographically. J Clin Dent 1999;10:135–138.

91 Sharma NC, Galustians HJ, Qaquish J, Galustians A, Rustogi KN, Petrone ME, Chaknis P, Garcia L, Volpe AR, Proskin HM: The clinical effectiveness of a dentifrice containing triclosan and a copolymer for controlling breath odor measured organoleptically twelve hours after toothbrushing. J Clin Dent 1999;10:131–134.

92 Sharma NC, Galustians HJ, Qaqish J, Galustians A, Rustogi K, Petrone ME, Chaknis P, García L, Volpe AR, Proskin HM: Clinical effectiveness of a dentifrice containing triclosan and a copolymer for controlling breath odor. Am J Dent 2007;20:79–82.

93 Hu D, Zhang YP, Petrone M, Volpe AR, Devizio W, Giniger M: Clinical effectiveness of a triclosan/copolymer/sodium fluoride dentifrice in controlling oral malodor: a 3-week clinical trial. Oral Dis 2005;11(suppl 1):51–53.

94 Niles HP, Hunter C, Vazquez J, Williams MI, Cummins D: The clinical comparison of a triclosan/copolymer/fluoride dentifrice vs a breath-freshening dentifrice in reducing breath odor overnight: a crossover study. Oral Dis 2005;11(suppl 1):54–56.

95 Sreenivasan PK, Furgang D, Zhang Y, DeVizio W, Fine DH: Antimicrobial effects of a new therapeutic liquid dentifrice formulation on oral bacteria including odorigenic species. Clin Oral Investig 2005;9:38–45.

96 Haraszthy VI, Zambon JJ, Sreenivasan PK: Evaluation of the antimicrobial activity of dentifrices on human oral bacteria. J Clin Dent 2010;21:96–100.

97 Sreenivasan P: The effects of a triclosan/copolymer dentifrice on oral bacteria including those producing hydrogen sulfide. Eur J Oral Sci 2003;111: 223–227.

98 Vazquez J, Pilch S, Williams MI, Cummins D: Clinical efficacy of a triclosan/copolymer/NaF dentifrice and a commercially available breath-freshening dentifrice on hydrogen sulfide-forming bacteria. Oral Dis 2005;11(suppl 1):64–66.

99 Fine DH, Furgang D, Markowitz K, Sreenivasan PK, Klimpel K, De Vizio W: The antimicrobial effect of a triclosan/copolymer dentifrice on oral microorganisms in vivo. J Am Dent Assoc 2006;137:1406–1413.

100 Raven S, Matheson J, Huntington E, Tonzetich J: The efficacy of a combined zinc and triclosan system in the prevention of oral malodour; in van Steenberghe D, Rosenberg M (eds): Bad Breath: A Multidisciplinary Approach. Leuven, Leuven University Press, 1996, pp 241–254.

101 Pilch S, Williams MI, Cummins D: Effect of a triclosan/PVM/MA copolymer/fluoride dentifrice on volatile sulfur compounds in vitro. Oral Dis 2005; 11(suppl 1):57–60.

102 Sharma NC, Galustians HJ, Qaqish J, Galustians A, Petrone ME, Rustogi KN, Zhang YP, DeVizio W, Volpe AR: The clinical efficacy of Colgate Total Plus Whitening Toothpaste containing a special grade of silica and Colgate Total Toothpaste for controlling breath odor twelve hours after toothbrushing: a single-use clinical study. J Clin Dent 2002;13:73–76.

103 Hu D, Zhang YP, DeVizio W, Proskin HM: A clinical investigation of the efficacy of two dentifrices for controlling oral malodor and plaque microflora overnight. J Clin Dent 2008;19:106–110.

104 Tonzetich J, Ng SK: Reduction of malodor by oral cleansing procedures. Oral Surg Oral Med Oral Pathol 1976; 42:172–181.

Marc Quirynen
Department of Periodontology, Catholic University of Leuven
Kapucijnenvoer 33
BE–3000 Leuven (Belgium)
E-Mail Marc.Quirynen@med.kuleuven.be

van Loveren C (ed): Toothpastes. Monogr Oral Sci. Basel, Karger, 2013, vol 23, pp 61–74
DOI: 10.1159/000350698

Anti-Calculus and Whitening Toothpastes

Cor van Loveren[a] · Ralph M. Duckworth[b]

[a]Department of Preventive Dentistry, Academic Center for Dentistry Amsterdam, Amsterdam, The Netherlands;
[b]Centre for Oral Health Research, School of Dental Sciences, Newcastle University, Newcastle upon Tyne, UK

Abstract

In terms of novel formulations, there seems to have been a shift in emphasis from anti-caries/anti-gingivitis to anti-calculus/whitening toothpastes in recent years. The anti-calculus and whitening effects of toothpastes are to some extent based on the same active ingredients: compounds of high affinity for tooth mineral. Due to this affinity, crystal growth may be hindered (anti-calculus) and chromophores be displaced (whitening). Besides these common ingredients, both types of toothpaste may contain agents specifically aimed at each condition. Clinical studies have shown that these active ingredients can be successfully formulated in fluoride toothpastes to give significant reductions in supragingival calculus and stain formation and facilitate their removal. Some of the ingredients are formulated in toothpastes that additionally contain anti-plaque and anti-gingivitis ingredients, making these toothpastes (together with the fluoride) truly multi-functional. The development of these products is not straightforward because of interaction between formulation components and because the active ingredients must maintain their beneficial characteristics during the shelf life of the paste. Neither a therapeutic benefit (in terms of less gingivitis or less caries) nor a societal benefit (in terms of less treatment demand) has been demonstrated as a result of the anti-calculus and whitening effects of toothpastes.

A significant proportion of the population experience dental calculus deposits [1]. The removal of calculus both for cosmetic and therapeutic reasons comprises a large percentage of the workload in today's dental practice [2]. Prevention of the formation of calculus may therefore have a major medical and societal impact. People have always had a strong desire for white teeth. Depending on the population examined, studies have shown that personal dissatisfaction with tooth colour ranges from 18 to 53% [3, 4]. To some extent, the anti-calculus and anti-stain effects of toothpastes are based on the same active ingredients. Therefore, there are toothpastes with comparable formulations that are either promoted as anti-calculus or as whitening. Besides these common ingredients, both types of toothpaste may contain agents specifically aimed at each condition. Anti-calculus agents include triclosan with zinc citrate, pyrophosphate or polyvinyl methyl ether (PVM)/maleic acid (MA) copolymer, and crystal growth inhibitors, including pyrophosphate with or without PVM/MA copolymer, zinc citrate, zinc chloride, sodium hexametaphosphate and polyaspartate. Whitening toothpastes may contain tailored abrasive systems and additional agents that augment the abrasive cleaning, such as peroxide, enzymes, citrate, pyrophosphate and hexametaphosphate (HMP), polyaspartate, or optical agents, e.g. covarine.

Calculus

Societal and Medical Impact
For adults, the prevalence of dental calculus deposits has been reported to vary from 42% to over 80% [1, 2, 5, 6]. The removal of calculus, both for cosmetic and therapeutic reasons, comprises a large percentage of the workload in today's dental practice [2]. Prevention of the formation of calculus may therefore have a great medical and societal impact. However, neither a therapeutic benefit (in terms of less gingivitis or less caries) nor a societal benefit (in terms of less treatment demand) has been demonstrated as a result of the use of anti-calculus toothpastes.

Calculus may develop supra- and subgingivally. For the teeth as a whole, significant associations have been demonstrated between clinical scores of supra- and subgingival calculus. For individual teeth, however, only a few teeth showed these associations [7]. An important reason for this distinction may be that the sources of calcium and phosphate to produce the two forms of calculus and the local environment differ. For the formation of supragingival calculus, calcium and phosphate are accumulated from saliva and for the formation of subgingival calculus from crevicular fluid.

Comparisons between populations where supra- and subgingival calculus may grow undisturbed without active professional intervention or home care, or when plaque and calculus are removed at regular intervals, are of interest. In Sri Lankan tea labourers, for example, both supra- and subgingival calculus formation started before the age of 14 years [8]. At 40 years of age, all participants and almost all teeth and tooth surfaces had calculus. Teeth with calculus showed a sig-

nificantly higher rate of loss of attachment than teeth that remained calculus free. For Norwegians who had enjoyed regular dental care throughout their lives, however, supragingival calculus did not increase in frequency from adolescence to their forties [8]. Approximately 70% of the interproximal surfaces were calculus free after 40–50 years of age. Subgingival calculus scores, although low, showed some increase with age. On average, each person had 0.4 interproximal surfaces with subgingival calculus as they approached 50 years of age. In this Norwegian population, subgingival calculus had no impact on loss of attachment. The difference between the two populations may not only be related to different standards of oral hygiene but also to the diet. It has been suggested that rice, which probably forms a staple part of the Sri Lankan diet, may contain amounts of silicon that could promote calculus formation [9, 10].

Dental calculus is often removed for therapeutic reasons. Dental calculus is, however, not a primary aetiological factor in the development of periodontal disease but, due to its porous structure, it may collect and retain pathogenic factors [11]. Vigorous control of supragingival plaque and calculus may result in a shift in pathogenic bacteria in associated shallow pockets [12], suggesting a beneficial effect on gingivitis. However, studies have shown no beneficial effects on gingivitis indices with less vigorous or partial elimination of dental calculus [13, 14]. Thorough removal of subgingival calculus by scaling and root planing has been proven to be effective in periodontal therapy. There is, however, no information on the effectiveness of less vigorous elimination techniques such as by chemical agents.

Duckworth and Huntington [15] showed in secondary analyses of 3 different types of clinical trial that caries prevalence is significantly lower in calculus-prone than in calculus-free subjects. The inverse relationship was demonstrated both at baseline and by the 3-year caries increment data for 11- to 13-year-old children in a clinical trial testing sodium monofluorophosphate (Na_2FPO_3) toothpastes with fluoride concentrations varying from 1,000 to 2,500 µg/g. Children classified as calculus formers at the start of the trial developed 30% fewer caries lesions on average than their initially calculus-free counterparts. Results from an epidemiological study showed that for 8-year-olds over a 6-year period, caries increments were significantly lower for children who had exhibited supra-gingival calculus at some time during the study than for those who were always calculus free. Data from a calculus formation study in adults showed that whilst the extent of caries and calculus experience were both positively linked to age, within specific age groups the relationship between the two dental conditions on an individual subject basis was clearly of an inverse nature. These results suggest a possible beneficial side effect of calculus in caries control.

Composition
Dental calculus is mainly composed of mineral with inorganic and organic components of bacterial, salivary and dietary origin. These can be incorporated during calcification or afterwards in the porosities of calculus deposits. Supragingival and subgingival calculus on extracted incisors and premolars have been found to contain on average 37% (range 16–51%) and 58% mineral (range 32–78%) by volume, respectively [16]. Brushite [DCPD (dicalcium phosphate dihydrate): $CaHPO_4 \cdot 2H_2O$], octacalcium phosphate [$Ca_8(PO_4)_4(HPO_4)_2 \cdot 5H_2O$], hydroxyapatite [HAP: $Ca_{10}(PO_4)_6(OH)_2$], and β-tricalcium phosphate or whitlockite [$(Ca,Mg)_3(PO_4)_2$] form the inorganic part of both supragingival and subgingival calculus [17]. Brushite is present only in the early stage of supragingival calculus [18]. Supersaturation of saliva, continued in plaque fluid, with respect to these calcium phosphate salts is the driving force for calculus formation. Plaque fluid, at or a little below physiological pH, is supersaturated with respect to these calcium phosphates [19], while saliva may

not be supersaturated with respect to the most soluble phase DCPD [20, 21]. Calculus formation begins with the deposition of kinetically favoured precursor phases of calcium phosphate, DCPD and octacalcium phosphate, which are gradually hydrolyzed and transformed into the less soluble HAP and whitlockite mineral phases [18].

Calculus Formation
Calculus formation can be induced in germ-free animals [22], suggesting the possibility of calcification without bacterial dental plaque. Thick plaque, however, is a better substrate for calculus formation due to the localised accumulation of calcium and phosphate, the degradation of salivary crystal growth inhibitors, the presence of crystal growth promoters and the presence of calcifying bacteria and bacterial components [23]. The mineral initially deposits in the matrix of plaque, while plaque micro-organisms gradually become calcified with increasing age of calculus [24].

Inhibitors and Promoters in Saliva and Plaque
Salivary inhibitors of crystal growth are proteins containing negatively charged sequences that may adsorb at active sites on the crystallite surfaces and thereby inhibit growth. Representative examples are: statherins, proline-rich proteins, some cystatins, histatin 1, immunoglobulins and albumins [25–29]. These calcification inhibitors can be degraded by proteases in saliva and plaque. Calculus levels have been found to be positively correlated with protease activity in saliva and dental plaque [30, 31]. In addition, the proteolytic breakdown of proteins by proteases may increase dental plaque pH [32], which would be expected to increase the relative supersaturation.

Pyrophosphate is a salivary component that is able to block adsorption sites available for crystal growth [33–35] and can also delay the initiation of conversion of DCPD to HAP [35]. Higher concentrations of pyrophosphate were noted in the parotid saliva and dental plaque of calculus non- and low-formers than in the saliva and plaque of (heavy) formers [36, 37].

Acid and alkaline (pyro)phosphatases hydro- lyze pyrophosphate, thereby favouring calculus formation. Such phosphatases are present in oral micro-organisms, dental plaque, dental cal- culus and saliva [38, 39]. Another indirect route by which phosphatases may promote crystal growth is when they hydrolyze phosphoproteins to produce inorganic phosphate ions [40].

The Role of Bacteria

A wide range of bacterial species, including *Streptococcus mutans* under non-pH-lowering conditions, may calcify in vitro when grown in a calcium-enriched broth or when incubated in calcium phosphate solutions [41, 42]. Compre- hensive information is available on calcifying *Corynebacterium matruchotii* strains [23]. The initiation of mineralisation is associated with acidic phospholipids in the membrane, when they bind calcium by their negatively charged groups. Inorganic phosphate can then associate with the bound calcium to form a Ca-phospho- lipid-phosphate complex. Apatite formation fol- lows when sufficient calcium and phosphate ions are present and the concentration of inhib- itors is low. Dead micro-organisms can induce calcification, which may be related to release of high intracellular phosphate concentrations [38, 43, 44]. This may explain the phenomenon that although chlorhexidine is a potent anti-plaque agent, it may cause an increase in the formation of supragingival calculus, fortunately without pathological consequences [45, 46]. Hydrolysis of urea by bacterial ureases may increase pH in dental plaque, which favours calcium phosphate precipitation [32, 47]. Son and Mühlemann [48] demonstrated that the urease inhibitor acetohy- droxamic acid inhibited supragingival calculus formation.

Anti-Calculus Strategies

The early strategies with chemotherapeutic agents focused on the removal of dental calculus from teeth were based on the belief that salivary mucins were essential in the attachment of calculus to the tooth structure. Destruction of these proteins would result in a reduction of calculus formation [34]. Amongst the enzyme preparations used were mucinase, pancreatic enzymes and enzymes de- rived from fungi [49]. The clinical effectiveness of these proteolytic enzymes was demonstrated in the 1950s and 1960s [34].

Early strategies also focused on chelating agents. These compounds dissolve calcium salts by se- questering Ca to form stable and soluble calcium complexes. As early as the 1940s, the chelating ca- pacity of sodium hexametaphosphate was success- fully examined for calculus control [50]. However, at that time it was not possible to formulate prod- ucts to compensate for unwanted decalcification effects on the tooth minerals [51]. Recent formula- tion techniques have overcome these problems and now effective anti-calculus toothpastes with sodium hexametaphosphate have been marketed [52–54]. Besides chelation, the mode of action is importantly based on blocking crystal growth [52].

Antimicrobial agents have also been used for calculus reduction. Early experiments with peni- cillin were not successful [55]. The use of chlorhexidine, as discussed above, may promote the development of calculus. Triclosan has been used successfully in anti-calculus toothpaste for- mulations with Zn citrate, pyrophosphate or with PVM/MA copolymer [56–58].

Since the 1970s, the major anti-calculus strate- gy has focused on inhibiting crystal growth and preventing development of mineralised plaque. For some time, anti-calculus toothpastes relied primarily on Zn salts and pyrophosphate. At pres- ent, anti-calculus agents include triclosan with zinc citrate, pyrophosphate or PVM/MA copoly- mer, and crystal growth inhibitors, including pyro- phosphate with or without PVM/MA copolymer, zinc citrate, zinc chloride, sodium hexametaphosphate and polyaspartate. All effective inhibitors have in common the ability to inhibit calcium phosphate nucleation and/or crystal growth processes and the transformation to more stable calcium phosphate phases. Clinical studies from 1972 to 1997 of anti-calculus toothpastes based on the above active ingredients have been comprehensively reviewed by Fairbrother and Heasman [54]. In general, clinical studies only evaluated the effect on supragingival calculus.

Zn Ions

Zn ions potentially have two mechanisms by which they can affect calculus formation. Firstly, they inhibit plaque growth [59–61], thereby reducing the base matrix for calculus. In addition, zinc can adsorb to the surface of the growing crystal and restrict the attachment of calcium ions [62]. Consequently, crystal growth is slowed or inhibited. Zinc ions may also affect the types and the degree of crystallinity of the calcium phosphate crystals [63, 64]. The binding of zinc is reversible and is itself inhibited by raising the local concentration of calcium [65]. This implies that calcium can compete for binding sites in the crystal lattice and displace zinc. Crystal growth sites occupied by zinc may also be 'over-grown' by mineralisation initiated at unoccupied sites [66]. The potential of zinc to modify crystal growth has been extensively reviewed by Le Geros et al. [63] and recently by Lynch [66]. Clinical studies have confirmed the effectiveness of both $ZnCl_2$ (0.2–2.0%) and Zn citrate (0.5–2.0%) in toothpastes; calculus reductions of 40–50% [67–69] and 14–50% [70–73], respectively, being recorded.

Triclosan

Triclosan is a non-ionic anti-microbial agent with a wide spectrum of activity against bacteria, fungi and yeasts. Triclosan has been used successfully in anti-calculus toothpaste formulations combined with Zn citrate, pyrophosphate and PVM/MA copolymer, respectively. All three adjuncts most likely contribute by themselves to the anti-calculus effect (see respective sections). The authors are not aware of a clinical study reporting an anti-calculus effect of toothpastes with triclosan as the only active anti-calculus ingredient.

Na_2FPO_3 toothpastes formulated with the combination of 0.2–0.3% triclosan and 0.5–0.75% zinc citrate were found to reduce calculus by up to 67% versus Na_2FPO_3 control pastes [56, 58, 74–77]. Toothpaste containing 0.3% triclosan with 5% pyrophosphate reduced calculus formation by approximately 18–25% [9, 58].

PVM/MA copolymer has been shown in in vitro studies to increase the uptake and retention of triclosan, and short-term studies in vivo demonstrated the potential of a formulation containing 0.3% triclosan and 2% copolymer to enhance plaque removal and improve gingival health [78, 79]. By itself, the copolymer has weak chelating and crystal growth inhibitory properties and can affect calculus formation [79]. The polymer adsorbed to saliva-coated HAP disks, and the adsorption was time and concentration dependent. Under exaggerated in vitro conditions, the copolymer (1%) did not damage or etch enamel surfaces at pH 7.5 and 5.5 [79]. It was effective against calculus formation in rats when applied topically as a 0.05% solution yielding a 54% reduction. In beagle dogs, it reduced calculus formation although not statistically significant over a period of 24–28 weeks when applied topically either as a rinse (0.05%) or as a toothpaste in combination with triclosan (2% PVM/MA) [79]. Collectively, the data indicated that the copolymer was an effective anti-calculus agent when applied topically in a solution or in a paste in the presence of triclosan [79].

The effects on calculus formation of triclosan and copolymer formulations have been substantiated by clinical studies. It was found that 0.3% triclosan and 2.0% PVM/MA copolymer in silica or alumina base toothpastes with NaF, Na_2FPO_3 or the combination NaF/Na_2FPO_3 significantly reduced the severity and occurrence of supragingival calculus after complete prophylaxis by 25–55% compared with control dentifrices [57, 58, 77, 80–82].

Pyrophosphate and Polyvinyl Methyl Ether/Maleic Acid Copolymer
Pyrophosphate at various concentrations has been widely used as an anti-calculus agent in dentifrices and mouthrinses [54, 83]. Pyrophosphate binds to calcium phosphate crystals preventing phosphate ions from adsorption onto the crystal, and thus crystal growth is inhibited. To inhibit crystal growth effectively, the concentration of pyrophosphate has to reach a critical level. Below this level, the addition of NaF can induce crystal growth [35]. These new crystals may overgrow the inhibitor and consequently generate new surfaces on which crystal growth may then proceed at rates comparable with those of inhibitor-free controls.

In addition to the inhibitory effect on crystal growth, pyrophosphate can also delay the initiation of conversion of DCPD to HAP by over threefold [84] and reduce acquired pellicle formation. It has been reported that pyrophosphate can desorb the acquired enamel pellicle due to its ability to displace anions and negatively charged macromolecules from tooth surfaces [85].

Pyrophosphate has limited hydrolytic stability and will be hydrolyzed in the oral cavity by bacterial and host phosphatases and pyrophosphatases in the presence of Mg [38, 86, 87]. The PVM/MA copolymer is believed to prevent hydrolysis of the pyrophosphate [88]. The proposed mechanism of action is that the copolymer binds tightly to magnesium ions which are a necessary substrate for alkaline phosphatase activity.

The addition of the copolymer to a pyrophosphate dentifrice could therefore be expected to have two effects. Firstly, the copolymer has an anti-calculus activity of its own (see above) and secondly, it stabilises pyrophosphate in saliva and thereby extends the time over which the pyrophosphate is active.

In more than 25 clinical studies, dentifrice containing 1.3–5% pyrophosphate either with or without 1–1.5% PVM/MA copolymer significantly inhibited the formation of supragingival calculus by 25–55% as compared with control fluoride (NaF, Na_2FPO_3 or NaF/Na_2FPO_3) dentifrices [54]. Three studies comparing dentifrices containing 1–3.3% pyrophosphate alone or in combination with 0.45–1% PVM/MA copolymer showed the PVM/MA-containing pastes to be more effective [89–91]. No difference in effect on caries was noticed between the pyrophosphate/copolymer/NaF mixture compared to NaF/Na_2FPO_3 dentifrices indicating that the pyrophosphate and copolymer system was not interfering with mineralisation of carious lesions [92].

Sodium Hexametaphosphate
Sodium hexametaphosphate is a polymer with 10–12 repeating pyrophosphate subunits, giving a stronger attraction to calcium HAP in enamel and dentine relative to other commonly used pyrophosphates [93]. This translates to greater coverage of the tooth surface and substantivity, increasing its potential to prevent calculus formation and stain adsorption. Similar to other polyphosphates, sodium hexametaphosphate has limited long-term stability in aqueous dentifrice vehicles. The toothpaste formulation including HMP involves a low-water system and a silica-based abrasive minimising the risk of hydrolysis before use. Reductions in the amount of calculus of 10–60% were reported after 6 months' use after baseline dental prophylaxis compared to various positive and negative control fluoride toothpastes [53, 94, 95]. These reductions, for concentrations of sodium hexametaphosphate which varied from 7 to 14%, suggest a dose-dependent effect.

Polyaspartate
A newly used agent is sodium polyaspartate. Polyaspartate is a polyanionic peptide used industrially to inhibit crystal growth, which could be used to reduce calculus formation [96, 97].

Table 1. Tooth-whitening agents by function adapted from Joiner [4]

Abrasive	Chemical	Optical
Hydrated silica	Hydrogen peroxide	Blue covarine
Calcium carbonate	Calcium peroxide	
Dicalcium phosphate dihydrate	Sodium citrate	
Calcium pyrophosphate	Sodium pyrophosphate	
Alumina	Sodium tripolyphosphate	
Perlite	Sodium hexametaphosphate	
Sodium bicarbonate	Papain	
	Papain and bromelain extracts	
	Sodium polyaspartate	

Polyaspartate was effective in controlling the formation of a bacterial biofilm when used in a toothpaste formulation in vitro [97]. However, in a 6-month clinical study, a toothpaste containing 2% polyaspartate and 0.45% Zn citrate had no effect on calculus deposition compared to a NaF control paste [98].

Whitening Toothpastes

The colour of the teeth is influenced by a combination of their intrinsic colour and the presence of any extrinsic stains that may form on the tooth surface [99, 100]. Intrinsic tooth colour depends on the light absorption and scattering properties of the enamel and dentine, with dentine playing a significant role in determining the overall tooth colour and with enamel playing mainly a role through scattering at wavelengths in the blue range causing a yellow to blue colour shift [101]. This 'enamel effect' aids the perception of tooth whiteness, giving the teeth their appreciated lustre.

The causes of extrinsic staining can be divided into two categories; those compounds which are incorporated into the pellicle and produce a stain as a result of their basic colour (direct staining), and those which lead to staining caused by chemical interaction at the tooth surface (indirect staining) [99]. Direct staining has a multi-factorial aetiology with chromophores derived from dietary or other sources. These organic chromophores are taken up by the pellicle, and the colour imparted is determined by the natural colour of the chromophore. Tobacco smoking and chewing are known to cause staining, as are particular beverages such as tea and coffee. Indirect extrinsic tooth staining is associated with cationic antiseptics (e.g. chlorhexidine) and metal ions (e.g. tin). The agent itself is colourless or has a different colour from the stain produced on the tooth surface. Poor toothbrushing facilitates staining as it allows accumulation of stained pellicle and coloured deposits.

In order to optimise the removal and control of extrinsic stain, toothpastes require a certain amount of abrasivity [102]. The evidence to date still suggests that the abrasive is the primary stain removal ingredient in toothpaste [103]. Abrasives continue to be developed to improve stain removal without being unduly abrasive [104–109]. Other toothpaste ingredients have been described in the literature for (facilitation of) removal and prevention of extrinsic stain including oxidising agents, surfactants, polyphosphates and enzymes (table 1). Recently, a toothpaste has been developed with blue covarine. This pigment mimics the 'enamel effect' by coating the tooth surface.

Oxidising Agents

Toothpastes containing oxidising agents such as peroxide, peroxide sources and sodium chlorite have been described [110, 111]. A 1–1.5% hydrogen peroxide/sodium bicarbonate toothpaste was shown to significantly decrease tooth yellowness and increase the lightness of tooth samples in vitro compared to a silica and sodium bicarbonate control toothpaste [112, 113]. A toothpaste containing 0.5% calcium peroxide (CP), 1,500 µg F (as Na_2FPO_3)/g in a precipitated calcium carbonate (PCC) base was compared to a second toothpaste containing 10% aluminium oxide and 1,500 µg F (as Na_2FPO_3)/g in a PCC base and to a fluoride control toothpaste without stain removal ingredients. After 6 weeks' use of their assigned products, those subjects in the CP/PCC toothpaste group and those subjects in the aluminium oxide/PCC toothpaste group demonstrated statistically significant improvements compared to the control group [114]. A toothpaste packaged into a dual-chambered container where one contained 1% hydrogen peroxide and the other was a formulation containing high-cleaning silica, phosphate salts and manganese gluconate, which can activate the peroxide during use, has been shown to be effective in extrinsic stain removal and intrinsic stain whitening in a series of in vitro studies [111]. A toothpaste delivering 1.0% hydrogen peroxide, 0.243% NaF and sodium tripolyphosphate in a high-cleaning silica base removed significantly more extrinsic stain, gave a greater reduction in mean tooth (Vita Shade Guide) score [115, 116] and significantly prevented extrinsic stain formation after dental prophylaxis compared to various (positive) control pastes [117]. In the EU, only a maximum of 0.1% peroxide is allowed, for safety reasons.

Enzymes

Enzymes such as proteases could help degrade the stained pellicles and facilitate their removal. Early clinical evidence in the 1960s demonstrated that a highly proteolytic mixture of enzymes of fungal origin formulated into toothpaste was effective at reducing extrinsic stain compared to a negative control toothpaste after 6 months of product use [118]. More recently, a toothpaste containing a mixture of the protease enzyme papain (from papaya), alumina and sodium citrate has been tested. Clinical studies have demonstrated the toothpaste to be effective at removing established stains [119, 120] and more effective at preventing and removing chlorhexidine-induced stain than a control toothpaste [121]. A clinical study comparing four commercially available dentifrices showed that the efficacy for preventing extrinsic tooth stain formation of this papain/alumina/sodium citrate paste was not significantly different from the negative control paste [122]. The two control whitening pastes, which contained Na_2FPO_3, sodium bicarbonate, CP, aluminium oxide, tetrasodium pyrophosphate and pentasodium triphosphate in a hydrated silica base, and NaF and sodium tripolyphosphate in a hydrated silica base, were (numerically) slightly more effective. Recently, the stain removal efficacy of a novel dentifrice containing papain and bromelain extracts (proteolytic enzymes from pineapple) has been demonstrated compared to NaF toothpaste in an in vitro study [123]. The enamel specimens were stained with a mixture prepared using tea, coffee, areca nut with tobacco and chlorhexidine.

Phosphates

The stain removal activity of phosphate compounds, such as pyrophosphate, tripolyphosphate (STP) and HMP, is based on their ability to displace anions, negatively charged macromolecules and acquired enamel pellicle from tooth surfaces (see above) [85, 124, 125]. Various toothpastes containing STP demonstrated significant extrinsic stain removal efficacy relative to baseline [126, 127]. A whitening toothpaste containing 0.243% sodium fluoride with PVM/MA copolymer, tetrasodium pyrophosphate and STP in a silica base has been shown to be effective in removing natural extrinsic stain compared control dentifrices [128–130]. This paste gave a significantly greater reduction of pre-existing extrinsic stain than a whitening toothpaste containing 0.243% sodium fluoride, baking soda, peroxide, tetrasodium pyrophosphate and STP, after 4 weeks' but not after 8 weeks' use [131]. Both products were significantly better than a regular silica toothpaste, yielding 45 and 28% less extrinsic tooth stain, respectively, after 4 weeks and approximately 30% (for both) after 8 weeks' use [131].

NaF (0.243%) toothpastes containing 7% sodium HMP or 3.5% HMP/1.25% soluble pyrophosphate were shown in clinical studies to significantly remove chlorhexidine/tea-induced stain by 30–40% after 3 and 6 weeks' product use [132–134]. Comparison with control toothpastes with dentine abrasivity values (RDA values) of 95 and 145 showed that both the 3.5% HMP/1.25% soluble pyrophosphate toothpaste (RDA 109) and the more abrasive alumina toothpaste significantly reduced stain from baseline by 40 and 35%, while no significant stain reduction was observed with a low abrasive paste [133]. This study demonstrates that following 6 weeks of treatment, sodium hexametaphosphate-containing dentifrices are effective in removing extrinsic tooth stain, with performance comparable to that seen with a more abrasive dentifrice. In vitro studies with a so-called powder stain prevention model have shown that pretreatment of HAP powder with HMP-containing toothpaste reduced the adsorption of tea chromogens onto HAP powder and discs [124].

HMP has been incorporated into other whitening toothpaste formulations, e.g. 11% sodium HMP with 0.243% NaF and 13% sodium HMP with 0.454% SnF_2, which have also been shown in clinical studies to give improved stain removal benefits [135–138]. Two studies did not report any extrinsic stain formation during 6 months' use of a 13% sodium HMP/0.454% SnF_2 toothpaste after professional prophylaxis [139, 140].

The same results were attained in these experiments with the control pastes being a 0.3% triclosan/2% Gantrez/0.243% NaF paste [139] and a 0.76% Na_2FPO_3 paste [140], respectively.

Polyaspartate
A newly used agent is sodium polyaspartate. Polyaspartate was effective in controlling the formation of a bacterial biofilm when used in a toothpaste formulation in vitro [97], as mentioned earlier. In a 3 months' clinical study, a whitening effect was observed when using a toothpaste containing 2% polyaspartate and 0.45% Zn citrate [98].

Blue Covarine
Blue covarine is a pigment that, like enamel, scatters wavelengths in the blue range resulting in a yellow-to-blue tooth colour shift of the surface it has been applied to. Following brushing extracted teeth in vitro, blue covarine has been shown to be deposited onto the tooth surface and to indeed give a yellow-to-blue colour shift with an overall improvement in measureable and perceivable tooth whitening [141]. In a clinical study, brushing once with a toothpaste containing blue covarine gave a significant and immediate reduction in tooth yellowness and an increase in tooth whiteness compared to baseline versus a clear gel negative control silica toothpaste, as measured by image analysis of digital photographs of the teeth [142].

Conclusions

To some extent, the anti-calculus and anti-stain effects of toothpastes are based on the same active ingredients. There are toothpastes with comparable formulations that are either promoted as anti-calculus or as whitening. Besides these common ingredients, both types of toothpaste may contain agents specifically aimed at each condition. Anti-calculus agents include triclosan with (or without) PVM/MA copolymer, and crystal growth inhibitors, including pyrophosphate with or without PVM/MA copolymer, zinc citrate, zinc chloride, sodium hexametaphosphate and polyaspartate. Whitening toothpastes may contain additional agents that augment abrasive cleaning, such as peroxide, enzymes, citrate, pyrophosphate and HMP, polyaspartate, or optical agents such as blue covarine. Clinical studies have shown that these active ingredients can be successfully formulated in fluoride toothpastes to give significant reductions in calculus and stain formation and to facilitate their removal. Some of the ingredients are formulated in toothpastes that additionally contain anti-plaque and anti-gingivitis ingredients, making these toothpastes (together with the fluoride) truly multi-functional. The development of these products is not straightforward because of interaction between formulation components and because the active ingredients must maintain their beneficial characteristics over a shelf life that can be years. Neither a therapeutic benefit (in terms of less gingivitis or less caries) nor a societal benefit (in terms of less treatment demand) has been demonstrated as a result of the anti-calculus and whitening effects of toothpastes per se. The development and promotion of these toothpastes fits into a switch in emphasis in dental practice and among patients to cosmetic dentistry and may therefore have an important function. However, the shift in emphasis from therapeutic anti-caries/ anti-gingivitis toothpastes to ones marketed for their cosmetic anti-calculus/whitening benefits should not lead to the notion that such cosmetic benefits are more important than the therapeutic ones.

References

1 Darby I, Phan L, Post M: Periodontal health of dental clients in a community health setting. Aust Dent J 2012;57:486–492.

2 Miller AJ, Brunelle JA, Carlos JP, Brown LJ, Löe H: Oral Health of United States Adults, the National Survey of Oral health in U.S. Employed Adults and seniors: 1985–1986. US Department of Health and Human Services, Public Health Service, National Institutes of Health NIH Publication No 87-2868, 1987.

3 Alkhatib MN, Holt R, Bedi R: Prevalence of self-assessed tooth discoloration in the United Kingdom. J Dent 2004;32: 561–566.

4 Joiner A: Whitening toothpastes: a review of the literature. J Dent 2010; 38(suppl 2):e17–e24.

5 Brown LJ, Brunelle JA, Kingman A: Periodontal status in the United States, 1988–1991: prevalence, extent, and demographic variation. J Dent Res 1996; 75:672–683.

6 Pilot T, Miyazaki H, Leclercq MH, Barmes DE: Profiles of periodontal conditions in older age cohorts, measured by CPITN. Int Dent J 1992;42:23–30.

7 Corbett TL, Dawes C: A comparison of the site-specificity of supragingival and subgingival calculus deposition. J Periodontol 1998;69:1–8.

8 Anerud A, Löe H, Boysen H: The natural history and clinical course of calculus formation in man. J Clin Periodontol 1991;18:160–170.

9 Gaare D, Rølla G, van der Ouderaa F: Comparison of the rate of formation of supragingival calculus in an Asian and a European population; in Ten Cate JM (ed): Recent Advances in the Study of Dental Calculus. Oxford, IRL Press, 1989, pp 115–122.

10 Damen JJM, ten Cate JM: Calcium phosphate precipitation is promoted by silicon; in Ten Cate JM (ed): Recent Advances in the Study of Dental Calculus. Oxford, IRL Press, 1989, pp 105–114.

11 Mandel ID, Gaffar A: Calculus revisited. A review. J Clin Periodontol 1986;13: 249–257.

12 McNabb H, Mombelli A, Lang NP: Supragingival cleaning 3 times a week. The microbiological effects in moderately deep pockets. J Clin Periodontol 1992; 19:348–356.

13 Koch G, Bergmann-Arnadottir I, Bjarnason S, Finnbogason S, Höskuldsson O, Karlsson R: Caries-preventive effect of fluoride dentifrices with and without anticalculus agents: a 3-year controlled clinical trial. Caries Res 1990;24:72–79.

14 Suomi JD, Horowitz HS, Barbano JP, Spolsky VW, Heifetz SB: A clinical trial of a calculus-inhibitory dentifrice. J Periodontol 1974;45:139–145.

15 Duckworth RM, Huntington E: Evidence for putting the calculus: caries inverse relationship to work. Community Dent Oral Epidemiol 2005;33:349–356.

16 Friskopp J, Isacsson C: A quantitative microradiographic study of mineral content of supragingival and subgingival dental calculus. Scand J Dent Res 1984; 92:25–32.

17 Le Geros RZ: Variations in the crystalline components of human dental calculus. I. Crystallographic and spectroscopic methods of analysis. J Dent Res 1974; 53:45–50.

18 Rowles SL: Biophysical studies on dental calculus in relation to periodontal disease. Dent Pract Dent Rec 1964;15: 2–7.

19 Carey C, Gregory T, Rupp W, Tatevossian A, Vogel GL: The driving force is human dental plaque fluid for demineralization and remineralization of enamel mineral; in Leach SA (ed): Factors Relating to Demineralization and Remineralization of the Teeth. Oxford, IRL Press, 1986, pp 163–173.

20 Lagerlöf F: Effects of flow rate and pH on calcium phosphate saturation in human parotid saliva. Caries Res 1983;17: 403–411.

21 Hay DI, Schluckebier SK, Moreno EC: Saturation of human salivary secretions with respect to calcite and inhibition of calcium carbonate precipitation by salivary constituents. Calcif Tissue Int 1986; 39:151–160.

22 Theilade J, Fitzgerald RJ, Scott DB, Nylen MU: Electron microscopic observations of dental calculus in germ-free rats and conventional rats. Arch Oral Biol 1964;9:97–100.

23 Boyan BD, Swain LD, Boskey AL: Mechanisms of microbial calcification; in Ten Cate JM (ed): Recent Advances in the Study of Dental Calculus. Oxford, IRL Press, 1989, pp 29–37.

24 Donald JW: Dental calculus: recent insight into occurrence, formation, prevention, removal and oral health effects of supragingival and subgingival deposits. Eur J Oral Sci 1997;105:508–522.

25 Hay DI, Smith DJ, Schluckebier SK, Moreno EC: Relationship between concentration of human salivary statherin and inhibition of calcium phosphate precipitation in stimulated human parotid saliva. J Dent Res 1984;63:857–863.

26 Johnsson M, Richardson CF, Bergey EJ, Levine MJ, Nancollas GH: The effects of human salivary cystatins and statherin on hydroxyapatite crystallization. Arch Oral Biol 1991;36:631–636.

27 Oppenheim FG, Yang YC, Diamond RD, Hyslop D, Offner GD, Troxler RF: The primary structure and functional characterization of the neutral histidine-rich polypeptide from human parotid saliva. J Biol Chem 1986;261:1177–1192.

28 Lindskog S, Friskopp J: Immunoglobulins in human dental calculus demonstrated with the peroxidase- antiperoxidase (PAP) method. Scand J Dent Res 1983;91:360–364.

29 Robinson C, Shore RC, Bonass WA, Brooks SJ, Boteva E, Kirkham J: Identification of human serum albumin in human caries lesions of enamel. The role of putative inhibitors of remineralization. Caries Res 1998;32:193–199.

30 Watanabe T, Toda K, Morishita M, Iwamoto Y: Correlations between salivary protease and supragingival or subgingival calculus index. J Dent Res 1982;61: 1048–1051.

31 Morita M, Watanabe T: Relation between the presence of supragingival calculus and protease activity in dental plaque. J Dent Res 1986;65:703–705.

32 Frostell G, Söder PÖ: The proteolytic activity of plaque and its relation to soft tissue pathology. Int J Dent 1970;20: 436–450.

33 Francis MD: The inhibition of calcium hydroxyapatite crystal growth by polyphosphates. Calcif Tissue Res 1969;3: 151–162.

34 Stookey GK, Jackson RD, Beiswanger BB, Stookey KR: Clinical efficacy of chemicals for calculus prevention; in Ten Cate JM (ed): Recent Advances in the Study of Dental Calculus. Oxford, IRL Press, 1989, pp 235–258.

35 Moreno EC, Aoba T, Gaffar A: Physical chemistry of calculus formation; in Ten Cate JM (ed): Recent Advances in the Study of Dental Calculus. Oxford, IRL Press, 1989, pp 129–142.

36 Vogel JJ, Amdur BH: Inorganic pyrophosphate in parotid saliva and its relation to calculus formation. Arch Oral Biol 1967;12:159–163.

37 Edgar WM, Jenkins GN: Inorganic pyrophosphate in human parotid saliva and dental plaque. Arch Oral Biol 1972;17: 219–223.

38 Pellat BP, Grand M: Inorganic pyrophosphatase activity in a plaque calcifying microorganism: Bacterionema matruchotii. J Biol Buccale 1986;14:223–228.

39 Bercy P, Vreven J: Correlation between calculus index and acid and alkaline pyrophosphatase activities of dental plaque and saliva. J Biol Buccale 1979;7:31–36.

40 Poirier TP, Holt SC: Acid and alkaline phosphatases of Capnocytophaga species. Isolation, purification and characterization of the enzymes from Capnocytophaga ochracea. Can J Microbiol 1983;29:1361–1368.

41 Ennever J, Vogel JJ, Brown LR Jr: Survey of microorganisms for calcification in a synthetic medium. J Dent Res 1972;51: 1483–1486.

42 Moorer WR, ten Cate JM, Buijs JF: Calcification of a cariogenic Streptococcus and of Corynebacterium (Bacterionema) matruchotii. J Dent Res 1993;72: 1021–1026.

43 Sidaway DA: A microbiological study of dental calculus. III. A comparison of the in vitro calcification of viable and nonviable microorganisms. J Periodontal Res 1979;14:167–172.

44 Sidaway DA: A microbiological study of dental calculus. IV. An electron microscopic study of in vitro calcified microorganisms. J Periodontal Res 1980;15: 240–254.

45 Löe H, Rindom-Schiött C, Karring G, Karring T: Two years oral use of chlorhexidine in man. I. General design and clinical effects. J Periodontal Res 1976;11:135–144.

46 Yates R, Jenkins S, Newcombe R, Wade W, Moran J, Addy M: A 6-month home usage trial of a 1% chlorhexidine toothpaste (1). Effects on plaque, gingivitis, calculus and toothstaining. J Clin Periodontol 1993;20:130–138.

47 Kleinberg I: Regulation of the acid-base metabolism of the dentogingival plaque and its relation to dental caries and periodontal disease. Int Dent J 1970;20:451–465.

48 Son S, Mühlemann HR: The effect of human supragingival calculus formation of acetohydroxamic acid. Helv Odontol Acta 1971;15(suppl 7):158–159.

49 Aleece AA, Forscher BK: Calculus reduction with a mucinase dentifrice. J Periodontol 1954;25:122–125.

50 Kerr DA, Filed H: Sodium hexametaphosphate as an aid in the treatment of periodontal disease. J Dent Res 1944;23: 313–316.

51 Weinstein E, Mandel ID: The present status of anticalculus agents. J Oral Ther Pharm 1964;1:327–334.

52 White DJ, Gerlach RW: Anticalculus effects of a novel, dual-phase polypyrophosphate dentifrice: chemical basis, mechanism, and clinical response. J Contemp Dent Pract 2000;15:1–19.

53 Schiff T, Saletta L, Baker RA, He T, Winston JL: Anticalculus efficacy and safety of a stabilized stannous fluoride/sodium hexametaphosphate dentifrice. Compend Contin Educ Dent 2005;26(suppl 1):29–34.

54 Fairbrother KJ, Heasman PA: Anticalculus agents. J Clin Periodontol 2000;27: 285–301.

55 Dossenbach WF, Mühlemann HR: Effect of penicillin and rincinoleate on early calculus formation. Helv Odont Acta 1961;5:25–28.

56 Svatun B, Saxton CA, Rölla G: Six-month study of the effect of a dentifrice containing zinc citrate and triclosan on plaque, gingival health, and calculus. Scand J Dent Res 1990;98:301–304.

57 Volpe AR, Schiff TJ, Cohen S, Petrone ME, Petrone D: Clinical comparison of the anticalculus efficacy of two triclosan-containing dentifrices. J Clin Dent 1992;3:93–95.

58 Fairbrother KJ, Kowolik MJ, Curzon ME, Müller I, McKeown S, Hill CM, Hannigan C, Bartizek RD, White DJ: The comparative clinical efficacy of pyrophosphate/triclosan, copolymer/triclosan and zinc citrate/triclosan dentifrices for the reduction of supragingival calculus formation. J Clin Dent 1997;8:62–66.

59 Fischman SL, Picozzi A, Cancro LP, Pader M: The inhibition of plaque in humans by two experimental oral rinses. J Periodontol 1973;44:100–102.

60 Skjorland K, Gjermo P, Rølla G: Effect of some polyvalent cations on plaque formation in-vivo. Scand J Dent Res 1978; 86:104–107.

61 Saxton CA, Harrap GJ, Lloyd AM: The effect of dentifrices containing zinc citrate on plaque growth and oral zinc levels. J Clin Periodontol 1986;13:301–306.

62 Gilbert RL, Ingram GS: The oral disposition of zinc following the use of an anticalculus toothpaste containing 0.5% zinc citrate. J Pharm Pharmacol 1988;40: 399–402.

63 Le Geros RZ, Bleiwas CB, Retino M, Rohanizadeh R, Le Geros JP: Zinc effect on the in vitro formation of calcium phosphates: relevance to clinical inhibition of calculus formation. Am J Dent 1999;12: 65–71.

64 Leskovar P, Hartung R: Inhibition of nucleation and growth of calcium oxalate crystals by aluminium, iron (II), lanthanum, cerium, neodynium, yttrium, europium, magnesium and zinc ions. Fortschr Urol Nephrol 1977;9:30–34.

65 Brudevold F, Steadman LT, Spinelli MA, Amdur BH, Gron P: A study of zinc in human teeth. Arch Oral Biol 1963;8: 135–144.

66 Lynch RJM: Zinc in the mouth, its interactions with dental enamel and possible effects on caries; a review of the literature. Int Dent J 2011;61(suppl 3):46–54.

67 Kohut B, Grossman E: The anticalculus effectiveness of an NaF-zinc containing dentifrice (abstract 951). J Dent Res 1986;65:275.

68 Rustogi KN, Volpe AR, Petrone ME: A clinical comparison of two anticalculus dentifrices. Compend Contin Educ Dent 1988;9:78–79.

69 Lobene RR, Soparker PM, Newman MB, Kohut BE: Reduced formation of supragingival calculus with the use of fluoride-zinc chloride dentifrice. J Am Dent Ass 1987;114:350–352.

70 Kazmierczak M, Mather M, Ciancio S, Fischman S, Cancro L: A clinical evaluation of anticalculus dentifrices. Clin Prev Dent 1990;12:13–17.

71 Lobene RR: A clinical comparison of the anticalculus effect of two commercially available dentifrices. Clin Prev Dent 1987;9:3–8.

72 Stephen KW, Burchell CK, Huntington E, Baker AG, Russell JI, Creanor SL: In vivo anticalculus effects of dentifrice containing 0.5% zinc citrate trihydrate. Caries Res 1987;40:380–384.

73 Segreto VA, Collins EM, D'Agostino R, Cancro LP, Pfeifer HJ, Gilbert RJ: Anticalculus effect of a dentifrice containing 0.5% zinc citrate trihydrate. Community Dent Oral Epidemiol 1991;19:29–31.

74 Svatun B, Saxton CA, Huntington E, Cummins D: The effects of three silica dentifrices containing Triclosan on supragingival plaque and calculus formation and on gingivitis. Int Dent J 1993; 43(suppl 1):441–452.

75 Svatun B, Saxton CA, Huntington E, Cummins D: The effects of a silica dentifrice containing Triclosan and zinc citrate on supragingival plaque and calculus formation and the control of gingivitis. Int Dent J 1993;43(suppl 1):431–439.

76 Stephen KW, Saxton CA, Jones CL, Ritchie JA, Morrison T: Control of gingivitis and calculus by a dentifrice containing a zinc salt and triclosan. J Periodontol 1990;61:674–679.

77 Bánóczy J, Sari K, Schiff T, Petrone M, Davies R, Volpe AR: Anticalculus efficacy of three dentifrices. Am J Dent 1995;8:205–208.

78 Nabi N, Mukerjee C, Schmid R, Gaffar A: In vitro and in vivo studies on triclosan/PVM/MA copolymer NaF combination as an anti-plaque agent. Am J Dent 1989;2:197–206.

79 Gaffar A, Esposito A, Afflitto J: In vitro and in vivo anticalculus effects of a triclosan/copolymer system. Am J Dent 1990;3:S37–S42.

80 Lobene RR, Battista GW, Petrone DM, Volpe AR, Petrone ME: Anticalculus effect of a fluoride dentifrice containing triclosan and a copolymer. Am J Dent 1990;3:S47–S49.

81 Lobene RR, Battista GW, Petrone DM, Volpe AR, Petrone ME: Clinical efficacy of an anticalculus fluoride dentifrice containing triclosan and a copolymer: a 6-month study. Am J Dent 1991;4:83–85.

82 Schiff T, Cohen S, Volpe AR, Petrone ME: Effects of two fluoride dentifrices containing triclosan and a copolymer on calculus formation. Am J Dent 1990;3:S43–S45.

83 Zacherl WA, Pfeiffer HJ, Swancar JR: The effect of soluble pyrophosphates on dental calculus in adults. J Am Dent Assoc 1985;110:737–738.

84 White DJ, Bowman WD, Nancollas GH: Physical-chemical aspects of dental calculus formation and inhibition: in vitro and in vivo studies; in Ten Cate JM (ed): Recent Advances in the Study of Dental Calculus. Oxford, IRL Press, 1989, pp 175–188.

85 Rykke M, Rölla G: Desorption of acquired enamel pellicle in vivo by pyrophosphate. Scand J Dent Res 1990;98: 211–214.

86 Mandel ID: Rinses for the control of supragingival calculus formation. Int Dent J 1992;42:270–275.

87 Francis MD: The inhibition of calcium hydroxyapatite crystal growth by polyphosphates. Calcif Tissue Res 1969;3: 151–162.

88 Gaffar A, Esposito A: Evaluation of a copolymer as an anticalculus agent (abstract 771). J Dent Res 1986;65:409.

89 Rosling B, Londhe J: The anticalculus efficacy of two commercially available anticalculus dentifrices. Compend Suppl 1987;8:S278–S282.

90 Schiff TG, Volpe AR, Gaffar A, Afflito J, Mitchell RL: Comparative anticalculus effect of dentifrices containing 1.30% soluble pyrophosphate with and without a copolymer. J Clin Dent 1990;2:48–52.

91 Singh SM, Petrone ME, Volpe AR, Rustogi KN, Norfleet J: Comparison of the anticalculus effect of two soluble pyrophosphate dentifrices with and without a copolymer. J Clin Dent 1990;2:53–55.

92 Gaffar A, Schmid R, Afflitto J, Coleman E: Effects of pyrophosphate/copolymer/NaF on dental calculus and caries formation in vivo. Compend Suppl 1987;8:S251–S255.

93 Baig A, He T: A novel dentifrice technology for advanced oral health protection: a review of technical and clinical data. Compend Contin Educ Dent 2005;26(suppl 1):4–11.

94 Liu H, Segreto V, Baker R, Vastola K, Ramsey L, Gerlach R: Anticalculus efficacy and safety of a novel whitening dentifrice containing sodium hexametaphosphate: a controlled six-month clinical trial. J Clin Dent 2002;13:25–28.

95 Winston JL, Fiedler SK, Schiff T, Baker R: An anticalculus dentifrice with sodium hexametaphosphate and stannous fluoride: a six-month study of efficacy. J Contemp Dent Pract 2007;8:1–8.

96 Sikes CS: Inhibition of mineral deposition by phosphorylated and related polyanionic peptides. US patent 5,051,401:1991.

97 Guan YH, Lath DL, Graaf T, Lilley TH, Brook AH: Moderation of oral bacterial adhesion on saliva-coated hydroxyapatite by polyaspartate. J Appl Microbiol 2003;94:456–461.

98 Jowett AK, Marlow I, Rawlinson A: A double blind randomised controlled clinical trial comparing a novel anti-stain and calculus reducing dentifrice with a standard fluoride dentifrice. J Dent, DOI: 10.1016/j.jdent.2012.12.005.

99 Watts A, Addy M: Tooth discoloration and staining: a review of the literature. Br Dent J 2001;190:309–316.

100 Joiner A: Tooth colour: a review of the literature. J Dent 2004;32(suppl 1):3–12.

101 Ten Bosch JJ, Coops JC: Tooth color and reflectance as related to light scattering and enamel hardness J Dent Res 1995;74:374–380.

102 Stookey KG, Barnhard TA, Schemehorn BR: In vitro removal of stain with dentifrices. J Dent Res 1982;61:1236–1239.

103 Joiner A: The cleaning of teeth; in Johansson I, Somasundaran P (eds): Handbook for Cleaning/Decontamination of Surfaces. Basel, Karger, 2007, vol 1, pp 371–405.

104 Rice DE, Dhabhar DJ, White DJ: Laboratory stain removal and abrasion characteristics of a dentifrice based upon a novel silica technology. J Clin Dent 2001;12:34–37.

105 Ayad F, Khalaf A, Chaknis P, Petrone ME, DeVizio W, Volpe AR, Proskin HM: Clinical efficacy of a new tooth whitening dentifrice. J Clin Dent 2002;13:82–85.

106 Singh S, Mankodi S, Chaknis P, Petrone ME, DeVizio W, Volpe AR, Proskin HM: The clinical efficacy of a new tooth whitening dentifrice formulation: a six-month study in adults. J Clin Dent 2002;13:86–90.

107 Collins LZ, Naeeni M, Schäfer F, Brignoli C, Schiavi A, Roberts J, Colgan P: The effect of a calcium carbonate/perlite toothpaste on the removal of extrinsic tooth stain in two weeks. Int Dent J 2005;55(suppl 1):S179–S182.

108 Joiner A, Philpotts CJ, Ashcroft AT, Laucello M, Salvaderi A: In vitro cleaning, abrasion and fluoride efficacy of a new silica based whitening toothpaste containing blue covarine. J Dent 2008; 36(suppl 1):S32–S37.

109 Nathoo S, Mateo LR, Delgado E, Zhang YP, DeVizio W: Extrinsic stain removal efficacy of a new dentifrice containing 0.3% triclosan, 2.0% PVM/MA copolymer, 0.243% NaF and specially-designed silica for sensitivity relief and whitening benefits as compared to a dentifrice containing 0.3% triclosan, 2% PVM/MA copolymer, 0.243% NaF and to a negative control dentifrice containing 0.243% NaF: a 6-week study. Am J Dent 2011;24:28A–31A.

110 Pontefract H, Sheen S, Addy M: The benefits of toothpaste – real or imagined? Review of its role in tooth whitening. Dent Update 2001;28:67–74.

111 Hoic D, Dixit N, Prencipe M, Subramanyam R, Cameron R, Malak RA: The technology behind Colgate Simply White toothpaste. J Clin Dent 2004;15:37–40.

112 Kleber CJ, Putt MS, Nelson BJ: In vitro tooth whitening by a sodium bicarbonate/peroxide dentifrice. J Clin Dent 1998;9:16–21.

113 Kleber CJ, Moore MH, Nelson BJ: Laboratory assessment of tooth whitening by sodium bicarbonate dentifrices. J Clin Dent 1998;9:72–75.

114 Ayad F, Arcuri H, Brevilieri E, Laffi S, Lemos AM, Yoshioka M, Baines E, Sheth J, DeVizio W: Efficacy of two dentifrices on removal of natural extrinsic stain. Am J Dent 1999;12:164–166.

115 Kakar A, Rustogi K, Zhang YP, Petrone ME, De Vizio W, Proskin HM: A clinical investigation of the tooth whitening efficacy of a new hydrogen peroxide-containing dentifrice. J Clin Dent 2004;15:41–45.

116 Soparkar P, Rustogi K, Zhang YP, Petrone ME, De Vizio W, Proskin HM: Comparative tooth whitening and extrinsic tooth stain removal efficacy of two tooth whitening dentifrices: six-week clinical trial. J Clin Dent 2004;15:46–51.

117 Sharma N, Galustians HJ, Qaqish J, Rustogi K, Zhang YP, Petrone ME, DeVizio W, Proskin HM: Comparative tooth whitening and extrinsic tooth stain prevention efficacy of a new dentifrice and a commercially available tooth whitening dentifrice: six-week clinical trial. J Clin Dent 2004;15:52–57.

118 Harrison WE, Salisbury GB, Abbott DD: Effect of enzyme-toothpastes upon oral hygiene. J Periodontol 1963;34:334–337.

119 Emling RC, Levin S, Shi X, Weinberg S, Yankell SL: Rembrandt toothpaste stain prevention with and without the use of Peridex. J Clin Dent 1992;3:59–65.

120 Lyon TC, Parker WA, Barnes GP: Evaluation of effects of application of a citroxain-containing dentifrice. J Esthet Dent 1991;3:51–53.

121 Emling RC, Shi X, Yankell SL: Rembrandt toothpaste: stain removal following the use of Peridex. J Clin Dent 1992;3:66–69.

122 Yankell SL, Emling RC, Petrone ME, Rustogi K, Volpe AR, DeVizio W, Chaknis P, Proskin HM: A six-week clinical efficacy study of four commercially available dentifrices for the removal of extrinsic tooth stain. J Clin Dent 1999;10:115–118.

123 Kalyana P, Shashidhar A, Meghashyam B, Sreevidya KR, Sweta S: Stain removal efficacy of a novel dentifrice containing papain and bromelain extracts – an in vitro study. Int J Dent Hyg 2011;9:229–233.

124 Baig AA, Kozak KM, Cox ER, Zoladz JR, Mahony L, White DJ: Laboratory studies on the chemical whitening effects of a sodium hexametaphosphate dentifrice. J Clin Dent 2002;13:19–24.

125 Baig A, He T, Buisson J, Sagel L, Suszcynsky-Meister E, White DJ: Extrinsic whitening effects of sodium hexametaphosphate – a review including a dentifrice with stabilized stannous fluoride. Compend Contin Educ Dent 2005;26(suppl 1):47–53.

126 Hughes N, Maggio B, Sufi F, Mason S, Kleber CJ: A comparative clinical study evaluating stain removal efficacy of a new sensitivity whitening dentifrice compared to commercially available whitening dentifrices. J Clin Dent 2009;20:218–222.

127 Walsh TF, Rawlinson A, Wildgoose D, Marlow I, Haywood J, Ward JM: Clinical evaluation of the stain removing ability of a whitening dentifrice and stain controlling system. J Dent 2005;33:413–418.

128 Ayad F, Demarchi B, Khalaf A, Petrone ME, Chaknis P, DeVizio W, Volpe AR, Proskin HM: A six-week clinical efficacy study of a new dentifrice for the removal of extrinsic tooth stain. J Clin Dent 1999;10:103–106.

129 Ayad F, Demarchi B, Khalaf A, Davies R, Ellwood R, Bradshaw B, Petrone ME, Chaknis P, DeVizio W, Volpe AR, Proskin HM: A six-week clinical tooth whitening study of a new calculus-inhibiting dentifrice formulation. J Clin Dent 2000;11:84–87.

130 Mankodi S, Sowinski J, Davies R, Ellwood R, Bradshaw B, Petrone ME, DeVizio W, Chaknis P, Volpe AR, Proskin HM: A six-week clinical efficacy study of a tooth whitening tartar control dentifrice for the removal of extrinsic tooth stain. J Clin Dent 1999; 10:99–102.

131 Ayad F, De Sciscio P, Stewart B, De Vizio W, Petrone ME, Volpe AR: The stain prevention efficacy of two tooth whitening dentifrices. Compend Contin Educ Dent 2002;23:733–736.

132 Gerlach RW, Liu H, Prater ME, Ramsey LL, White DJ: Removal of extrinsic stain using a 7.0% sodium hexametaphosphate dentifrice: a randomized clinical trial. J Clin Dent 2002; 13:6–9.

133 Gerlach RW, Ramsey LL, White DJ: Extrinsic stain removal with a sodium hexametaphosphate-containing dentifrice: comparisons to marketed controls. J Clin Dent 2002;13:10–14.

134 Gerlach RW, Ramsey LL, Baker RA, White DJ: Extrinsic stain prevention with a combination dentifrice containing calcium phosphate surface active builders compared to two marketed controls. J Clin Dent 2002;13:15–18.

135 Li Y, He T, Sun L, Zhang Y, Li X, Wang Y, Zhao S, Tang R: Extrinsic stain removal efficacy of a dual-phase dentifrice. Am J Dent 2007;20:227–230.

136 He T, Baker R, Bartizek RD, Biesbrock AR, Chaves E, Terezhalmy G: Extrinsic stain removal efficacy of a stannous fluoride dentifrice with sodium hexametaphosphate. J Clin Dent 2007; 18:7–11.

137 Terezhalmy G, Chaves E, Bsoul S, Baker R, He T: Clinical evaluation of the stain removal efficacy of a novel stannous fluoride and sodium hexametaphosphate dentifrice. Am J Dent 2007; 20:53–58.

138 Terezhalmy G, Biesbrock AR, Farrell S, Barker ML, Bartizek RD: Tooth whitening through the removal of extrinsic stain with two sodium hexametaphosphate-containing whitening dentifrices. Am J Dent 2007;20: 309–314.

139 Schiff T, Saletta L, Baker RA, He T, Winston JL: Anticalculus efficacy and safety of a stabilized stannous fluoride/ sodium hexametaphosphate dentifrice. Compend Contin Educ Dent 2005; 26(suppl 1):29–34.

140 Mankodi S, Bartizek RD, Winston JL, Biesbrock AR, McClanahan SF, He T: Anti-gingivitis efficacy of a stabilized 0.454% stannous fluoride/sodium hexametaphosphate dentifrice. J Clin Periodontol 2005;32:75–80.

141 Joiner A, Philpotts CJ, Alonso C, Ashcroft AT, Sygrove NJ: A novel optical approach to achieving tooth whitening. J Dent 2008;36:S8–S14.

142 Collins LZ, Naeeni M, Platten SM: Instant tooth whitening from a silica toothpaste containing blue covarine. J Dent 2008;36(suppl 1):S21–S25.

Prof. Dr. Cor van Loveren, DDS, PhD
Department of Preventive Dentistry, Academic Center for Dentistry Amsterdam
University of Amsterdam and VU University Amsterdam
Gustav Mahlerlaan 3004, NL–1081 LA Amsterdam (The Netherlands)
E-Mail C.van.loveren@acta.nl

van Loveren C (ed): Toothpastes. Monogr Oral Sci. Basel, Karger, 2013, vol 23, pp 75–87
DOI: 10.1159/000350477

The Role of Toothpaste in the Aetiology and Treatment of Dentine Hypersensitivity

M. Addy · N.X. West

School of Oral and Dental Science, University of Bristol, Bristol, UK

Abstract

Dentine hypersensitivity (DH) is a common, painful dental condition with a multi-factorial aetiology. The hydrodynamic mechanism theory to explain dentine sensitivity also appears to fit DH: lesions exhibiting large numbers of open dentinal tubules at the surface and patent to the pulp. By definition, DH can only occur when dentine becomes exposed (lesion localisation) and tubules opened (lesion initiation), thus permitting increased fluid flow in tubules on stimulation. Erosion, particularly from dietary acids appears to play a dominant role in both processes. Toothbrushing with most toothpaste products alone cause clinically insignificant wear of enamel but are additive, even synergistic, to erosive enamel loss. Additionally, toothbrushing with toothpaste is implicated in 'healthy' gingival recession. Toothbrushing with most toothpastes removes the smear layer to expose tubules and again can exacerbate erosive loss of dentine. These findings thereby implicate toothbrushing with toothpaste in the aetiology of DH. Management of the condition should have secondary prevention at the core of treatment and therefore, must consider first and foremost the aetiology. Fluoride toothpaste at present appears to provide little primary or secondary preventive benefits to DH; additional ingredients can provide therapeutic benefits. Potassium-based products to block pulpal nerve response have caused much debate and are considered by many as unproven, which should not translate to ineffective. Several toothpaste technologies formulated to block tubules are from studies in vitro, in situ and controlled clinical trials considered proven for the treatment of DH.

Many years have passed and much researched, published and reviewed since Johnson and co-workers stated in 1982 that: 'DH is an enigma being frequently encountered yet ill-understood' [1]. Given the plethora of writings on dentine hypersensitivity (DH), it would not be unreasonable to suggest that a great deal more is known of the condition, but with much still to be learnt. This said, it appears that DH remains 'ill-understood' by many dental professionals around the world [2], which must limit primary and secondary prevention, diagnosis and management of the condition. Arguably, this arises through a lack of understanding of the aetiology of the condition particularly in respect of dentine exposure through enamel loss and gingival recession [for reviews see 3, 4]. As a result, countries have published guidelines on DH for dissemination to their dental professionals [2, 5], and very recently, media advertising of sensitivity toothpastes provide important snippets of information on the condition and the mode of action of products: clearly educational for the profession and public alike.

The aim of this chapter is to summarise what is known about DH and use this as a basis to discuss toothpaste as a possible aetiological agent in the condition and, conversely, as a factor in a preventive-based management programme. Some overlap with other chapters in the monograph occurs, notably with the chapter Toothpaste and Erosion by Ganss et al. [6].

Overview of Dentine Hypersensitivity

A brief summary of our present knowledge of DH will be given here to set the scene for a discussion of the possible role of toothbrushing and toothpaste in the condition [for reviews see 3, 7–10].

Definition

An international meeting [11] proposed the following definition for DH: 'short sharp pain arising from exposed dentine in response to stimuli, typically thermal, evaporative, tactile, osmotic or chemical, and which cannot be ascribed to any other form of dental defect or pathology. Thus, DH is a specific dental defect, which needs to be distinguished from other causes of dentine sensitivity [10] and in particular root sensitivity, a term adopted by the European Federation of Periodontology to describe sensitivity associated with periodontal disease and treatment [12].

Sensitivity Mechanism

The hydrodynamic mechanism proposed in 1900 [13] and much later proven to explain the sensitivity of dentine [for reviews see 14–17] is also considered to apply to DH [for review see 10]. Thus, appropriate stimuli applied to exposed dentine cause an increased inward or outward flow of dentinal fluid in the tubule network to stimulate, by a mechano-receptor action, A-beta and A-delta nerve fibres in and around the dentine pulp border. Theoretically, because of pressure change related, streaming potentials created when fluid flow occurs in tubes, pulp nerve stimulation could also be electrical [18, 19].

The Lesion

Histological, dye penetration and replica studies have shown that exposed dentine on teeth exhibiting DH have many more and wider open tubules than exposed dentine on non-sensitive teeth [20–22]. Since fluid flow in tubes obeys Poiseuille's law, fluid flow across dentine in DH would be directly proportional to the number of tubules and to the power four of the tubule radius: simple mathematics allow an appreciation of the probable huge difference in potential fluid flow and therefore pressure change across sensitive compared to non-sensitive dentine.

Aetiology of Dentine Hypersensitivity: The Possible Role of Toothbrushing and Toothpaste

Unfortunately, evidence concerning the aetiology of DH has been drawn from studies in vitro and in situ, clinical anecdote, case reports and epidemiological studies. The epidemiological data nevertheless, have provided associations between variables, which although circumstantial, in some aspects of the complex pathogenesis of the condition, are quite compelling.

Exposure of Dentine (Lesion Localisation)

By definition [11], dentine must first be exposed for DH to occur. Such exposure can come about by loss of enamel and or gingival recession (with loss of cementum). Loss of enamel, outside acute trauma, is a tooth wear process involving attrition, abrasion and erosion, often in combination. Abfraction (cervical tensile stress) may also be involved [for review see 23] since it is hypothesised that stress may render cervical enamel more susceptible to abrasion and or erosion: the jury is still out on this possible aetiological factor in DH.

Attrition

Wear of teeth by attrition particularly on occlusal surfaces can be quite rapid, and in individuals with para-functional habits, such as bruxism, may expose dentine at a relatively young age. Thus, based on studies in vitro, abrasion combined with attrition appears to increase wear, whereas erosion combined with attrition decreases wear [for review see 24]. Since occlusal DH is uncommon, and the interaction of toothpaste abrasion with attrition in enamel loss unreported to date, it would seem more appropriate to the aims of this chapter to consider loss of cervical enamel through erosion and abrasion: accepting of course that some malocclusions can produce labial and cervical enamel loss through attrition, thereby acting as a co-factor in lesion localisation.

Erosion

Dental erosion has been the subject of much research in recent years, including a monograph devoted to the subject [25] to which the interested reader is referred. Only a brief summary of the salient details of enamel erosion will be given here. Acids from intrinsic and particularly extrinsic dietary sources have two interrelated effects on enamel: dissolution and 'softening'. The former is irreversible, but the latter reversible by rehardening, albeit over time. Unfortunately, softened enamel is extremely fragile and can be removed by relatively minimal traumas: an issue most relevant to the interplay of erosion and abrasion. Extrapolations from studies in situ indicate that, depending on individual susceptibility, soft drinks imbibed at 1 litre per day can remove 1 mm of enamel in 2–20 years, highlighting the susceptibility of the cervical area of teeth to dentine exposure through erosion. Several chemical and physical characteristics of acid solutions and their intake appear to influence erosion of enamel both in a positive and negative direction [for reviews see 26–28].

Abrasion

The following two sections involve a discussion of relative dentine abrasivity (RDA), and the reader is referred to the more detailed chapter on the subject by Gonzales-Cabezas et al. [29]. Abrasion is a three-body wear process where a vehicle carries an abrasive substance over a substrate. Although abrasion of enamel could and has occurred through abrasive materials rubbed over the tooth surface, by virtue of common habitual use, the issue here is abrasion of enamel through toothbrushing with toothpaste. Over many years, dental textbooks have referred to buccal cervical wear facets of a variety of shapes as 'cervical abrasion lesions' and strongly implicated toothbrushing with toothpaste as the main, if only, aetiological factor. This section is concerned with enamel loss only and begs the question whether brushing with toothpaste abrades enamel and if so how much. If one summarises and extrapolates the data derived from studies in vitro using realistic brushing forces and toothpaste that conforms to the International Standards Organisation and British Standards Institute standards for dentifrices, the resounding conclusion must be that toothbrushing with toothpaste would cause minimal, even miniscule, wear of enamel in a lifetime of normal brushing. The explanation is straightforward, in that most toothpaste abrasives are softer than enamel. The exception is non-hydrated alumina, but even the few pastes containing this abrasive cause very limited abrasion to enamel. Thus far, it must be concluded that toothpaste abrasion to enamel alone would play a clinically insignificant role in lesion localisation in DH.

Abrasion-Erosion Interaction

Over the last 30 years, a number of studies in vitro and in situ have reported that toothbrushing, with or without toothpaste, of enamel previously exposed to dietary acids, causes additive if not synergistic tissue loss [for review see 24]. This occurs because the enamel softened by acid, alluded to earlier, is highly susceptible to abrasion [30]. Indeed, there are data which show that softened enamel can be removed by the abrasive action of the tongue [31]. The apparent positive interaction of abrasion and erosion begs the question and opens debate on the timing of toothbrushing to food and drink intake: before or after? Arguably, the present authors consider that toothpaste has mostly preventive rather than therapeutic actions and by definition should be used prior to any expected or potential insult. Thus, in individuals identified to have dental erosion, brushing before acid intake would be ideal or at least divorcing toothbrushing for a few hours after acid intake. Although unproven, it may also be prudent to recommend the use of low RDA toothpaste.

Gingival Recession

Exposure of dentine through loss of gingival and periodontal tissues can usefully be classified as 'unhealthy' or 'healthy' gingival recession, the aetiology of the former being well understood and of the latter poorly explained. Thus, unhealthy gingival recession can occur through acute and chronic periodontal diseases, and surgical and non-surgical periodontal procedures. Gingival recession in otherwise healthy tissues has been described as an enigma albeit, at the same time, implicating chronic trauma, in particular toothbrushing, as a major factor in the pathogenesis of the condition [for reviews see 4, 32]. Support for this theory comes from case reports of factitious injury or abusive toothbrushing habits and epidemiological associations of recession, positive in respect of particular tooth surfaces, type and site, and negative in respect of plaque [33]: evidence which is rather circumstantial but nevertheless compelling. Most of the debate concerning toothbrushing and gingival recession has centred around brush head characteristics: filament stiffness, filament end rounding, etc. Supportive evidence so far has been drawn only from recording numbers of gingival lacerations and excoriations caused by different toothbrushes, often without the use of toothpaste. This apparent lack of interest in toothpaste as a co-factor with the toothbrush in gingival recession is somewhat surprising given what is known about toothbrush-toothpaste interactions in tooth wear [34, 35]. Thus, although brush head and filament characteristics modulate the abrasivity of toothpaste, it is the paste that is the major factor in tooth wear. Therefore, it is not a great leap in faith to suggest that toothpaste could play a role in gingival recession. Such a role could be both physical, through abrasion, and chemical, through cytotoxicity of ingredients such as detergents to soft tissues.

Opening of Dentine Tubules (Lesion Initiation)
This section will consider briefly erosion and toothbrush and toothpaste abrasion, alone or combined in exposing dentinal tubules. Non-sensitive dentine reveals few if any open dentinal tubules at the surface [21], and it is assumed, but as yet surprisingly not proven that the tubules are covered by a 'smear layer' consisting of collagen and hydroxyapatite [for review see 36]; it is unlikely to be cementum as a study of early recession lesions revealed an absence of this tissue [37]. To initiate DH, this layer has to be removed, and studies in vitro and in situ strongly implicate erosion, the smear layer being acid labile [38, 39]. Indeed, body dentine itself appears twice as susceptible as enamel to erosion [40]. Toothbrushes alone have clinically insignificant effects on the smear layer [38], although they can accelerate erosion [for review see 41]. Toothpaste can produce a variety of effects on dentine, although from studies in vitro and in situ, most if not all, remove the smear layer [39, 42], probably by a combined abrasive/detergent action [for review see 43]. Subsequent to tubule exposure, toothpaste may produce narrowing of tubule orifices

by secondary abrasive smearing or deposition of toothpaste constituents onto the dentine surface and into tubules.

Management of Dentine Hypersensitivity: Toothpaste in Primary and Secondary Prevention

More recent reviews point out that the management of DH in the past has been treatment orientated without consideration of aetiological factors, highlighting the limitations of such an approach [for reviews see 8–10, 44, 45]. The same reviews suggest a management strategy based on aetiology to which the reader is referred. Discussion thus far strongly implicates erosion as a major aetiological factor in DH both from the point of view of enamel loss to expose dentine and removal of the dentine smear layer to open dentinal tubules. Toothbrushing with toothpaste appears as a co-aetiological factor as alone it is implicated in gingival recession and exposure of dentinal tubules, and, perhaps more importantly, when combined with erosion, exacerbates loss of enamel and dentine. In this knowledge, management of DH ideally should have a biological basis with prevention at the core.

As with all diseases and conditions, primary prevention directed towards the aetiology would be ideal. In the case of DH, a primary preventive strategy at present would require controlling erosive and abrasive effects to hard and soft tissues to prevent dentine exposure (lesion localisation), directed in particular at diet and tooth cleaning. The difficulties of this approach are obvious: firstly, good oral hygiene, using toothbrushes and fluoride toothpaste form the basis of prevention of gingivitis, periodontal diseases and caries; secondly, diets considered healthy are relatively high in acidic foods and drinks. Dental professionals, however, should advise moderation to limit erosive/abrasive loss of enamel and abrasive gingival recession. Unfortunately, our present lack of understanding of individual susceptibility limits recommendations to sensible rather than scientific levels, namely: limiting the frequency and duration of dietary acid intake; dissociating tooth cleaning from acid intake, by recommending brushing before dietary intake or to a few hours after acid intake; advising gentle but efficient toothbrushing practices. Several reviews make detailed recommendations for the prevention of dental erosion, particularly in those individuals already showing signs of erosive tooth wear [46–48]. Such recommendations are also relevant to the secondary prevention of DH and dovetail nicely with treatment planning approach recommended for the condition [9, 44], namely:

1 Correct diagnosis based on a history, clinical examination and compatibility with the definition of DH.
2 Differential diagnosis to identify alternative or additional causes of dentinal pain, which if found should be treated first by appropriate methods.
3 Identification of aetiological and predisposing factors particularly dietary and oral hygiene habits relevant to erosion, abrasion and gingival recession. If tooth wear appears associated with regurgitation or vomiting, appropriate referral to medical colleagues is recommended in the first instance.
4 Elimination, reduction or modification of aetiological factors through oral hygiene and dietary advice.
5 Provision/recommendation of proven efficacious treatments based upon individual needs.

The question arises whether there are agents that could be placed in toothpaste to at least protect enamel against erosion. As such, these agents would act as a primary preventive for dentine exposure and therefore DH: the answer is presented in the appropriate chapter [6], and here only fluoride will be considered. Reviews indicate that fluoride can offer some protection to enamel against erosion, but greatest benefits appear to arise from topically applied fluoride solutions or gels, combination fluoride regimens, or fluoride salts as yet not formulated into toothpaste, for example titanium fluoride, rather than everyday fluoride toothpaste products [6, 26, 48].

Finally in this section, given that erosion and toothpaste abrasion alone and combined can initiate DH by removing the smear layer to expose tubules, could toothpaste protect the smear layer? In the sense of primary prevention, the answer must be no. From the available data [for review see 3], all toothpastes readily remove the smear layer probably by a combined physical action of abrasives and chemical action of detergents [49]. Also, dentine smear layers exposed briefly to dietary acids are readily removed by a toothbrush alone [38]. This said and to be discussed, other ingredients in toothpaste products can be deposited on the dentine surface and in the tubules to protect against erosion.

Toothpaste in the Treatment of Dentine Hypersensitivity

In all branches of Medicine and Dentistry, proof of efficacy of treatments for diseases and conditions, for several decades has relied on randomised controlled clinical trials (RCTs) which conform to the criteria for good clinical practice (GCP). Both RCTs and GCP are large subject areas in themselves and beyond the scope of this chapter. Nevertheless, interested readers are referred to a publication specific to clinical trials on DH [11] and standard texts on GCP [50]. Additionally, the reader should be aware of the many factors that can confound RCTs in DH, and for that matter all clinical studies on pain, most notable of which are regression to the mode and the placebo response [for reviews see 10, 44, 51].

Treatment approaches to DH using toothpaste fall into two categories, namely: (1) modify or block pulp nerve response; (2) occlude dentinal tubules.

Historically [for review see 52], a surprisingly large number of physically and chemically diverse agents have been recommended for the treatment of DH, some of which could be or were formulated into toothpaste. Unfortunately, relatively few were subjected to the rigours of RCTs, leading one author to state that 'many reports on treatments for DH belong in the realms of testimonials' [for review see 52]. In keeping with the theme for this chapter, home-use, desensitising toothpaste products will mainly be discussed, with emphasis on those for which the present authors consider there is good evidence, drawn from RCTs, in some cases supported by studies in vitro and in situ, for efficacy in treating DH.

Toothpaste Products to Block Pulp Nerve Response: Potassium Salts

A number of potassium salts have been formulated into toothpaste for the treatment of DH, on the principle that the potassium ion will diffuse along the tubules and accumulate at the pulp dentine border to block the neural response of A-beta and A-delta nerve fibres. It would appear that most toothpaste manufacturers have at least one potassium-based desensitising product. Few manufacturers have subjected their products to RCTs and presumably, based on potassium availability data, 'piggyback' claims from those manufacturers who have, not unlike the situation with fluoride toothpastes. It is important to state, however, that there are conflicting scientific opinions and data for the efficacy of potassium toothpaste, which can be summarised under 'for' and 'against' headings [for reviews see 10, 53–55]:

For potassium:

1 Animal studies showed that potassium solutions held, on dentine, close to the pulp blocked neural responses.

2 A number of RCTs showed significant differences in favour of potassium versus control toothpaste.

3 The FDA issued a monograph supporting the safety and efficacy of potassium nitrate toothpaste in the treatment of DH.

Against potassium:

1 Animal experiments did not remotely simulate potassium delivery in the mouth, particularly in respect of vehicle, contact time and distance from the pulp.
2 Potassium ion diffusion is over several millimetres and against the direction of fluid flow in tubules: diffusion would be just as likely away from dentine and into saliva, gingival or mucous membranes.
3 Biologically, potassium ions are tissue labile and would be unlikely to accumulate in the pulp.
4 Several RCTs reported no significant difference between potassium and control toothpastes.
5 There are no studies of potassium salts in aqueous solutions versus water and two mouth rinse studies reported no difference from controls.
6 Reviews, including two Cochrane systematic reviews [56, 57], have concluded the evidence is equivocal or unproven for potassium toothpaste.

This unproven status of potassium toothpaste creates a further debate, namely how does potassium achieve an effect at the pulp? Arguments against tubule penetration and tissue lability of potassium are physiologically strong, particularly since apparent benefits take many days to accrue. One hypothesis, propounded by the present authors, and which, would fit the time scale described, is absorption of potassium into body dentine, eventually forming a depot at the pulp dentine border.

The fact that there is such a debate on the efficacy of potassium toothpaste raises issues in respect of controls for clinical trials. Some RCTs, including recently, have used potassium toothpaste as the only control for a test product, implying, against many contrary opinions [11], that there are positive or 'gold standard' controls for DH clinical studies. The 'unproven' status quo for potassium toothpaste renders the findings of such direct comparisons meaningless, emphasising need for other controls, such as a 'benchmark', normal use toothpaste product [for review of control definitions see 58].

Toothpaste Products to Block Tubules
As discussed, many agents have been used in toothpastes for the treatment of DH and purported, directly or indirectly, to occlude tubules. Of the earlier agents, delivered in simple solutions in vitro, including sodium fluoride and sodium monofluorophosphate, few, such as tin and zinc salts, left significant occluding deposits and in the case of zinc the deposit was water soluble [59]. Here, only those agents which, alone or when contained in toothpaste, have been shown to occlude tubules in vitro and or in situ will be discussed, together with the outcome of related RCTs [for reviews see 9, 53–55].

Strontium (Chloride and Acetate)
Arguably, strontium chloride was the first toothpaste ingredient thought to occlude tubules based on an often misinterpreted study in vitro using radio-labelled strontium and auto-radiography [60]. The auto-radiographs published could only have shown the presence of strontium on or in dentine: not whether tubules were occluded. A scanning electron microscopic (SEM) study failed to show tubule occlusion by strontium chloride solutions [59]. A later SEM study, with the original strontium chloride toothpaste, revealed a deposit on dentine but which was clearly the diatomaceous earth abrasive system [61]. The same study in vitro running parallel to an RCT showed that three artificial silica-based toothpastes, two with strontium acetate alone or combined with fluoride and one without either, coated the dentine surface and occluded the tubules: the occluding agent being the artificial silica, which was not water or acid labile [61]. Interestingly, the parallel clinical study showed all three artificial silica formulations were similar and significantly better than the original strontium chloride and a formalin-based toothpaste in the treatment of DH [62]. The resulting strontium acetate/artificial silica

(Sr/Si) product has again been shown in studies in vitro and in situ to occlude tubules with an acid-resistant silica/strontium-containing deposit, although the role of the strontium in the substantivity of the deposit cannot be teased out [39, 42, 63–66]. At least one review [54] has quite rightly commented as to why a considerable number of today's toothpaste which contain similar artificial silica abrasives do not occlude tubules or appear effective in DH. One explanation may lie in the use of sodium lauryl sulphate (SLS) as detergent in most toothpastes but the inability to formulate it with strontium-containing desensitising pastes due to mutual inactivation. Being anionic SLS in artificial silica-containing toothpaste would compete with the hydroxyl groups on silica for attachment to dentine.

Not all RCTs have reported differences in favour of the Sr/Si product compared to a variety of control products, although none has reported negative results against controls and some have reached significance in favour [67]. Interestingly, for many years, the present authors, in light of laboratory and later in situ studies already cited, have recommended, without supportive RCTs, the use of twice-daily brushing with the Sr/Si product with evening finger topical application to teeth. Such a recommendation appears to have been re-invented recently by the manufacturers of this and other tubule-occluding technologies.

Arginine and Calcium Carbonate

Clinical evidence for the beneficial effects of arginine and calcium carbonate (A/C) in DH and root sensitivity has been reviewed [55], and initially came from an in-office-applied prophylactic paste. The treatment effects were immediate and thought to be due to tubule occlusion by calcium phosphate. Studies in vitro on A/C prophylactic paste and toothpaste confirmed the deposit was indeed largely calcium and phosphate [68, 69]. The use of a variety of controls indicated that the A/C combination was essential to tubule oc-

clusion. There are conflicting data to be discussed as to the acid solubility of the deposit, probably arising from differences in the acid challenges employed. Given the nature of the deposit, effectively similar to hydroxyapatite, it would be expected that the deposit would be labile to any reasonable dietary acid challenge. This of course may not matter whilst the A/C toothpaste is in regular use: any deposit dissolved by acid being replaced at the next brushing. Clinical efficacy data first came from RCTs on the A/C prophylactic paste and revealed immediate and 4-week benefits significantly greater than controls [70, 71]. Subsequently, a number of RCTs of varying duration comparing A/C toothpaste with a variety of controls reported, for the most part, superior treatment effects immediately and up to 8 weeks of A/C toothpaste [72–79].

Stannous Fluoride with and without Sodium Hexametaphosphate

Evidence from studies in vitro already cited reveal that, stannous salt solutions precipitate onto dentine, block tubules and the deposit is water and acid resistant [59]. More recent studies, using stannous fluoride gel, reported the same observations [80] and further indicated a protective effect of the dentine smear layer against acid erosion [81]. Consistent with the findings in vitro, clinical studies reported efficacy of stannous fluoride gel or solutions in the treatment of DH [82–84], and the ADA issued a seal of acceptance for a 0.4% stannous fluoride gel in this application. More recently, RCTs have reported that hexametaphosphate-stabilised sodium hexametaphosphate (SnF_2) toothpaste provided immediate, 4- and 8-week benefits in the treatment of DH, which were significantly greater than appropriate control toothpaste products [85–88].

Calcium Sodium Phosphosilicate

Calcium sodium phosphosilicate (CSPS) is a bioglass first used in bone regeneration, but more recently formulated into an anhydrous toothpaste product for the treatment of DH [for reviews see 89–91]. Essentially, CSPS, in an aqueous environment, is attracted to dentine collagen, reacting to form a deposit or precipitate made up of calcium, phosphate and silica. A number of studies in vitro, when summarised, essentially show that CSPS in solution or toothpaste interacts on the dentine surface and forms a deposit over the dentine and in the tubules [91–94]. This tubule-blocking deposit appears water and acid insoluble and mechanically resistant. The deposit has a hydroxyapatite appearance but also contains silica and when derived from toothpaste vehicle, titanium. A number of RCTs comparing CSPS toothpaste with a variety of controls and extending up to 8 weeks overall showed significantly greater benefits for the CSPS product in the treatment of DH [95–98]. None of the cited studies had a measurement for the immediate benefits of CSPS toothpaste after the first brushing or for the paste topically applied; given the data in vitro, such an immediate effect might be predicted.

Tubule Occlusion: Toothpaste Product Comparisons

The literature reviewed thus far concerning the four toothpaste technologies formulated to occlude tubules and thereby treat DH, in the opinion of the present authors, provide sufficient data to support efficacy of each. This conclusion has been reached based on the balance of available evidence, with the caveat that this is not a systematic review, and as far as the present authors are aware, no such systematic reviews of the above products exist. Thus, studies in vitro and in situ indicate that the Sr/Si-, A/C-, SnF_2- and CSPS-containing toothpastes all occlude tubules; for the Sr/Si product the role of Sr in the deposit is unclear, and for the A/C product the acid stability is open to question. These points made, the data suggest that with twice-daily use, in particular with additional topical application, all four products would be expected to bring about rapid and considerable relief of symptoms during product use. Additionally, the benefits of each product would be expected to be similar, thereby providing the profession and the consumer with a choice of efficacious toothpaste products for the treatment of DH.

Product comparison studies however, are not entirely consistent with this biological, even logical conclusion. Comparative studies in vitro, whilst not all encompassing, with one part exception [99], again suggest that deposits from Sr/Si, SnF_2 and CSPS are more resistant to dietary acid than from A/C [64, 65]. A study in situ also demonstrated that the deposit on dentine from CSPS was more acid resistant than from A/C [100]. Chemically, this difference in solubility could be predicted given the nature of the respective deposits. To reiterate, however, such differences in acid solubility may not be reflected in clinical efficacy when products are in regular daily use, leading the present authors to expect similar outcomes from direct comparisons in RCTs. Such comparisons available to date do not entirely fit the above conclusion; rather, they throw the picture into confusion as follows: one study reported SnF_2 significantly better than A/C [88], one study showed CSPS better than SnF_2 up to 4 weeks but no difference at 12 weeks [101], one study reported no difference between Sr/Si and A/C [102] and three studies reported A/C significantly better than Sr/Si [103–105].

Conclusions

1 Toothbrushing with toothpaste alone is unlikely to expose dentine through abrasion of enamel but can potentiate erosion by removing softened enamel.
2 Erosion of enamel is a major aetiological factor in exposing dentine, particularly at cervical areas, and agents such as fluoride in toothpaste afford limited or no protection in the long term. Any chemical benefit would likely be vitiated by toothpaste abrasivity if used after an erosive challenge.

3   Circumstantial but arguably compelling evidence links toothbrushing with toothpaste in gingival recession.

4   Erosion is a dominant factor in loss of dentine and exposure of tubules to initiate DH. Toothbrushing with toothpaste can expose tubules by removal of the smear layer and can exacerbate loss of dentine by erosion. Fluoride in toothpaste affords little if any clinically meaningful protection to dentine against erosion.

5   Management of DH must be based on secondary prevention with consideration of aetiological factors including dietary and toothbrushing practices of the individual.

6   Treatment of DH should use products of proven efficacy from RCTs, and if possible supported by studies in vitro and/or in situ.

Arguably, toothpastes are the first-choice treatment, containing actives which could block neural activity in pulp nerves such as potassium or block dentinal tubules.

7   The efficacy of potassium-based toothpastes is much debated and considered by many as unproven: this does not translate to ineffective.

8   Tubule occlusion technologies in toothpaste products include Sr/Si, A/C, SnF_2 and CSPS for which data from studies in vitro and in situ support their mode of action and RCTs their efficacy in the treatment of DH. Available evidence at present suggests that these products should be considered equally effective, and can be recommended for use in this condition. Hopefully, more studies will be published to permit systematic reviews to be performed.

References

1   Johnson RH, Zulgar-Nairn BJ, Kovall JJ: The effectiveness of an electro-ionising toothbrush in the control of dentinal hypersensitivity. J Periodont 1982;53: 353–359.

2   Canadian Advisory Board on Dentine Hypersensitivity: Consensus-based recommendations for the diagnosis and management of dentine hypersensitivity. J Can Dent Assoc 2003;69:221–228.

3   Addy M: Tooth brushing, tooth wear and dentine hypersensitivity – are they associated? Int J Dent 2005;55(suppl 4):261–267.

4   Smith RG: Gingival recession. Reappraisal of an enigmatic condition and a new index for monitoring. J Clin Periodontol 1997;24:201–205.

5   Rao CB, Kohli A, Addy M: Dentine hypersensitivity: information document for Indian dental professionals. Dental Council of India, 2010.

6   Ganss C, Schulze K, Schlueter N: Toothpaste and Erosion; in van Loveren C (ed): Toothpastes. Monogr Oral Sci. Basel, Karger, 2013, vol 23, pp 88–95.

7   Addy M: Dentine hypersensitivity: definition, prevalence, distribution and aetiology; in Addy M, Embery G, Edgar WM, Orchardson R (eds): Tooth Wear and Sensitivity. London, Martin Dunitz, 2000, pp 239–248.

8   Addy M: Dentine hypersensitivity: new perspectives on an old problem. Int Dent J 2002;52(suppl 5):367–375.

9   Addy M, Smith SR: Dentin hypersensitivity: an overview on which to base tubule occlusion as a management concept. J Clin Dent 2010;21:25–30.

10 West NX: Dentine hypersensitivity; in Lussi A (ed): Dental Erosion. Monogr Oral Sci. Basel, Kager, 2006, vol 20, pp 173–189.

11 Holland GR, Nahri MN, Addy M, Gangarosa L, Orchardson R: Guidelines for the design and conduct of clinical trials on dentine hypersensitivity. J Clin Periodontol 1997;24:808–813.

12 Sanz M, Addy M: Group D summary. J Clin Periodontol 2002;29(suppl 3):195–196.

13 Gysi A: An attempt to explain the sensitiveness of dentine. Br J Dent Sci 1900; 43:865–868.

14 Brannstrom M: A hydrodynamic mechanism in the transmission of pain-produced stimuli through the dentine; in Anderson DJ (ed): Sensory Mechanisms in Dentine. Oxford, Pergamon Press, 1963, pp 73–79.

15 Brannstrom M: The sensitivity of dentine. Oral Surg Oral Med Oral Path 1966; 21:517–526.

16 Anderson DJ, Hannam AG, Matthews B: Sensory mechanisms in mammalian teeth and their supporting structures. Physiol Rev 1970;59:171–176.

17 Narhi MVO: Response of pulpal nociceptors to tissue injury and inflammation: in Addy M, Embery G, Edgar WM, Orchardson R (eds): Tooth Wear and Sensitivity. London, Martin Dunitz, 2000, pp 257–266.

18 Anderson DJ, Matthews B: Osmotic stimulation of human dentine and the distribution of pain thresholds. Arch Oral Biol 1967;12:417–426.

19 Griffiths H, Morgan G, Williams K, Addy M: The measurement in vitro of streaming potentials with fluids flow across dentine and hydroxyapatite. J Periodont Res 1993;28:59–65.

20 Ishikawa S: A clinico-histological study on the hypersensitivity of dentine (in Japanese). Kokubyo Gakkai Zasshi 1969; 36:278–298.

21 Absi EG, Addy M, Adams D: Dentine hypersensitivity: a study of the patency of dentinal tubules in sensitive and non sensitive cervical dentine. J Clin Periodontol 1987;14:280–284.

22 Absi EG, Addy M, Adams D: Dentine hypersensitivity: the development and evaluation of a replica technique to study sensitive and nonsensitive cervical dentine. J Clin Periodontol 1989;16:190–196.

23 Grippo JO: Abfractions: a new classification of hard tissue lesions of teeth. J Esthet Dent 1991;3:14–19.

24 Addy M, Shellis RP: Interaction between attrition, abrasion and erosion in tooth wear; in Lussi A (ed): Dental Erosion. From Diagnosis to Therapy. Monogr Oral Sci. Basel, Karger, 2006, vol 20, pp 17–31.

25 Lussi A (ed): Dental Erosion. From Diagnosis to Therapy. Basel, Karger, 2006, pp 1–214.

26 Lussi A, Jaeggi T: Chemical factors; in Lussi A (ed): Dental Erosion. From Diagnosis to Therapy. Monogr Oral Sci. Basel, Karger, 2006, vol 20, pp 77–87.

27 Zero DT, Lussi A: Etiology of enamel erosion: intrinsic and extrinsic factors; in Addy M, Embery G, Edgar WM, Orchardson R (eds): Tooth Wear and Sensitivity. London, Martin Dunitz, 2000, pp 121–140.

28 Zero DT, Lussi A: Behavioral factors; in Lussi A (ed): Dental Erosion. From Diagnosis to Therapy. Monogr Oral Sci. Basel, Karger, 2006, vol 20, pp 100–105.

29 Gonzales-Cabezas C, Hara A, Hefferen J, Lippert F: Abrasives in toothpastes, problems in measuring RDA; in van Loveren C (ed): Toothpastes. Monogr Oral Sci. Basel, Karger, 2013, vol 23, pp 96–103.

30 Eisenburger M, Shellis P, Addy M: Scanning electron microscopy of softened enamel. Caries Res 2004;38:67–74.

31 Gregg T, Mace S, West NX, Addy M: A study in vitro of the abrasive effect of the tongue on enamel and dentine softened by acid erosion. Caries Res 2004; 38:557–560.

32 Watson PJC: Gingival recession. J Dent 1984;12:29–35.

33 Addy M, Mostafa P, Newcombe R: Dentine hypersensitivity: the distribution of recession, sensitivity and plaque. J Dent 1987;15:242–250.

34 Phaneuf EA, Harrington JH, Dale PP, Shklar G: Automatic toothbrush: a new reciprocating action. J Am Dent Assoc 1962;65:12–25.

35 Dyer D, Addy M, Newcombe RG: Studies in vitro of abrasion by different manual toothbrush heads and a standard toothpaste. J Clin Periodontol 2000;27:99–103.

36 Pashley DH: Smear layer: physiological considerations. Operative Dent 1984; 9(suppl 3):13–29.

37 Bevenius J, Lindskog S, Hultenby K: The micromorphology in vivo of the buccocervical region of premolar teeth in young adults. A replica study by scanning electron microscopy. Acta Odontol Scand 1994;52:323–334.

38 Absi EG, Addy M, Adams D: Dentine hypersensitivity. The effects of toothbrushing and dietary compounds on dentine in vitro: a SEM study. J Oral Rehab 1992;19:101–110.

39 Banfield N, Addy M: Dentine hypersensitivity: development and evaluation of a model in situ to study tubule patency. J Clin Periodontol 2004;31:325–335.

40 Hunter ML, West NX, Hughes JA, Newcombe RG, Addy M: Erosion of deciduous and permanent dental hard tissues in the oral environment. J Dent 2000;28:257–264.

41 Addy M, Hunter ML: Can tooth brushing damage your health? Effects on oral and dental tissues. Int Dent J 2003; 53(suppl 3):177–186.

42 Absi EG, Addy M, Adams D: Dentine hypersensitivity: uptake of toothpastes onto dentine and effects of brushing, washing and dietary acid. J Oral Rehab 1995;22:175–182.

43 Dababneh RH, Khouri AT, Addy M: Dentine hypersensitivity – an enigma? A review of terminology, epidemiology, mechanisms, aetiology and management. Br Dent J 1999;187:606–611.

44 Addy M, West NX: Dentinal hypersensitivity; in Daniel SJ, Harfst SA, Wilder RS (eds): Dental Hygiene: Concepts, Cases and Competences. St Louis, Mosby, 2008, chapter 33, pp 623–640.

45 Orchardson R: Strategies for the management of dentine hypersensitivity; in Addy M, Embery G, Edgar WM, Orchardson R (eds): Tooth Wear and Sensitivity. London, Martin Dunitz, 2000, pp 315–326.

46 Lussi A, Hellwig E: Risk assessment and preventive measures; in Lussi A (ed): Dental Erosion. From Diagnosis to Therapy. Monogr Oral Sci. Basel, Karger, 2006, vol 20, pp 190–199.

47 Lussi A, Jaeggi T, Zero D: The role of diet in the aetiology of dental erosion. Caries Res 2004;38:34–44.

48 Zero D, Lussi A: Erosion – chemical and biological factors of importance to the dental practitioner. Int Dent J 2005;55:285–290.

49 Moore C, Addy M: Wear of dentine in vitro by toothpaste abrasive and detergents alone and combined. J Clin Periodontol 2005;32:1242–1246.

50 International Conference on Harmonisation for Good Clinical Practice. http://ichgcp.net/; retrieved 29th November 2012.

51 Curro FA, Friedman M, Leight RS: Design and conduct of clinical trials on dentine hypersensitivity; in Addy M, Embery G, Edgar WM, Orchardson R (eds): Tooth Wear and Sensitivity, London, Martin Dunitz, 2000, pp 299–314.

52 Addy M, Dowell P: Dentine hypersensitivity – a review. II. Clinical and in vitro evaluation of treatment agents. J Clin Periodontol 1983;10:356–363.

53 Jackson RJ: Potential treatment modalities for dentine hypersensitivity: Home use products; in Addy M, Embery G, Edgar WM, Orchardson R (eds): Tooth Wear and Sensitivity. London, Martin Dunitz, 2000, pp 327–338.

54 Cummins D: Recent advances in dentin hypersensitivity: clinically proven treatments for instant and lasting sensitivity relief. Am J Dent 2010;23:3–13.

55 Cummins D: Advances in the clinical management of dentin hypersensitivity: a review of recent evidence for the efficacy of dentifrices in providing instant and lasting relief. J Clin Dent 2011;22:100–107.

56 Poulsen S, Errboe M, Hovgaard O, Worthington HW: Potassium nitrate toothpaste for dentine hypersensitivity. Cochrane Database Syst Rev 2001;CD001476.

57 Poulsen S, Errboe M, Lescoy Mevil Y, Glenny AM: Potassium containing toothpastes for dentine hypersensitivity. Cochrane Database Syst Rev 2006;CD001476.

58 Addy M, Moran J: Chemical supragingival plaque control; in Lindhe J (ed): Clinical Periodontology and Implantology. Oxford, Backwell Munksgaard, 2007, chapter 36, pp 734–765.

59 Addy M, Mostafa P: Dentine hypersensitivity 1. Effects produced by the uptake in vitro of metal ions, fluoride and formaldehyde onto dentine. J Oral Rehab 1988;15:575–585.

60 Kun L: Etude biophysique des modifications des tissues dentaires provoquées par l'application totale de Strontium. Schweiz Monatschr Zahnheilk 1976;86:661–676.

61 Addy M, Mostafa P: Dentine hypersensitivity 11. Effects produced by the uptake in vitro of toothpastes onto dentine. J Oral Rehab 1989;16:35–48.

62 Addy M, Mostafa P, Newcombe RG: Dentine hypersensitivity: a comparison of five toothpastes used during a 6-week period. Br Dent J 1989;163:45–50.

63 Claydon NCA, Addy M, Macdonald EL, West NX, Maggio B, Barlow A, Parkinson C, Butler A: Development of an in situ methodology for the clinical evaluation of dentine hypersensitivity occlusion ingredients. J Clin Dent 2009;20:158–166.

64 Parkinson CR, Wilson RJ: A comparative in vitro study investigating the occlusion and mineralization properties of commercial toothpastes in a four-day dentin disc model. J Clin Dent 2011;22:74–81.

65 Parkinson CR, Butler A, Wilson RJ: Development of an acid challenge-based in vitro dentin disc occlusion model. J Clin Dent 2010;21:31–36.

66 Earl JS, Ward MB, Langford RM: Investigation of dentinal tubule occlusion using FIB-SEM milling and EDX. J Clin Dent 2010;21:37–41.

67 Mason S, Hughes N, Sufi F, Bannon L, Maggio B, North M, Holt J: A comparative clinical study investigating the efficacy of a dentifrice containing 8% strontium acetate and 1040 ppm fluoride in a silica base and a control dentifrice containing 1,450 ppm fluoride in a silica base to provide immediate relief of dentin hypersensitivity. J Clin Dent 2010;21:42–48.

68 Petrou I, Heu R, Stanick M, Lavender S, Zaidel L, Cummins D, Sullivan RJ, Hsueh C, Gimzewski JK: A breakthrough therapy for dentin hypersensitivity: how dental products containing 8% arginine and calcium carbonate work to deliver effective relief of sensitive teeth. J Clin Dent 2009;20:23–31.

69 Lavender SA, Petrou I, Heu R, Stranick MA, Cummins D, Kilpatrick-Liverman L, Sullivan RJ, Santarpia RP: Mode of action studies on a new desensitizing dentifrice containing 8% arginine, a high cleaning calcium carbonate system and 1,450 ppm fluoride. Am J Dent 2010;23: 14–19.

70 Hamlin D, Williams KP, Delgado E, Zhang YP, DeVizio W, Mateo LR: Clinical evaluation of the efficacy of a desensitizing paste containing 8.0% arginine and calcium carbonate for the in-office relief of dentin hypersensitivity associated with dental prophylaxis. Am J Dent 2009;22:16–20.

71 Schiff T, Delgado E, Zhang YP, Cummins D, DeVizio W, Mateo LR: Clinical evaluation of the efficacy of a desensitizing paste containing 8.0% arginine and calcium carbonate in providing instant and lasting relief of dentin hypersensitivity. Am J Dent 2009;22:8–15.

72 Ayed F, Ayad N, Delgado E, Zhang YP, DeVizio W, Cummins D, Mateo LR: Comparing the efficacy in providing instant relief of dentin hypersensitivity of a new toothpaste containing 8.0% arginine, calcium carbonate and 1,450 ppm fluoride to a sensitive toothpaste containing 2% potassium ion and 1,450 ppm fluoride and to a control toothpaste with 1,450 ppm fluoride: a three-day clinical study in Mississauga, Canada. J Clin Dent 2009;20:115–122.

73 Nathoo S, Delgado E, Zhang YP, DeVizio W, Cummins D, Mateo LR: Comparing the efficacy in providing instant relief of dentin hypersensitivity of a new toothpaste containing 8.0% arginine, calcium carbonate and 1,450 ppm fluoride relative to a sensitive toothpaste containing 2% potassium ion and 1,450 ppm fluoride and to a control toothpaste with 1450 ppm fluoride: a three-day clinical study in New Jersey. J Clin Dent 2009;20:123–130.

74 Ayed F, Ayad N, Zhang YP, DeVizio W, Cummins D, Mateo LR: Comparing the efficacy in reducing dentin hypersensitivity of a new toothpaste containing 8.0% arginine, calcium carbonate and 1,450 ppm fluoride to a commercial sensitive toothpaste containing 2% potassium ion: an eight-week clinical study on Canadian adults. J Clin Dent 2009;20:10–16.

75 Docimo R, Montesami L, Maturo P, Costacurta M, Bartolino M, DeVizio W, Zhang YP, Cummins D, Dibart S, Mateo LR: Comparing the efficacy in reducing dentin hypersensitivity of a new toothpaste containing 8.0% arginine, calcium carbonate and 1450 ppm fluoride to a commercial sensitive toothpaste containing 2% potassium ion: an eight-week clinical study in Rome. J Clin Dent 2009; 20:17–22.

76 Docimo R, Montesami L, Maturo P, Costacurta M, Bartolino M, Zhang YP, Zhang YP, DeVizio W, Delgado E, Cummins D, Dibart S, Mateo LR: Comparing the efficacy in reducing dentin hypersensitivity of a new toothpaste containing 8.0% arginine, calcium carbonate and 1,450 ppm fluoride to a benchmark commercial sensitive toothpaste containing 2% potassium ion: an eight-week clinical study in Rome. J Clin Dent 2009; 20:137–143.

77 Fu Y, Lin L, Que K, Wang M, Hu D, Mateo LR, DeVizio W, Zhang YP: Instant dentin hypersensitivity relief of a new desensitizing toothpaste containing 8.0% arginine, a high cleaning calcium carbonate system and 1450 ppm fluoride: a three-day clinical study in Chengdu, China. Am J Dent 2010;23:20–27.

78 Que K, Fu Y, Lin L, Hu D, Zhang YP, Panagakos FS, DeVizio W, Mateo LR: Dentin hypersensitivity reduction of a new toothpaste containing 8.0% arginine, a high cleaning calcium carbonate system and 1,450 ppm fluoride: an eight-week clinical study on Chinese adults. Am J Dent 2010;23:28–35.

79 Schiff T, Delgado E, Zhang YP, Cummins D, DeVizio W, Mateo LR: A clinical investigation of the efficacy of a dentifrice containing 8.0% arginine, calcium carbonate and 1450 ppm fluoride in providing instant relief of dentin hypersensitivity: the effect of a single direct topical application using a cotton swab applicator versus the use of a fingertip. J Clin Dent 2009;20: 131–136.

80 von Koppenfels RL, Kozak KM, Duschner H, White DJ, Goetz H, Taylor E, Zoladz JR: Stannous fluoride effects on dentinal tubules (abstract 93). J Dent Res 2005;84.

81 White DJ, Lawless MA, Fatade A, Baig A, von Koppenfels R, Duschner H, Gotz H: Stannous fluoride/sodium hexametaphosphate dentifrice increases resistance to tubule exposure in vitro. J Clin Dent 2007;18:55–59.

82 Blong MA, Volding B, Thrash WJ, Jones DL: Effects of a gel containing 0.4% stannous fluoride on dentinal hypersensitivity. Dent Hyg 1985;59:489–492.

83 Snyder RA, Beck FM, Horton JE: The efficacy of a 0.4% stannous fluoride gel on root surface hypersensitivity. J Dent Res 1985;62:201, abstr 237.

84 Thrash WJ, Dodds WJ, Jones DL: The effect of stannous fluoride on dentine hypersensitivity. Int Dent J 1994; 44(suppl 1):107–118.

85 Schiff T, He T, Sagel L, Baker RJ: Efficacy and safety of a novel stabilized stannous fluoride and sodium hexametaphosphate dentifrice for dental hypersensitivity. J Contemp Dent Pract 2006;7:1–8.

86 Schiff T, Saletta L, Baker RA, Winston JL, He T: Desensitizing effect of a stabilized stannous fluoride/sodium hexametaphosphate dentifrice. Compend Contin Educ Dent 2005;26(suppl 1):35–40.

87 He T, Barker ML, Qaqish J, Sharma N: Fast onset sensitivity relief of a 0.454% stannous fluoride dentifrice. J Clin Dent 2011;22:46–50.

88 He T, Cheng R, Biesbrock AR, Chang A, Sun L: Rapid desensitizing efficacy of a stannous-containing sodium fluoride dentifrice. J Clin Dent 2011;22:40–45.

89 Greenspan DC: NovaMin and tooth sensitivity-an overview. J Clin Dent 2010; 21:61–65.

90 Gendreau L, Barlow APS, Mason S: Overview of the clinical evidence for the use of NovaMin in providing relief from the pain of dentin hypersensitivity. J Clin Dent 2011;22:90–95.

91 Layer TM: Development of a fluoridated, daily-use toothpaste containing NovaMin technology for the treatment of dentin hypersensitivity. J Clin Dent 2011;22:59–61.

92 LaTorre G, Greenspan DC: The role of ionic release of NovaMin (calcium sodium silicophosphate) in tubule occlusion: an exploratory in vitro study using radio-labeled isotopes. J Clin Dent 2010; 21:72–76.

93 Earl JS, Leary RK, Muller KH, Langford RM, Greenspan DC: Physical and chemical characterization of surface layers formed on dentin following treatment with a fluoridated toothpaste containing NovaMin. J Clin Dent 2011;22:68–73.

94 Earl JS, Topping N, Elle J, Langford RM, Greenspan DC: Physical and chemical characterization of dentin surface following treatment with NovaMin technology. J Clin Dent 2011;22: 62–67.

95 Du Min Q, Bian Z, Jiang H, Greenspan DC, Burwell AK, Zhong J, Tai BJ: Clinical evaluation of a dentifrice containing calcium sodium phosphosilicate (NovaMin) for the treatment of dentin hypersensitivity. Am J Dent 2008;21: 210–214.

96 Pradeep AR, Anuj SJ: Comparison of the clinical efficacy of a dentifrice containing calcium sodium phosphosilicate with a dentifrice containing potassium nitrate and a placebo on dentinal hypersensitivity. J Periodont 2010;81: 1167–1173.

97 Litkowski L, Greenspan DC: A clinical study of the effect of calcium sodium phosphosilicate on dentin hypersensitivity – proof of principle. J Clin Dent 2010;21:77–81.

98 Salian S, Thakur S, Kulkarni S, LaTorre G: A randomized controlled clinical study evaluating the efficacy of two desensitizing dentifrices. J Clin Dent 2010;21:82–87.

99 Patel R, Chopra S, Vandeven M, Cummins D: Comparison of the effects on dentin permeability of two commercially available sensitivity relief dentifrices. J Clin Dent 2011;22:108–112.

100 West NX, Macdonald EL, Jones SB, Claydon NCA, Hughes N, Jeffery P: Randomized in situ clinical study comparing the ability of two new desensitizing toothpaste technologies to occlude patent dentin tubules. J Clin Dent 2011;22:82–89.

101 Sharma N, Roy S, Kakar A, Greenspan DC, Scott R: A clinical study comparing oral formulations containing 7.5% calcium sodium phosphosilicate (NovaMin), 5% potassium nitrate and 0.4% stannous fluoride for the management of dentin hypersensitivity. J Clin Dent 2010;21:88–92.

102 Hughes N, Mason S, Jeffrey P, Welton H, Tobin M, O'Shea C, Browne M: A comparative clinical study investigating the efficacy of a test dentifrice containing 8% strontium acetate and 1,040 ppm sodium fluoride versus a marketed control dentifrice containing 8% arginine, calcium carbonate and 1,450 ppm sodium monofluorophosphate in reducing dentinal hypersensitivity. J Clin Dent 2010;21:49–55.

103 Li Y, Lee S, Zhang YP, Delgado E, DeVizio W, Mateo LR: Comparison of the clinical efficacy of three toothpastes in reducing dentin hypersensitivity. J Clin Dent 2011;22:113–120.

104 Docimo R, Perugia C, Bartilino M, Maturo P, Montesani L, Zhang YP, DeVizio W, Mateo LR, Dibart S: Comparative evaluation of the efficacy of three commercially available toothpastes on dentin hypersensitivity reduction: an eight-week study. J Clin Dent 2011;22:121–127.

105 Schiff T, Mateo LR, Delgado E, Cummins D, Zhang YP, DeVizio W: Clinical efficacy in reducing dentin hypersensitivity of a dentifrice containing 8.0% arginine, calcium carbonate and 1,450 ppm fluoride compared to a dentifrice containing 8% strontium acetate and 1,040 ppm fluoride under consumer usage conditions before and after switch-over. J Clin Dent 2011;22:128–138.

Martin Addy
The Willows
3 Manor Way
Failand, Bristol, BS8 3UY (UK)
E-Mail Martin.Addy@bristol.ac.uk

van Loveren C (ed): Toothpastes. Monogr Oral Sci. Basel, Karger, 2013, vol 23, pp 88–99
DOI: 10.1159/000350475

Toothpaste and Erosion

Carolina Ganss · Katja Schulze · Nadine Schlueter

Department of Conservative and Preventive Dentistry, Dental Clinic, Justus Liebig University, Giessen, Germany

Abstract

Dental erosion develops from the chronic exposure to non-bacterial acids resulting in bulk mineral loss with a partly demineralised surface of reduced micro-hardness. Clinical features are loss of surface structures with shallow lesions on smooth surfaces and cupping and flattening of cusps; already in early stages, coronal dentine often is exposed. Not only enamel, but also dentine is therefore an important target tissue for anti-erosion strategies. The main goal of active ingredients against erosion is to increase the acid resistance of tooth surfaces or pellicles. The challenge with toothpastes is that abrasives, otherwise beneficial in terms of cleaning properties, may counteract the effects of active ingredients. Fluoride toothpastes offer a degree of protection, but in order to design more effective formulations, active ingredients in addition to, or other than, fluorides have been suggested. Polyvalent metal cations, Ca/P salts in nano-form, phosphates, proteins, and various biopolymers, e.g. chitosan, are substances under study. The complex combined action of active ingredients and abrasives on the dental hard tissues, and the role of excipients of complex toothpaste formulations are not yet fully understood. Current evidence is flawed by the diversity of experimental designs, and there is no knowledge from clinical studies with patients so far. However, research results indicate that there is potential to develop effective toothpastes in this field. As the prevalence of initial erosive lesions particularly in younger age groups is high in some countries, such strategies would be of great importance for maintaining oral health.

Toothpastes are established part of oral hygiene practices and are used all over the world. Not only are they carriers of active ingredients and facilitate tooth cleaning by abrasives and other ingredients, but make oral hygiene attractive by fancy packages, and the variety of flavours and colours. Requirements for toothpastes are that they have anti-caries efficacy, which could be accompanied by other benefits like antibacterial properties. The use of toothpastes needs to be safe in terms of wear and other side effects like discoloration or mucosal irritation. In the last years, almost all companies market a toothpaste claiming to deliver special protection against dental erosion. As the prevalence of erosive lesions is high in some countries, specifically in younger age groups [1], effective toothpastes for erosion prevention would significantly contribute to oral health.

The potential of conventional or special toothpastes in this field has been increasingly investigated, but there is still limited knowledge available about the role of toothpastes in the context of dental erosion. Evidence is currently constituted from in vitro and in situ research with healthy volunteers, but there is no clinical study with patients published; evidence from epidemiological studies is lacking.

The present chapter starts with a brief description of the clinical and histological feature of the condition and describes the underlying pathomechanism. It further aims to provide an overview over what is known about the effects of toothpastes and to describe new concepts and approaches in the field.

Erosion and the Dental Hard Tissues

Understanding the effects of toothpastes on eroded dental hard tissues requires understanding the pathomechanism of the condition as well as its histological features and physical properties.

Dental erosion by definition is caused by the exposure of tooth surfaces by extrinsic or intrinsic acids not related to bacterial metabolism. In other words, acids directly interact with clean tooth surfaces. Under the condition that the acidic liquid surrounding of the tooth surface is undersaturated with respect to tooth minerals, erosive demineralisation can occur [2]. When the acid exposure continues, clinically visible lesions are likely to develop. Initially, the natural lustre of sound enamel disappears followed by the development of distinct lesions. On smooth surfaces, these defects are located coronal from the cemento-enamel junction often with a gingival band of sound enamel. They are shallow in shape and their width exceeds their depth. On occlusal surfaces, the morphological structures flatten and the crowns increasingly loose height [3]. Importantly, dentine is often exposed already in initial stages, for instance at the cervical

area where the enamel covering is relatively thin. Therefore, not only enamel, but also dentine is an important target tissue for strategies aiming to prevent erosion progression and in particular for considerations regarding toothpaste effects.

Sound enamel mainly consists of calcium and phosphate arranged in the form of crystallites building up a prismatic structure. The mineral is densely packed and the mineral content of enamel is around 87 vol% [4]. When acids act on the enamel surface under erosive conditions, mineral dissolves from the outermost enamel surface. With continuing erosive demineralisation, mineral is dissolved layerwise resulting in a bulk tissue loss; the remaining enamel surface is partly demineralised. The surface structure is similar to an etching pattern [5, 6] (fig. 1); on cross-sections, this partial surface demineralisation appears as a less dense band on the surface which is a few microns in thickness [7]. This histological feature means that active ingredients, in particular fluoride in combination with polyvalent metal cations, do not act as agents for remineralising a subsurface lesion, but interact with the eroded enamel surface in order to make it less susceptible to subsequent erosive acid attacks. This can be achieved by the precipitation of mineral salts on the surface (e.g. CaF_2-like material, various more acid-resistant Sn-containing salts [8–10], or Ti-containing glaze-like precipitates [11, 12]) or by the incorporation of Sn in the outermost few microns of enamel [7]. The partial loss of mineral on the surface is accompanied by a loss of microhardness, which makes eroded enamel more prone to wear from physical impacts [13]. This is of importance because toothpastes are applied via toothbrushing. The loss of microhardness depends on the severity of the erosive impact; a 1-min erosion with an erosive beverage (Sprite Light) can reduce the microhardness of enamel by 12% and a 15-min erosion by 31%. The result is a 4- and 13-fold increase in abrasive loss, respectively [13]. Similar results were reported after immersion in 1% citric acid for 3

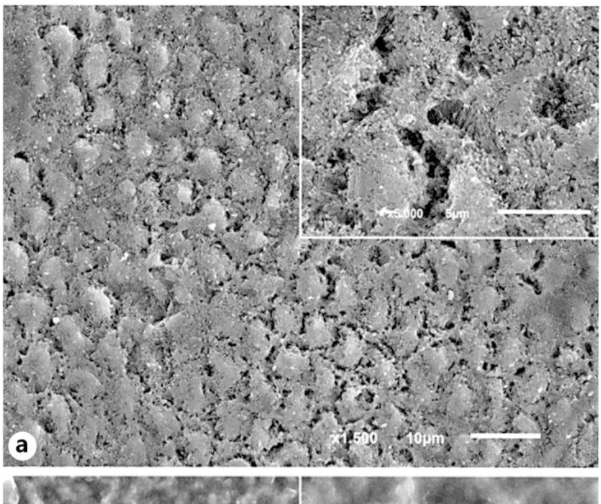

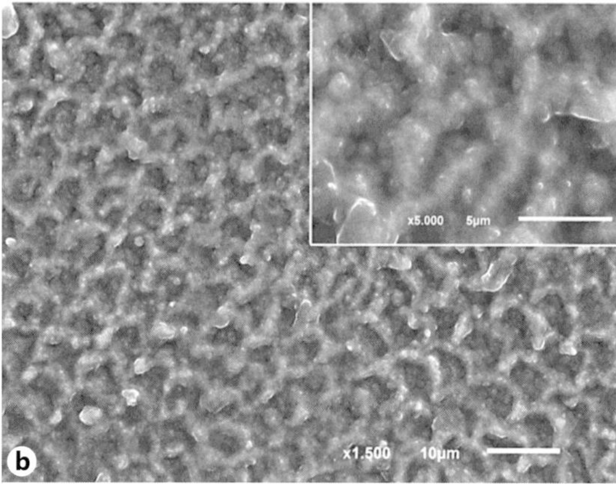

Fig. 1. a Enamel specimen from an in vitro experiment (10 days, 0.5% citric acid pH 2.7, 6 × 2 min/day). Twice daily, the specimen was immersed in NaF toothpaste slurry for 2 min and brushed within this time for 15 s with a brushing machine (load 200 g). **b** Enamel specimen from an in situ study (7 days, 0.5% citric acid pH 2.7, 6 × 2 min/day extra-orally). Twice daily, the specimen was intra-orally exposed to the saliva/NaF toothpaste mixture for 2 min and was intra-orally brushed within this time with a powered toothbrush for 5 s (load 250 g). In both studies, the last intervention was brushing. Under both experimental conditions, an etching pattern is clearly visible even after the brushing procedure. On the specimen from the in situ study, the glaze-like appearance indicates the presence of the pellicle.

min, with a reduction of microhardness of approximately 10% [14].

Dentine has a much more complex structure and reacts substantially differently under erosive conditions. The mineral content of the tissue is lower, whereas its organic content is higher (47 and 21 vol%, respectively), and it contains much water (21 vol%) [4]. Generally, the mineral also is hydroxyapatite (HA), but the crystallites are much smaller than in enamel. They are relatively densely packed in the peritubular regions and are arranged in the intertubular regions with the collagen fibrils [15], which is important for considerations about the mode of action of active ingredients.

Due to its complex structure, the hardness of dentine is difficult to measure, but overall, it is much lower than that of enamel. Due to its higher mineral content, the peritubular areas are harder than the intertubular regions [16]. Similar to enamel, erosive demineralisation in dentine is a centripetal process. While the mineral component of the tissue is dissolving, the organic portion is not degraded from clinically relevant acid impacts. Instead, demineralised collagen persists on the surface (fig. 2), and can reach considerable thickness at least under in vitro and in situ conditions [17]. It can be degraded by various proteolytic enzymes, for instance collagenases [18, 19], but, importantly, is considerably resistant against physical impacts [20–22] (fig. 2). Though the histological structure of eroded dentine from in vitro erosion has been clearly described, little is known about its in vivo histology. Samples eroded in vitro or in situ appear soft and resilient after a certain time of erosive demineralisation. Clinically, even severe erosive lesions appear hard when scratched with a probe indicating that the in vivo histology of such lesions might differ from that of experimental erosion. The organic surface material may have significant effects on erosion progression [19, 23], brushing impacts [20–22] or the action of active ingredients [24]. Therefore, the histological feature of experimental dentine erosion needs to be considered when choosing measuring methods and experimental designs for interpreting study outcomes and for transferring research results into recommendations for patients.

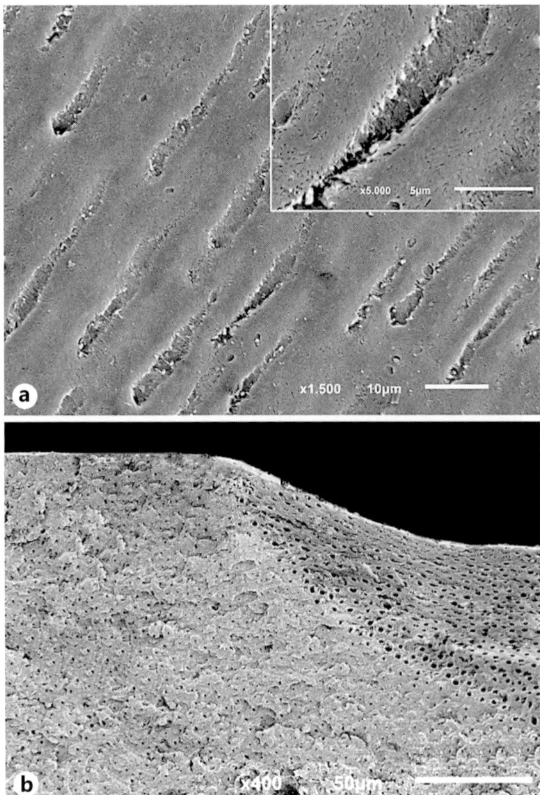

Fig. 2. Surface (**a**) and cross-section (**b**) of eroded and brushed dentine specimens. The specimens were eroded (HCl; pH 1.6, 6 × 2 min/day, 9 days) twice daily; the specimen was brushed with a powered toothbrush and fluoride-free toothpaste for 15 s (load 200 g). **a** No structural alteration of the demineralised organic matrix was found on the surface. **b** On the cross-section, it is clearly visible that a broad zone of demineralised collagen has survived the brushing procedure.

Effects of Toothpastes on Eroded Dental Hard Tissues – The Role of Active Ingredients

There is some evidence that fluoride toothpastes generally deliver a certain degree of protection against erosion. Table 1 summarises studies retrieved from a PubMed search using the MeSH terms 'toothpaste AND erosion' and 'dentifrice AND erosion'. Only profilometric and pH-cycling studies were included.

Generally, fluorides play a major role in erosion prevention, but the mode of action differs substantially from that in the frame of caries prevention. It is well known that CaF_2-like mineral salts are deposited on the tooth surfaces under certain conditions [25]; these precipitates are relatively soluble in acids, which is important for protection against caries, but is less effective in the case of erosion. Anyhow, compared to placebo, toothpastes containing sodium or amine fluoride were reported to deliver a degree of protection in enamel, but much less information is available about the role of such toothpastes in preventing dentine erosion. Overall, effects of conventional sodium fluoride toothpastes compared to fluoride-free controls appear to range between no effect and 37% protection in enamel and between no effect and 32% protection in dentine (table 1). Controversial results were reported for highly concentrated formulations. An in vitro study comparing a 1,100 and a 5,000 ppm sodium fluoride formulation revealed a protection compared to placebo of 26 and 53%, respectively, when applied with brushing and of 27 and 57%, respectively, when applied as slurry [26]; an in situ experiment demonstrated a 55% increase in protection of the 5,000 ppm formulation compared to a product with 1,450 ppm F [27] when applied as slurry without brushing. Other in situ experiments, however, found no significant benefit of the highly concentrated toothpaste with respect to protecting enamel and dentine against erosion and abrasion [28, 29].

Searching for more effective approaches for prevention in patients with dental erosion, cations other than sodium or amine being assumed to establish more acid-resistant precipitates came into play. It has been shown that polyvalent metal ions like the stannous or the titanium ion have promising erosion-inhibiting properties [30]. Titanium tetrafluoride has been investigated as solution, gel, and lacquer [31], but so far there is no information whether this compound is suitable as ingredient in toothpastes. Stannous fluoride

Table 1. Compilation of profilometric pH-cycling studies investigating the effects of toothpastes with various active ingredients in vitro and in situ

Reference	Days	Erosion	Intervention	Brushing force and mode	Active ingredients	Controls	Order of tissue loss, µm	Effects of abrasion[1]	Effect size[2]
In vitro *Enamel*									
[89]	–	5 × 5 min Sprite Diet	5 × 18.5 min brushing (5,000 strokes) slurry preparation: 1 part TP:2 parts distilled water (w/w)	300 g brushing machine	A: NaF, 1,500 ppm F⁻ B: MFP, 1,500 ppm F⁻ (baking soda) C: MFP, 1,500 ppm F⁻ (whitening) D: MFP, 1,100 ppm F⁻ (tartar control)	distilled water	2.3–2.5	–	no significant effects
[35]	15	1 × 20 min/day orange juice	1 min slurry/day slurry preparation: 3 g TP:10 ml water	–	A: NaF B: SnF₂ F⁻ conc. not given	water	19–56	–	A: 18% B: 67%
[26]	7	4 × 5 min/day Sprite	4 × 15 s slurry/day or 4 × 15 s slurry + brushing/day slurry preparation: 1 g TP:3 ml water	30 g powered toothbrush	A: NaF, 1,100 ppm F⁻ B: NaF, 5,000 ppm F⁻ C: NaF, 500 ppm F⁻ + 3% TMP	placebo	1.3–4.6	38%	slurry: A: 27%, B: 57%, C: 62% slurry +brushing: A: 26%, B: 53%, C: 51%
[37]	10	6 × 2 min/day 1% citric acid	2 × 2 min slurry/day or 2 × 2 min slurry + 2 × 15 s brushing/day slurry preparation: 1 part TP:3 parts mineral salt solution (w/w)	200 g brushing machine	A: NaF, 1,450 ppm F⁻ B: 1% Zn-carbonate-HA-nanoparticles, no F C: chitosan, no F D: SnF₂/NaF, 1,450 ppm F⁻, 3,436 ppm Sn²⁺	slurry: erosion only slurry + brushing: no F⁻ TP	16.8–37.1	29%	slurry: A: 23% B: n.s. C: 29% D: 55% slurry + brushing A–D: n.s.
[90]	7	4 × 2 min/day cola	2 × 15 s slurry/day or 2 × 15 s slurry + brushing/day slurry preparation: 1 part TP:3 parts water	1.5 N powered toothbrush	A: 10% xylitol B: NaF, 1,030 ppm F⁻ + 10% xylitol C: NaF, 1,030 ppm F⁻	placebo	3.1–7.3	30%	slurry: A: n.s. B: 39% C: 25% slurry + brushing: A: 33% B: 47% C: 37%
[38]	10	6 × 2 min/day 0.5% citric acid	2 × 2 min slurry + 2 × 15 s brushing/day slurry preparation: 1 part TP:3 parts mineral salt solution (w/w)	200 g brushing machine	A: NaF, 1,400 ppm F⁻ B: AmF/SnF₂, 1,400 ppm F⁻, 3,280 ppm Sn²⁺ C: AmF/NaF/SnCl₂, 1,400 ppm F⁻, 3,500 ppm Sn²⁺ D: AmF/NaF/SnCl₂/chitosan, 1,400 ppm F⁻, 3,500 ppm Sn²⁺	placebo according to A	4.6–20.2	40%	A: n.s. B: 33% C: 39% D: 67%
Dentine [91]	–	5 × 5 min Sprite Diet	5 × 18.5 min brushing (5,000 strokes) slurry preparation: 1 part TP:2 parts distilled water (w/w)	300 g brushing machine	A: NaF, 1,500 ppm F⁻ B: MFP, 1,500 ppm F⁻ (baking soda) C: MFP, 1,500 ppm F⁻ (whitening) D: MFP, 1,100 ppm F⁻ (tartar control)	distilled water	2.2–17.6	–	increase compared to negative control: A: 452% B: 637% C: 593% D: 798%
[92]	–	5 × 40 min orange juice	5 × 10 s slurry or 5 × 10 s slurry + brushing slurry preparation: 3 g TP:10 ml water	200 g brushing machine	A: TP with F⁻ B: TP no F⁻ F⁻ conc. not given	slurry: erosion only slurry + brushing: water	21.5–27.7	9%, n.s.	slurry: A: n.s. B: – slurry and brushing: A: 23% B: n.s.

Reference	Days	Erosion	Intervention	Brushing force and mode	Active ingredients	Controls	Order of tissue loss, µm	Effects of abrasion[1]	Effect size[2]
In situ									
Enamel									
[93]	3	2 × 90 s/day Sprite Light extra-orally	2 × 40 strokes/day slurry preparation: 1 part TP:3 parts distilled water (w/w)	manual tooth-brush, extra-orally	A: NaF, 1,500 ppm F⁻ hydrated silica (whitening) B: MFP, 1,500 ppm F⁻, silica and calcium carbonate (regular)	–	2.6–2.9	–	A, B: n.s.
[35]	15	4 × 10 min/day orange juice extra-orally	2 × 1 min slurry rinse/day slurry preparation: 3 g TP:10 ml water	–	A: NaF B: SnF$_2$ F⁻ conc. not given	mineral water	0.95–3.2	–	A: 30% B: 71%
[94]	7	4 × 5 min/day cola extra-orally	4 × 30 brushing strokes/day undiluted TP	manual tooth-brush extra-orally	A: NaF, 1,098 ppm F⁻	placebo	5.4–6.8	–	A: 21%
[28]	7	4 × 1 min/day cola extra-orally	4 × 30 s slurry/day or 4 × 30 s slurry + brushing/day slurry preparation: 1 g TP:3 ml deionised water	powered tooth-brush extra-orally	A: NaF, 1,100 ppm F⁻ B: NaF, 5,000 ppm F⁻	placebo according to B	3.5– 5.1	20%	erosion: A, B: n.s. erosion + abra-sion: A, B: n.s.
[39]	4	3 × 5 min/day 1% citric acid extra-orally	2 × 2 min slurry + 10 strokes brushing/day slurry preparation: 1 part TP:3 parts demi-water	brushing machine 150 g	A: SnF$_2$, 1,050 ppm F⁻, AmF, 350 ppm F⁻ B: SnF$_2$, 1,100 ppm F⁻, NaF, 350 ppm F⁻ C: NaF, 1,450 ppm F⁻	water	15–25	–	A: 34% B: 26% C: n.s.
[27]	5	4 × 10 min/day orange juice intra-orally	2 × 1 min slurry rinse/day slurry preparation: 3 g TP:10 ml distilled water	–	A: NaF, 5,000 ppm F⁻ B: NaF, 1,450 ppm F⁻	–	5.7–12.6	–	A: 5.7 µm B: 12.6 µm
Dentine									
[93]	3	2 × 90 s/day Sprite Light extra-orally	2 × 40 strokes/day slurry preparation: 1 part TP:3 parts distilled water (w/w)	manual tooth-brush, extra-orally	A: NaF, 1,500 ppm F⁻ hydrated silica (whitening) B: MFP, 1,500 ppm F⁻, silica and calcium carbonate (regular)	–	3.1–4.4	–	A, B: n.s.
[29]	7	4 × 1 min/day cola extra-orally	4 × 30 s slurry/day or 4 × 30 s slurry + brushing/day slurry preparation: 1 g TP:3 ml water	powered tooth-brush extra-orally	A: NaF, 1,100 ppm F⁻ B: NaF, 5,000 ppm F⁻	placebo according to B	2.5–3.9	8% n.s.	slurry: A: 32% B: 28% slurry and brush-ing: A: 25% B: 26%
[40]	15	3 × 2 min/day orange juice extra-orally	3 × 15 slurry + 3 × 4 s brushing/day undiluted TP	powered tooth-brush extra-orally	A: NaF, 1,100 ppm F⁻ B: SnF$_2$, 1,100 ppm F⁻	–	12–23	–	A: 12.4±1.8 µm B: 22.5±1.8 µm

TP = Toothpaste; MFP = sodium monofluorophosphate; TMP = trimetaphosphate.

[1] Percent increase in tissue loss from brushing in the control group compared to erosion/control groups without brushing.

[2] Percent reduction in tissue loss compared to controls.

has been used already at the beginnings of fluoride toothpastes [32]. Sn^{2+}- and F^--containing toothpastes play a role in the frame of gingivitis prevention [33] and are considered as erosion prevention formulations. When applied as slurries, promising results were found for enamel [34–37] ranging between 55 and 95% reduction of tissue loss compared to a control. When such toothpastes were applied with brushing, however, the protecting effects decreased markedly to the order of conventional NaF toothpastes [37, 38]. This was found for formulations with different sources of the stannous ion (SnF_2 or $SnCl_2$) and different additional fluoride compounds (amine fluoride or NaF or combination of both) as well as different amounts of available Sn [38]. One in situ study revealed superiority of two SnF_2-containing products over an NaF product, which had no significant effect over a water control [39].

A relatively simple explanation is that the physical action of the abrasive particles at the solid/liquid interface disturbs the precipitation of Sn salts on the surface or removes established Sn-enriched enamel surface structures. This is supported by the finding that an SnF_2 gel with a similar Sn concentration as Sn toothpastes but without abrasives provided strong protection even under relatively severe erosive conditions whether with or without brushing (75 and 78%, respectively) [37].

Almost nothing is known about the efficacy of Sn-containing toothpastes in dentine. A recent randomised in situ trial revealed that a SnF_2-containing product caused even more wear than a NaF formulation [40], but the latter had a much lower relative dentine abrasion (RDA) value, which makes the results difficult to compare.

Anorganic compounds other than fluoride or stannous ions have been introduced in toothpastes claiming to exhibit particular anti-erosion/abrasion prevention properties. HA in nanocrystalline form was used in formulations with and without fluoride. Nano-HA has been investigated with respect to its potential to remineralise enamel [41] and dentine caries lesions [42], and its capability to infiltrate fully demineralised dentine [43]. It is clear that precipitation of these minerals can occur as soon as there is (super)saturation with respect to respective Ca/P mineral salts. As soon as pH drops, however, the concept behind these strategies is not clear. So far, there is no evidence that HA in its nano-crystalline form behaves differently than that occurring in dental hard tissues. Correspondingly, the very few investigations published on the issue revealed that nano-HA is much less effective than NaF in a pH-cycling caries model [44] and has no effect under erosive conditions [37]. When combined with fluoride, nano-HA may decrease the available fluoride. A respective product showed effects similar to conventional sodium fluoride formulations [37], but its low amount of available fluoride could result in insufficient protection against caries.

Deduced from caries research, another approach is to supplement fluoride toothpastes with phosphates, e.g. trimetaphosphate, in order to enhance mineral precipitation on the tooth surfaces. Little is known about the efficacy of such formulations though there are first promising results published [26].

Besides anorganic components, organic substances have been investigated. It is assumed that polymers like mucin or carboxymethylcellulose can form protective layers on the tooth surface or can strengthen the protecting properties of the pellicle. These substances have been mostly investigated as solutions or as additive to erosive fluids [45–49]. Some of them are frequent ingredients in toothpastes, e.g. hydroxyethylcellulose, carboxymethylcellulose, alginate, xanthan gum or polyethyleneglycol compounds. Sodium fluoride toothpastes with the same fluoride content have been shown to vary with respect to their erosion-inhibiting properties, and it is well conceivable that these substances may be one explaining factor for this variation in effects.

One biopolymer that has been investigated as active ingredient in toothpastes is chitosan, a cationic polysaccharide obtained by the deacetylation of chitin. Chitosan is widely used in industrial and medical fields [50, 51], e.g. as scaffold for tissue engineering or for drug delivery. For applications in the oral cavity, it has interesting properties such as its capability to act against oral bacteria [52–56] and to enhance tissue regeneration [57, 58]. A property making it specifically suitable as anti-erosion substance is that it has a strong positive charge at low pH [50]. It is then capable of adsorbing to solid structures with negative zeta potentials [59], such as enamel [60]. Chitosan has been further shown to potentially follow a multilayer adsorption behaviour [61], particularly with mucin [62, 63], and can adsorb to the pellicle [64]. The resulting layer is relatively stable against the anionic surfactant sodium dodecyl sulfate [62, 65] used in many toothpaste formulations.

From these properties, it can be deduced that chitosan might form a protective layer on enamel and might enhance pellicle structures in situ. It has indeed been shown that a fluoride-free toothpaste containing chitosan revealed protecting effects in the order of NaF toothpastes when applied as slurry without brushing [37]. A further promising finding was that the addition of chitosan has increased the in vitro efficacy of an Sn-containing toothpaste distinctly [38].

Milk-derived proteins have also been investigated as erosion-inhibiting compounds, and have shown protective potential when applied in solutions [66]. For applications of casein phosphopeptide (CPP) in combination with amorphous calcium phosphate (ACP) as a cream with or without fluoride, conflicting results have been published [67–71], and so far, there is no evidence that CCP/ACP adds effects over those of fluorides as such. CPP/ACP has been formulated in tooth creams, which are not intended to replace a toothpaste. A recent study investigating in vitro and in situ the effects of toothpastes containing casein, various enzymes, and IgG, in two different concentrations, showed some promise for the prevention of erosion [72].

Effect of Abrasives in Toothpastes on Eroded Dental Hard Tissues

The abrasion effects from toothpastes on sound tissues have been intensively investigated. In sound enamel, abrasion from toothpastes is generally very low [73], but under erosive pH-cycling conditions, brushing can increase the substance loss distinctly (table 1). From the histological feature of the eroded enamel surface, it was assumed that the weakened surface crystallites are easily abraded even by the friction of the oral soft tissues [74, 75], and more so by the action of the toothbrush and of the abrasives. The partly demineralised surface enamel, however, is not completely removed by brushing with toothpaste [76] (fig. 1) or by ultrasonication [6], indicating that at least deeper demineralised layers are more resistant against physical impacts. Similar to sound enamel, it seems to be the action of toothpaste abrasives rather than the toothbrush itself that causes tissue loss [77, 78].

This leads to the question how the abrasivity of toothpaste impacts the loss of eroded enamel, but there are only very few studies available systematically studying this issue. A study with experimental fluoride-free toothpastes without abrasives, and with variations in calcium pyrophosphate particles (relative enamel abrasion, REA, of 2, 6 and 9), revealed the most striking effect between the presence and absence of abrasives. The difference of tissue loss between REA 6 and 9 was only significant when a hard brush (bristle diameter 0.25 mm) was used [77]. Similar results were found in a study comparing fluoride-free experimental toothpastes with silica and with a REA of 3.8, 5.8 and 8.9 [79].

When active ingredients come into play, effects on the surface properties of the eroded enamel surface in terms of microhardness can be expected. In the case of fluorides as active agents, this could occur through the precipitation of mineral salts. From single applications of toothpaste slurries, however, only limited effects on microhardness recovery were observed. After a decrease in hardness of 10% after in vitro erosion, the immersion in slurries from various NaF toothpastes and an amine fluoride/SnF$_2$ formulation did not led to a significant increase of hardness [14]. Only limited effects were found in an in situ study investigating two different NaF toothpastes. After an erosion impact, the Knoop indentation length increased by around 30%, indicating loss of surface hardness, but after slurry immersion decreased only by <10% [80]. The interaction of fluoride and abrasivity has rarely been systematically studied. It could be expected that physical impacts could hamper the precipitation of minerals; this could be more pronounced with formulations with high abrasivity. One study indeed revealed that the REA value plays a more pronounced role in the presence than in the absence of fluoride [79].

On dentine, abrasion generally has a greater impact as the tissue is much softer than enamel. Several factors influence the abrasivity of a toothpaste such as the kind of abrasives [81, 82] and toothbrush [81], the dilution and the diluent [82, 83], the temperature [82], the kind of detergents [84], and the presence of the pellicle [85]. In principle, toothpastes with a higher RDA value cause more abrasion [86]. The impact of the abrasivity of toothpaste on eroded dentine was investigated with the same study design as mentioned above for enamel [77]. Experimental fluoride-free toothpaste formulations with an RDA of 10, 20, 50 and 100 were used. A clear relation between RDA and dentine loss, however, was only demonstrated when the toothpastes were applied with a soft brush (bristle diameter 0.15 mm) [87]. The authors assumed that bristles with a small diameter are more flexible and might have a greater contact area with the dentine surface than bristles

with a greater diameter and thus increase the quantity of abrasives moving across the surface. Further, the soft brush might have retained greater amounts of abrasives due to its higher number of bristles. Another study, however, revealed clear positive relation between dentine loss and toothpaste abrasivity (RDA 15, 56, and 117) regardless of the presence or absence of fluoride [79]. It was speculated that abrasivity is a dominant factor in dentine wear and thus had counteracted the protective potential of fluoride. Other studies also demonstrated higher loss values with higher RDA values [86, 40], or an impact of brushing in general, but only a minor relation to RDA [88]; these studies, however, compared commercial products with different composition and kind of active ingredients, which makes the interpretation of the results difficult.

Conclusion

Toothpastes are complex formulations, and their action in the frame of dental erosion is currently not fully understood. In caries prevention, active ingredients act in an environment which is relatively protected against physical impacts (i.e. the subsurface lesion and the approximal surface), and abrasives add to the beneficial effects of toothpastes due to their cleaning properties. In the case of erosion, which is a phenomenon occurring on plaque-free smooth surfaces and the occlusal areas, specific active ingredients offer protection, but the abrasive component is a counteracting factor here, and the interplay of both is not fully elucidated. There is evidence that fluoride toothpastes offer a degree of protection, but erosive lesions develop despite the widespread use of fluoride toothpastes. Therefore, research focuses on substances other than fluoride in order to make the dental hard tissues more resistant against erosive demineralisation and also against physical impacts, or on strategies to improve the protective properties of the pellicle.

Promising results indicate that polyvalent metal cations, phosphates or biopolymer additives could play a role in the future. Even though an essential breakthrough has not yet been made, there is great potential to develop effective toothpastes in this field. As the prevalence of initial erosive lesions particularly in younger age groups is high in some countries, such strategies would be of great importance for maintaining oral health.

A difficulty with interpreting results from published studies is that there is still no generally approved study design available. Experimental procedures vary substantially with respect to the preparation of toothpaste slurries, the order of tissue loss, the erosion and abrasion procedures, the balance between erosive and abrasive impacts, and the controls. Future research strategies might benefit from considerations put forward at the workshop Methodology and Models in Erosion Research [95].

References

1 Jaeggi T, Lussi A: Prevalence, incidence and distribution of erosion. Monogr Oral Sci 2006;20:44–65.
2 Larsen MJ: Chemical events during tooth dissolution. J Dent Res 1990;69:575–580.
3 Ganss C, Lussi A: Diagnosis of erosive tooth wear. Monogr Oral Sci 2006;20:32–43.
4 Nikiforuk G: Understanding Dental Caries. Basle, Karger, 1985.
5 Meurman JH, Frank RM: Progression and surface ultrastructure of in vitro caused erosive lesions in human and bovine enamel. Caries Res 1991;25:81–87.
6 Eisenburger M, Shellis RP, Addy M: Scanning electron microscopy of softened enamel. Caries Res 2004;38:67–74.
7 Schlueter N, Hardt M, Lussi A, Engelmann F, Klimek J, Ganss C: Tin-containing fluoride solutions as anti-erosive agents in enamel: an in vitro tin-uptake, tissue-loss and scanning electron micrograph study. Eur J Oral Sci 2009;117:427–434.
8 Babcock FD, King JC, Jordan TH: The reaction of stannous fluoride and hydroxyapatite. J Dent Res 1978;57:933–938.
9 Hercules DM, Craig NL: Fluorine and tin uptake by enamel studied by x-ray photoelectron spectroscopy (ESCA). J Dent Res 1976;57:296–305.
10 Krutchkoff DJ, Jordan JH, Wei SH, Nordquist WD: Surface characterization of the stannous fluoride-enamel interaction. Arch Oral Biol 1972;17:923–930.
11 Mundorff SA, Little MF, Bibby BG: Enamel dissolution. II. Action of titanium tetrafluoride. J Dent Res 1972;51:1567–1571.

12 Wei SHY, Sobodroff DM, Wefel JS: Effects of titanium tetrafluoride on human enamel. J Dent Res 1976;55:426–431.
13 Attin T, Koidl U, Buchalla W, Schaller HG, Kielbassa AM, Hellwig E: Correlation of microhardness and wear in differently eroded bovine dental enamel. Arch Oral Biol 1997;42:243–250.
14 Lussi A, Megert B, Eggenberger D, Jaeggi T: Impact of different toothpastes on the prevention of erosion. Caries Res 2008;42:62–67.
15 Weatherell JA, Robinson C: The inorganic composition of teeth; in Zipkin I (ed): Biological Mineralization. New York, John Wiley and Sons, 1973, pp 43–74.
16 Kinney JH, Balooch M, Marshall SJ, Marshall GWJ, Weihs TP: Hardness and Young's modulus of human peritubular and intertubular dentine. Arch Oral Biol 1996;41:9–13.
17 Lussi A, Schlueter N, Rakhmatullina E, Ganss C: Dental erosion – an overview with emphasis on chemical and histopathological aspects. Caries Res 2011;45:2–12.
18 Klont B, ten Cate JM: Susceptibility of the collagenous matrix from bovine incisor roots to proteolysis after in vitro lesion formation. Caries Res 1991;25:46–50.
19 Ganss C, Klimek J, Starck C: Quantitative analysis of the impact of the organic matrix on the fluoride effect on erosion progression in human dentine using longitudinal microradiography. Arch Oral Biol 2004;49:931–935.
20 Ganss C, Schlueter N, Hardt M, von Hinckeldey J, Klimek J: Effects of toothbrushing on eroded dentine. Eur J Oral Sci 2007;115:390–396.

21 Ganss C, Hardt M, Blazek D, Klimek J, Schlueter N: Effects of tooth brushing force on the mineral content and demineralised organic matrix of eroded dentine. Eur J Oral Sci 2009;117:255–260.
22 Schlueter N, Glatzki J, Klimek J, Ganss C: Erosive-abrasive tissue loss in dentine under simulated bulimic conditions. Arch Oral Biol 2012;57:1176–1182.
23 Hara AT, Ando M, Cury JA, Serra MC, Gonzalez-Cabezas C, Zero D: Influence of the organic matrix on root dentine erosion by citric acid. Caries Res 2005;39:134–138.
24 Ganss C, Lussi A, Sommer N, Klimek J, Schlueter N: Efficacy of fluoride compounds and stannous chloride as erosion inhibitors in dentine. Caries Res 2010;44:172–176.
25 ten Cate JM: Review on fluoride, with special emphasis on calcium fluoride mechanisms in caries prevention. Eur J Oral Sci 1997;105:461–465.
26 Moretto MJ, Magalhaes AC, Sassaki KT, Delbem AC, Martinhon CC: Effect of different fluoride concentrations of experimental dentifrices on enamel erosion and abrasion. Caries Res 2010;44:135–140.
27 Ren YF, Liu X, Fadel N, Malmstrom H, Barnes V, Xu T: Preventive effects of dentifrice containing 5000 ppm fluoride against dental erosion in situ. J Dent 2011;39:672–678.
28 Rios D, Magalhaes AC, Polo RO, Wiegand A, Attin T, Buzalaf MA: The efficacy of a highly concentrated fluoride dentifrice on bovine enamel subjected to erosion and abrasion. J Am Dent Assoc 2008;139:1652–1656.

29 Magalhaes AC, Rios D, Moino AL, Wiegand A, Attin T, Buzalaf MA: Effect of different concentrations of fluoride in dentifrices on dentin erosion subjected or not to abrasion in situ/ex vivo. Caries Res 2008;42:112–116.

30 Magalhaes AC, Wiegand A, Rios D, Buzalaf MA, Lussi A: Fluoride in dental erosion. Monogr Oral Sci 2011;22:158–170.

31 Wiegand A, Magalhaes AC, Attin T: Is titanium tetrafluoride (TiF4) effective to prevent carious and erosive lesions? A review of the literature. Oral Health Prev Dent 2010;8:159–164.

32 Caplan DJ, Slade GD, Biesbrock AR, Bartizek RD, McClanahan SF, Beck JD: A comparison of increment and incidence density analyses in evaluating the anticaries effects of two dentifrices. Caries Res 1999;33:16–22.

33 Paraskevas S, Van der Weijden GA: A review of the effects of stannous fluoride on gingivitis. J Clin Periodontol 2006;33:1–13.

34 Young A, Thrane PS, Saxegaard E, Jonski G, Rölla G: Effect of stannous fluoride toothpaste on erosion-like lesions: an in vivo study. Eur J Oral Sci 2006;114:180–183.

35 Hooper SM, Newcombe RG, Faller R, Eversole S, Addy M, West NX: The protective effects of toothpaste against erosion by orange juice: studies in situ and in vitro. J Dent 2007;35:476–481.

36 Faller RV, Eversole SL, Tzeghai GE: Enamel protection: a comparison of marketed dentifrice performance against dental erosion. Am J Dent 2011;24:205–210.

37 Ganss C, Lussi A, Grunau O, Klimek J, Schlueter N: Conventional and anti-erosion fluoride toothpastes: effect on enamel erosion and erosion-abrasion. Caries Res 2011;45:581–589.

38 Ganss C, von Hinckeldey J, Tolle A, Schulze K, Klimek J, Schlueter N: Efficacy of the stannous ion and a biopolymer in toothpastes on enamel erosion/abrasion. J Dent 2012;40:1036–1043.

39 Huysmans MC, Jager DH, Ruben JL, Unk DE, Klijn CP, Vieira AM: Reduction of erosive wear in situ by stannous fluoride-containing toothpaste. Caries Res 2011;45:518–523.

40 West NX, Hooper SM, O'Sullivan D, Hughes N, North M, Macdonald EL, Davies M, Claydon NC: In situ randomised trial investigating abrasive effects of two desensitising toothpastes on dentine with acidic challenge prior to brushing. J Dent 2012;40:77–85.

41 Huang S, Gao S, Cheng L, Yu H: Remineralization potential of nano-hydroxyapatite on initial enamel lesions: an in vitro study. Caries Res 2011;45:460–468.

42 Tschoppe P, Zandim DL, Martus P, Kielbassa AM: Enamel and dentine remineralization by nano-hydroxyapatite toothpastes. J Dent 2011;39:430–437.

43 Besinis A, van Noort R, Martin N: Infiltration of demineralized dentin with silica and hydroxyapatite nanoparticles. Dent Mater 2012;28:1012–1023.

44 Huang SB, Gao SS, Yu HY: Effect of nano-hydroxyapatite concentration on remineralization of initial enamel lesion in vitro. Biomed Mater 2009;4:034104.

45 Barbour ME, Shellis RP, Parker DM, Allen GC, Addy M: An investigation of some food-approved polymers as agents to inhibit hydroxyapatite dissolution. Eur J Oral Sci 2005;113:457–461.

46 Gracia LH, Brown A, Rees GD, Fowler CE: Studies on a novel combination polymer system: in vitro erosion prevention and promotion of fluoride uptake in human enamel. J Dent 2010;38:S4–S11.

47 Cheaib Z, Lussi A: Impact of acquired enamel pellicle modification on initial dental erosion. Caries Res 2011;45:107–112.

48 Hemingway CA, White AJ, Shellis RP, Addy M, Parker DM, Barbour ME: Enamel erosion in dietary acids: inhibition by food proteins in vitro. Caries Res 2010;44:525–530.

49 Scaramucci T, Sobral MA, Eckert GJ, Zero DT, Hara AT: In situ evaluation of the erosive potential of orange juice modified by food additives. Caries Res 2012;46:55–61.

50 Li Q, Dunn ET, Grandmaison EW, Goosen MFA: Applications and properties of chitosan. J Bioact Compat Pol 1992;7:370–397.

51 Ravi Kumar MNV, Muzzarelli RAA, Muzzarelli C, Sashiwa H, Domb AJ: Chitosan chemistry and pharmaceutical perspectives. Chem Rev 2004;104:6017–6084.

52 Tarsi R, Muzzarelli RA, Guzman CA, Pruzzo C: Inhibition of *Streptococcus mutans* adsorption to hydroxyapatite by low-molecular-weight chitosans. J Dent Res 1997;76:665–672.

53 Sano H, Shibasaki K, Matsukubo T, Takaesu Y: Effect of chitosan rinsing on reduction of dental plaque formation. Bull Tokyo Dent Coll 2003;44:9–16.

54 Decker EM, von Ohle C, Weiger R, Wiech I, Brecx M: A synergistic chlorhexidine/chitosan combination for improved antiplaque strategies. J Periodontal Res 2005;40:373–377.

55 Bae K, Jun EJ, Lee SM, Paik DI, Kim JB: Effect of water-soluble reduced chitosan on *Streptococcus mutans*, plaque regrowth and biofilm vitality. Clin Oral Investig 2006;10:102–107.

56 Verkaik MJ, Busscher HJ, Jager D, Slomp AM, Abbas F, van der Mei HC: Efficacy of natural antimicrobials in toothpaste formulations against oral biofilms in vitro. J Dent 2011;39:218–224.

57 Galler KM, D'Souza RN, Hartgerink JD, Schmalz G: Scaffolds for dental pulp tissue engineering. Adv Dent Res 2011;23:333–339.

58 Xu C, Lei C, Meng L, Wang C, Song Y: Chitosan as a barrier membrane material in periodontal tissue regeneration. J Biomed Mater Res B Appl Biomater 2012;100:1435–1443.

59 Claesson PM, Ninham BW: pH-dependent interactions between adsorbed chitosan layers. Langmuir 1992;8:1406–1412.

60 Young A, Smistad G, Karlsen J, Rölla G, Rykke M: Zeta potentials of human enamel and hydroxyapatite as measured by the Coulter DELSA 440. Adv Dent Res 1997;11:560–565.

61 Guo C, Gemeinhart RA: Understanding the adsorption mechanism of chitosan onto poly(lactide-co-glycolide) particles. Eur J Pharm Biopharm 2008;70:597–604.

62 Dedinaite A, Lundin M, Macakova L, Auletta T: Mucin-chitosan complexes at the solid-liquid interface: multilayer formation and stability in surfactant solutions. Langmuir 2005;21:9502–9509.

63 Svensson O, Lingh L, Cardenas M, Arnebrant T: Layer-by-layer assembly of mucin and chitosan – Influence of surface properties, concentration and type of mucin. J Colloid Interface Sci 2006;299:608–616.

64 van der Mei HC, Engels E, de Vries J, Dijkstra RJ, Busscher HJ: Chitosan adsorption to salivary pellicles. Eur J Oral Sci 2007;115:303–307.

65 Pettersson T, Dedinaite A: Normal and friction forces between mucin and mucin-chitosan layers in absence and presence of SDS. J Colloid Interface Sci 2008;324:246–256.

66 White AJ, Gracia LH, Barbour ME: Inhibition of dental erosion by casein and casein-derived proteins. Caries Res 2011;45:13–20.
67 Wang X, Megert B, Hellwig E, Neuhaus KW, Lussi A: Preventing erosion with novel agents. J Dent 2011;39:163–170.
68 Wegehaupt FJ, Attin T: The role of fluoride and casein phosphopeptide/amorphous calcium phosphate in the prevention of erosive/abrasive wear in an in vitro model using hydrochloric acid. Caries Res 2010;44:358–363.
69 Rees J, Loyn T, Chadwick B: Pronamel and tooth mousse: an initial assessment of erosion prevention in vitro. J Dent 2007;35:355–357.
70 Ranjitkar S, Rodriguez JM, Kaidonis JA, Richards LC, Townsend GC, Bartlett DW: The effect of casein phosphopeptide-amorphous calcium phosphate on erosive enamel and dentine wear by toothbrush abrasion. J Dent 2009;37: 250–254.
71 Turssi CP, Maeda FA, Messias DC, Neto FC, Serra MC, Galafassi D: Effect of potential remineralizing agents on acid softened enamel. Am J Dent 2011;24: 165–168.
72 Jager DH, Vissink A, Timmer CJ, Bronkhorst E, Vieira AM, Huysmans MC: Reduction of erosion by protein-containing toothpastes. Caries Res 2012; 47:135–140.
73 Addy M, Hunter ML: Can tooth brushing damage your health? Effects on oral and dental tissues. Int Dent J 2003; 53(suppl):177–186.
74 Gregg T, MAce S, West NX, Addy M: A study in vitro of the abrasive effect of the tongue on enamel and dentine softened by acid erosion. Caries Res 2004; 38:557–560.
75 Vieira A, Overweg E, Ruben JL, Huysmans MC: Toothbrush abrasion, simulated tongue friction and attrition of eroded bovine enamel in vitro. J Dent 2006;34:336–342.

76 Rios D, Honorio HM, Magalhaes AC, Silva SM, Delbem AC, Machado MA, Buzalaf MA: Scanning electron microscopic study of the in situ effect of salivary stimulation on erosion and abrasion in human and bovine enamel. Braz Oral Res 2008;22:132–138.
77 Wiegand A, Schwerzmann M, Sener B, Magalhaes AC, Roos M, Ziebolz D, Imfeld T, Attin T: Impact of toothpaste slurry abrasivity and toothbrush filament stiffness on abrasion of eroded enamel – an in vitro study. Acta Odontol Scand 2008;66:231–235.
78 Voronets J, Lussi A: Thickness of softened human enamel removed by toothbrush abrasion: an in vitro study. Clin Oral Invest 2010;14:251–256.
79 Hara AT, Gonzales-Cabezas C, Creeth J, Parmar M, Eckert GJ, Zero DT: Interplay between fluoride and abrasivity of dentifrices on dental erosion-abrasion. J Dent 2009;37:781–785.
80 Hara AT, Kelly SA, Gonzales-Cabezas C, Eckert GJ, Barlow AP, Mason SC: Influence of fluoride availability of dentifrices on eroded enamel remineralization in situ. Caries Res 2009;43:57–63.
81 Harte DB, Manly RS: Effect of toothbrush variables on wear of dentin produced by four abrasives. J Dent Res 1975;54:993–998.
82 Harte DB, Manly RS: Four variables affecting magnitude of dentifrice abrasiveness. J Dent Res 1976;55:322–327.
83 Franzò D, Philpotts CJ, Cox TF, Joiner A: The effect of toothpaste concentration on enamel and dentine wear in vitro. J Dent 2010;38:974–979.
84 Moore C, Addy M: Wear of dentine in vitro by toothpaste abrasives and detergents alone and combined. J Clin Periodontol 2005;32:1242–1246.
85 Joiner A, Schwarz A, Philpotts CJ, Cox TF, Huber K, Hannig M: The protective nature of pellicle towards toothpaste abrasion on enamel and dentine. J Dent 2008;36:360–368.

86 Macdonald E, North A, Maggio B, Sufi F, Mason S, Moore C, Addy M, West NX: Clinical study investigating abrasive effects of three toothpastes and water in an in situ model. J Dent 2010;38:509–516.
87 Wiegand A, Kuhn M, Sener B, Roos M, Attin T: Abrasion of eroded dentin caused by toothpaste slurries of different abrasivity and toothbrushes of different filament diameter. J Dent 2009;37:480–484.
88 Hooper S, West NX, Pickles MJ, Joiner A, Newcombe RG, Addy M: Investigation of erosion and abrasion on enamel and dentine: a model in situ using toothpastes of different abrasivity. J Clin Periodontol 2003;30:802–808.
89 Turssi CP, Messias DC, De Menezes M, Hara AT, Serra MC: Role of dentifrices on abrasion of enamel exposed to an acidic drink. Am J Dent 2005;18:251–255.
90 Rochel ID, Souza JG, Silva TC, Pereira AF, Rios D, Buzalaf MA, Magalhaes AC: Effect of experimental xylitol and fluoride-containing dentifrices on enamel erosion with or without abrasion in vitro. J Oral Sci 2011;53:163–168.
91 De Menezes M, Turssi CP, Hara AT, Messias DC, Serra MC: Abrasion of eroded root dentine brushed with different toothpastes. Clin Oral Investig 2004; 8:151–155.
92 Ponduri S, Macdonald E, Addy M: A study in vitro of the combined effects of soft drinks and tooth brushing with fluoride toothpaste on the wear of dentine. Int J Dent Hyg 2005;3:7–12.
93 Turssi CP, Faraoni JJ, Rodrigues Jr AL, Serra MC: An in situ investigation into the abrasion of eroded dental hard tissues by a whitening dentifrice. Caries Res 2004;38:473–477.
94 Magalhaes AC, Rios D, Delbem AC, Buzalaf MA, Machado MA: Influence of fluoride dentifrice on brushing abrasion of eroded human enamel: an in situ/ex vivo study. Caries Res 2007;41:77–79.
95 Methodology and Models in Erosion Research. Caries Res 2011;45(suppl 1):1–77.

Carolina Ganss
Dental Clinic, Department of Conservative and Preventive Dentistry
Schlangenzahl 14
DE–35392 Giessen (Germany)
E-Mail carolina.ganss@dentist.med.uni-giessen.de

van Loveren C (ed): Toothpastes. Monogr Oral Sci. Basel, Karger, 2013, vol 23, pp 100–107
DOI: 10.1159/000350476

Abrasivity Testing of Dentifrices – Challenges and Current State of the Art

Carlos González-Cabezas[a] · Anderson T. Hara[b] · John Hefferren[c] · Frank Lippert[b]

[a]Department of Cariology, Restorative Sciences and Endodontics, University of Michigan, School of Dentistry, Ann Arbor, Mich., [b]Department of Preventive and Community Dentistry, Indiana University School of Dentistry, Indianapolis, Ind., and [c]Department of Pharmaceutical Chemistry, University of Kansas, Lawrence, Kans., USA

Abstract

Abrasivity potential of dentifrices is assessed mostly in vitro due to practical, scientific, and ethical reasons. The two most used evaluation methods are based on the measurement of radioactive dentin release or dentin surface profile changes, after simulation of toothbrushing with dentifrices. The radiotracer method known as radioactive or relative dentin abrasivity (RDA) was developed decades ago and is the most frequently used today (the 'gold standard' for many). The RDA is a reasonably robust method considered a useful tool for the determination of the relative abrasive level of dentifrices and abrasive powders. Studying the level of abrasivity of dentifrices under laboratory conditions is important to develop new formulations, to evaluate quality control of production, and to obtain a rough estimate of its potential clinical abrasivity. However, it is inappropriate to use RDA values alone to determine clinical safety when considering that dental wear is multifactorial and in vitro dentifrice abrasivity level is only one of the variables potentially affecting this outcome. It is important to remember that individuals present significant behavioral differences when brushing that could dramatically affect the potential of abrasion of a particular dentifrice. RDA values should be just one of the multiple variables being taken into consideration by professionals when providing recommendations to prevent dental wear.

In most cases, toothbrushing is performed with the use of a toothbrush and an abrasive-containing dentifrice. The original concept of dentifrice was to have a mechanical abrasive that was softer than enamel, but able to break up and remove the accumulated dental stain on the tooth which was less organized and generally softer than human enamel. Detergents and humectants were added to support the removal process initiated by the abrasive system. Dental wear is a natural physiological process that results from the tooth interaction with its environment. Tooth wear increases with age [1]; however, during the last two centuries, tooth wear rate has diminished as a result of the dietary shift that humans incurred after the industrial revolution. On the other hand, lifespan and tooth retention has increased dramatically in the last century, and the current percentage of adults presenting severe tooth wear is high. Wear has been estimated to increase from 3% of the population at the age of 20 years to 17% at the age of 70 years [1]. Dental wear is affected by numerous variables, and toothbrushing abrasion has been identified as an important factor that might accelerate the process, particularly in cervical areas [2]. The level of abrasiveness varies significantly among dentifrices and therefore their potential to contribute to dental wear.

Because of its potential to affect dental wear and its role in cleaning efficacy, testing the abrasivity of dentifrices has been a topic of great interest by clinicians and manufacturers for decades. In vivo assessment of the abrasivity of dentifrices on tooth structure under randomized controlled conditions would be the ideal testing conditions. However, there is lack of adequate methods to assess accurately small amounts of wear in vivo within a reasonable length of time [3]. Additionally, it would be unethical to expose volunteers to irreversible and preventable loss of healthy tooth structure to evaluate the abrasiveness of a dentifrice. Other in vivo methods to evaluate dentifrice abrasion potential have been investigated with limited success by placing enamel and dentin samples or other substrates such as acrylic intraorally (i.e. in situ) [4, 5]. As a result of these clinical challenges, development of laboratory models and the testing of dentifrice abrasivity in vitro have received more attention historically and continue to be of great interest and importance nowadays.

Historically, the relative hardness relationship between harder human enamel, softer dentifrice abrasive and dental stain, considered as the softest of the three materials, was the basis for the selection of abrasives to be included in the dentifrice formulation. A wide variety of generally recognized as safe and perceived as biologically safe materials have been evaluated historically as dentifrice abrasives with the essential criteria that dentifrice must be softer than dental enamel to avoid any damage to enamel during normal dentifrice use.

Early studies on the abrasivity of dentifrice ingredients were focused on human enamel. Laboratory studies quickly showed that human enamel was resistant to early food grade materials such as chalk and calcium phosphate which were consequently selected as dentifrice abrasives primarily based on their relative hardness to human enamel. The following phase in this selection process was to document the absence of small hard particles, frequently called 'clinkers'. These smaller, very hard particles could scratch human enamel, so glass was used as surrogate for human enamel and a silver coin used to rub back and forth on a glass microscope slide with a 25 g weight. This method was able to predict human enamel surface change, but today we know that the degree of enamel scratching does not correlate well with enamel abrasion data. While this method is not widely used today, it remains in use in China.

Considering the physical and mechanical differences between enamel and dentin, the next significant factor influencing the evolution of dentifrice abrasion tests came with the inclusion of human dentin in the tests, which is significantly softer than enamel. While enamel was difficult to abrade, dentin would easily lose measurable amounts (by weight) during a simulated period of dentifrice use and became the preferred substrate for abrasion assessment that continues today. However, since dentin is a hydrate and measuring weight change was less accurate than desired, new measuring methods were developed. Measuring dentin changes after brushing with a dentifrice using a scintillation counter and radioactive dentin or a profilometer and an optically flat portion of dentin became the two most used methods for measuring dentin abrasivity of dentifrices and are included in the latest ISO specification (ISO 11609).

Brushing without toothpaste has no deleterious effects on the integrity of sound enamel since the hard tissue loss is mainly attributed to the abrasive content of the dentifrice [6, 7]. Extrapolations based on studies using intraoral models have shown that the amount of enamel surface wear due to lifetime toothbrushing is probably negligible [8–10], supporting the use of dentin as a preferable substrate for evaluation of dentifrice abrasivity. Exception is made for demineralized enamel as it presents decreased mechanical properties. It has been previously shown that the wear resistance of erosion-softened enamel is significantly reduced [11]. Similarly, incipient carious lesions tend to have softer surfaces [12] and lower mechanical properties [13] compared to sound enamel. Kielbassa et al. [14] showed that surface loss values of artificial enamel caries lesions were twice as high as those of sound enamel; suggesting that lesion surface layer removal could take place under the effect of toothpaste abrasives. Despite the evidence of the higher susceptibility of surface-softened enamel to the abrasiveness of dentifrices, there is no standard method to evaluate it.

Dentin has shown to be considerably more susceptible to abrasion than sound enamel [9] and has become the main parameter to determine the relative abrasive level of dentifrices and the focus of most investigations in the area. The radiotracer method mentioned above, known as radioactive dentin abrasivity (RDA), was developed more than five decades ago [15, 16] and is the method most frequently used today. It is one of the two methods described in the ISO specification (11609) for testing the abrasivity of dentifrices and for many the current 'gold standard'. In this test, the abrasivity level of dentifrices (RDA value) is calculated in relation to a standard abrasive, which is given an arbitrary value of 100. To obtain comparable RDA data from different dentifrices, it is very important to use the specific reference standard described in the ISO specification; different reference standards will produce different RDA values. Although originally used to describe the radiotracer method, the term 'RDA' has also been used as an abbreviation for 'relative' dentin abrasivity [17]. This modified meaning has been incorporated in the latest ISO 11609 specification and allows for a broader use of the term RDA, which could accommodate both the

radiotracer and an alternative method (surface profile) described in the specification. The radiotracer method is not an easy method to set up. The method requires that the laboratory team has access to a research reactor and regulatory clearance for isotope use, which clearly reduces the number of laboratories that can use the method. Surface profile methods are easier to set up and represent the method of choice for in situ studies.

RDA values are not intended and should not be used as a prediction tool of dental abrasion, since it does not reproduce the complex multifactorial nature of the toothbrushing abrasion process clinically. Therefore, it is not surprising that some studies using intraoral models have shown a good correlation between the rate of dentin wear and RDA value of dentifrices [9, 18, 19], while other studies have not been able to differentiate the dental surface loss of two dentifrices with distinct RDA values (90 vs. 204) [5, 20]. The radiotracer method was developed trying to reduce and control the number of variables, and important behavioral, chemical, mechanical and biological aspects involved in the clinical toothbrushing procedure were purposefully not included in the original method [16]. For instance, brushing the dentin surfaces for 1,500–2,000 strokes continuously, which is done to allow for proper sensitivity on the evaluation method, carries no clinical application. However, it takes into consideration that the rate of brushing affects the rate of substrate loss; shorter more rapid brushing reduces total substrate loss. Similarly, the lack of saliva impacts the characteristics of the slurry, most importantly its acidity and viscosity control [21]. There is no question that human saliva will alter the observed abrasivity, but use of pooled fresh saliva in this type of laboratory studies is not practical, and using simulated saliva (i.e., artificial saliva) without the comprehensive salivary milieu will have a significantly reduced effect. Furthermore, the presence of the dental acquired pellicle, which has shown to directly affect the abrasive wear in in situ studies reproducing specific clinical conditions [20], is not considered

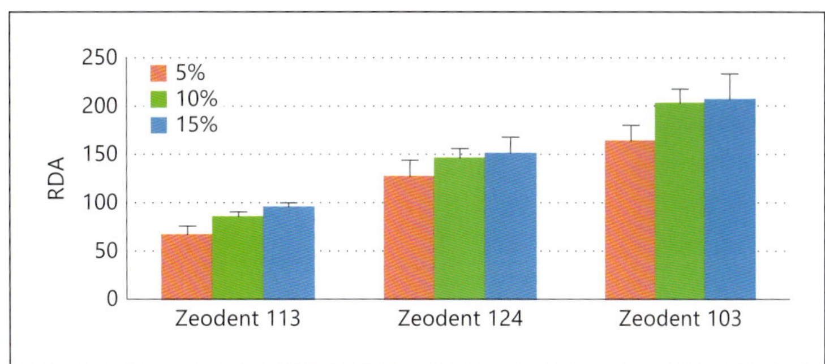

Fig. 1. RDA values of different abrasives at different concentrations. T bars indicate standard deviations.

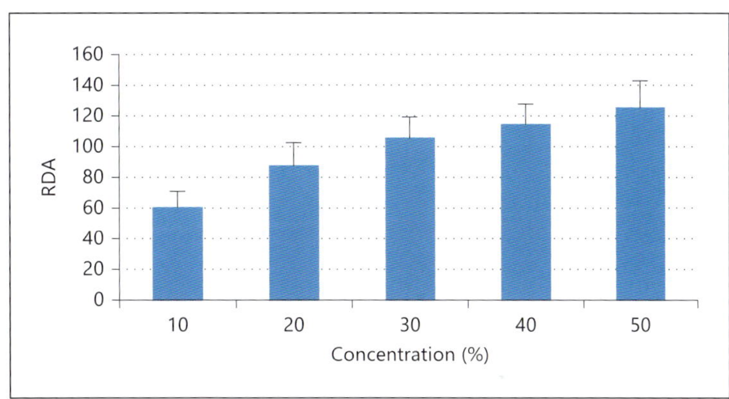

Fig. 2. RDA values of a CaCO₃ abrasive at different concentrations. T bars indicate standard deviations.

in the RDA method. In order to address these and other clinical aspects, more elaborated in vitro and in situ models are recommended, as it will be later discussed in this chapter.

The oral care industry and researchers have made efforts to arbitrarily rank dentifrices' abrasive levels based on RDA values, suggesting that a high-abrasive paste would be in the range of about 151–250, a moderate in the range of 70–150 and a low-abrasive dentifrice below 70 [22]. However, based on the limitations previously mentioned, caution should be taken when directly extrapolating the RDA results to the clinical situation. Nonetheless, it seems important that at least the upper set limit (2.5× the reference material) be considered for safety reasons, although more clinical data are still needed to support it. Above

this abrasivity level, no increase in cleaning ability of the dentifrice can be observed in vitro [16].

Despite the many limitations preventing it from being a good predictor of the clinical abrasive wear, RDA can be considered a useful tool for the determination of the relative abrasive level of dentifrices and abrasive powders [17]. Figure 1 shows RDA values of three different types of hydrated silica (kindly provided by J.M. Huber Corporation) tested at three different concentrations (5, 10, 15%). The RDA outcomes clearly differentiate between abrasive types, being also able to show a fairly good response for their concentrations. Similar dose-response also can be observed using a different class of abrasive, CaCO₃ (kindly provided by Colgate-Palmolive Company; fig. 2). This allows experimental den-

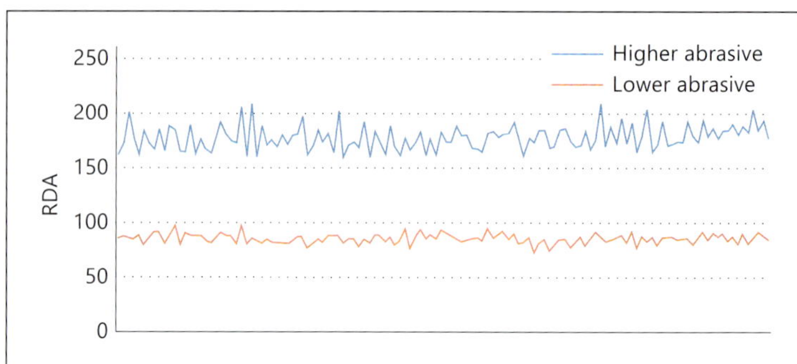

Fig. 3. RDA values of high- and low-abrasivity dentifrice controls, from 128 tests.

tifrice formulations to be extensively tested during their development in a relatively fast and cost-effective manner.

The interpretation of the RDA values requires some understanding of the intra- and inter-test variations. It is common to see RDA values published as an absolute number, without any measure of variation such as standard deviation. While this may be acceptable when differences are obvious (50%), it can be misleading for less distinct values. As illustrated in figure 3, data of two dentifrice controls (high and low abrasivity levels) from 128 RDA tests performed at the Oral Health Research Institute (Indiana University) have shown that variability between 15 and 20% should be expected for the same product tested at different times. Most of this variability can be explained by the biological variations of the test, mostly related to inherent differences in the dentin substrate. The test is reasonably robust showing little variability when used by different well-trained personnel [17].

Current research in dentifrice abrasion is focusing on the development of more clinically relevant study models and also the standardization of the surface profile method. It is clear that there is a gap between the RDA results obtained by the radiotracer and surface profilometry methods and those obtained from clinical observations that deserves a deeper look. This gap of information potentially could be fulfilled by in situ or sophisticated in vitro models. However, given the multitude of factors involved in toothbrushing abrasion, it seems rather impossible to have a standard model covering all aspects of the process. Therefore, RDA should be kept as a test purely measuring the abrasivity level of dentifrices, and other specific models should be developed to study additional factors. These models should look not only at the abrasivity of the dentifrice and their effects on dentin, but also at modulating factors, involving behavioral (frequency, force, length, etc.), chemical/physical (fluoride, detergents, pH, temperature, etc.), mechanical (abrasive, toothbrush) and biological (type and condition of the substrate, saliva and dental pellicle) aspects, as well as any particular interaction among these factors. Some of these parameters have been investigated in vitro. Parry et al. [23] developed a toothbrushing simulator capable of controlling variables of significant impact on tooth wear studies, including brushing force, brushing temperature (impact on slurry viscosity and particle suspension) and brushing speed. The influence of dentifrice abrasivity on softened substrates has also been tested in erosion-abrasion in vitro models [24], as well as their interactions with other brushing factors [25, 26]. These studies have shown that these modulating factors are important and can affect the abrasive wear caused by the toothpaste. They should, therefore, closely match specific clinical conditions under investigation.

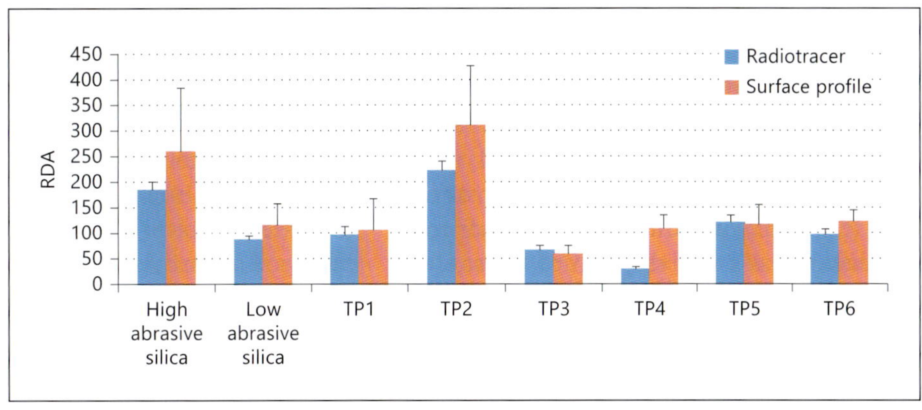

Fig. 4. RDA mean values by the radiotracer and surface profile methods. T bars indicate standard deviations.

The above-mentioned laboratory models have shown to be valuable to better understand some particularities of the dynamics of toothbrushing abrasion. However, relevant behavioral (brushing frequency, duration force and acidic dietary patterns) and biological aspects (saliva, acquired dental pellicle) can be simulated only to some extent with in vitro studies. These parameters seem to be more adequately mimicked with in situ models. In situ models have been developed to test the effects of dentifrice on dental surface abrasive wear. They can be characterized based on the mechanism of insertion and exposure of the dental specimen (enamel or dentin) to the oral environment, as well as on the evaluation method. Dental specimens have been allocated to gold circumferential clasps cemented to lower premolars [27], into the labial surface of upper incisor porcelain crown [28], intraoral appliances [29] and full dentures [30]. Enamel surface loss can be quantitatively evaluated by surface profilometry and by the measurement of changes on the geometry of Knoop indentation [31]. Longitudinal measurements during the experiment are also possible, by creating replicas of the specimens using impression technique.

Currently used methods to obtain RDA data while still very useful could be further developed to better meet today's research environment and expectations. The use of radiation is particularly worth mentioning. Although rigid quality control is applied to ensure the safety of all people involved, the interest for the development of alternative radiation-free methods is growing. The use of surface profilometry for the measurement of dentin loss has been proposed as an environmentally friendly alternative, which has gained more attention especially with the development of high-resolution optical scanners able to generate tridimensional images of the scanned tooth surface. The profilometry method was recently incorporated in the ISO standard for dentifrices (11609), even though it had been described in the British standards (BSI 5137) since 1981 and by Hefferren in 1976 [16]. Besides not involving radiation, the surface profilometry has the advantage of directly measuring the tooth surface loss, compared to the indirect measurement provided by the radiotracer method. A comparative study was recently conducted at Indiana University testing and calculating the RDA values of commercially available dentifrices and abrasives with both the radiotracer and surface profile methods (fig. 4). The results of this study showed that the radiotracer method provides lower mean values and variation compared to the surface profile method, suggesting it is a more robust test method. Some changes in ranks were also observed, in the lower end of the RDA range. These results corroborate those from a previous study comparing both methods that also showed poor correlation [32], with significantly different values for the same abrasives and different precision levels. It seems evident that the surface profilometry technique still has to be better developed and refined. Because of its historical seniority and the very large body of research data, it has been recommended to give precedence to the RDA radiotracer method when discrepancy between the two methods arises [33].

In conclusion, studying the level of abrasivity of a dentifrice under laboratory conditions is important to develop new formulations, to evaluate quality control of production, and to obtain a rough estimate of its potential clinical abrasivity. However, it is inappropriate to use this value alone to determine clinical safety when considering that dental wear is multifactorial and in vitro dentifrice abrasivity level is only one of the variables potentially affecting this outcome. It is important to remember that individuals present significant behavioral differences when brushing that could dramatically affect the potential of abrasion of a particular dentifrice. RDA values should be just one of the multiple variables being taken into consideration by the professional when providing recommendations to patients for preventing dental wear, as it was recently recommended by a group of experts [33].

References

1 Van't Spijker A, Rodrigues JM, Kreulen CM, Bronkhorst EM, Bartlett DW, Creugers NHJ: Prevalence of tooth wear in adults. Int J Prosthodont 2009;22: 35–42.
2 Hattab FN, Yassin OM: Etiology and diagnosis of tooth wear: a literature review and presentation of selected cases. Int J Prosthodont 2000;13:101–107.
3 Huysmans MCDNJM, Chew HP, Ellwood RP: Clinical studies of dental erosion and erosive wear. Caries Res 2011; 45(suppl 1):60–68.
4 Facq JM, Volpe AR: In vivo actual abrasiveness of three dentifrices against acrylic surfaces of veneer crowns. J Am Dent Assoc 1970;80:317–323.
5 Pickles MJ, Joiner A, Weader E, Cooper YL, Cox TF: Abrasion of human enamel and dentine caused by toothpastes of differing abrasivity determined using an in situ wear model. Int Dent J 2005; 55(suppl 1):188–193.
6 Absi EG, Addy M, Adams D: Dentine hypersensitivity – the effect of toothbrushing and dietary compounds on dentine in vitro: an SEM study. J Oral Rehabil 1992;19:101–110.
7 Sangnes G: Traumatization of teeth and gingiva related to habitual tooth cleaning procedures. J Clin Periodontol 1976; 3:94–103.
8 Addy M, Hunter ML: Can tooth brushing damage your health? Effects on oral and dental tissues. Int Dent J 2003;53: 177–186.
9 Hooper S, West NX, Pickles MJ, Joiner A, Newcombe RG, Addy M: Investigation of erosion and abrasion on enamel and dentine: a model in situ using toothpastes of different abrasivity. J Clin Periodontol 2003;30:802–808.
10 Philpotts CJ, Weader E, Joiner A: The measurement in vitro of enamel and dentine wear by toothpastes of different abrasivity. Int Dent J 2005;55:183–187.
11 Attin T, Koidl U, Buchalla W, Schaller HG, Kielbassa AM, Hellwig E: Correlation of microhardness and wear in differently eroded bovine dental enamel. Arch Oral Biol 1997;42:243–250.
12 Arends J, Jongebloed W, Ogaard B, Rolla G: SEM and microradiographic investigation of initial enamel caries. Scand J Dent Res 1987;95:193–201.
13 Arends J, Christoffersen J: The nature of early caries lesions in enamel. J Dent Res 1986;65:2–11.
14 Kielbassa AM, Gillmann L, Zantner C, Meyer-Lueckel H, Hellwig E, Schulte-Monting J: Profilometric and microradiographic studies on the effects of toothpaste and acidic gel abrasivity on sound and demineralized bovine dental enamel. Caries Res 2005;39:380–386.
15 Grabenstetter RJ, Broge RW, Jackson FL, Radike AW: The measurement of the abrasion of human teeth by dentifrice abrasives: a test utilizing radioactive teeth. J Dent Res 1958;37:1060–1068.
16 Hefferren JJ: A laboratory method for assessment of dentifrice abrasivity. J Dent Res 1976;55:563–573.
17 González-Cabezas C: Determination of the abrasivity of dentifrices on human dentin using the radioactive (also known as relative) dentin abrasion (RDA) method. J Clin Dent 2010; 21(suppl):S9–S10.
18 Addy M, Hughes J, Pickles MJ, Joiner A, Huntington E: Development of a method in situ to study toothpaste abrasion of dentine. Comparison of 2 products. J Clin Periodontol 2002;29: 896–900.

19 Macdonald E, North A, Maggio B, Sufi F, Mason S, Moore C, Addy M, West NX: Clinical study investigating abrasive effects of three toothpastes and water in an in situ model. J Dent 2010;38:509–516.

20 Joiner A, Schwarz A, Philpotts CJ, Cox TF, Huber K, Hannig M: The protective nature of pellicle towards toothpaste abrasion on enamel and dentine. J Dent 2008;36:360–368.

21 Imfeld T: Standard operation procedures for the relative dentin abrasion (RDA) method used at the University of Zurich. J Clin Dent 2010;21(suppl):S11–S12.

22 Giles A, Claydon NC, Addy M, Hughes N, Sufi F, West NX: Clinical in situ study investigating abrasive effects of two commercially available toothpastes. J Oral Rehabil 2009;36:498–507.

23 Parry J, Harrington E, Rees GD, McNab R, Smith AJ: Control of brushing variables for the in vitro assessment of toothpaste abrasivity using a novel laboratory model. J Dent 2008;36:117–124.

24 Wiegand A, Attin T: Design of erosion/abrasion studies – insights and rational concepts. Caries Res 2011;45(suppl 1): 53–59.

25 Wiegand A, Kuhn M, Sener B, Roos M, Attin T: Abrasion of eroded dentin caused by toothpaste slurries of different abrasivity and toothbrushes of different filament diameter. J Dent 2009; 37:480–484.

26 Turssi CP, Messias DC, Hara AT, Hughes N, Garcia-Godoy F: Brushing abrasion of dentin: effect of diluent and dilution rate of toothpaste. Am J Dent 2010;23:247–250.

27 Cowell CR: An appliance for the study of tooth tissue in vivo. Br Dent J 1974;137: 61–62.

28 Davis WB: The cleaning, polishing and abrasion of teeth by dental products; in Breuer MM (ed): Cosmetic Science. London, Academic Press, 1978, vol 1, pp 39–81.

29 Kodaka T, Kuroiwa M, Okumura J, Mori R, Hirasawa S, Kobori M: Effects of brushing with a dentifrice for sensitive teeth on tubule occlusion and abrasion of dentin. J Electron Microsc 2001;50: 57–64.

30 Joiner A, Pickles MJ, Tanner C, Weader E, Doyle P: An in situ model to study the toothpaste abrasion of enamel. J Clin Periodontol 2004;31:434–438.

31 Jaeggi T, Lussi A: Toothbrush abrasion of erosively altered enamel after intra-oral exposure to saliva: an in situ study. Caries Res 1999;33:455–461.

32 Hefferren JJ, Kingman A, Stookey GK, Lehnhoff R, Muller T: An international collaborative study of laboratory methods for assessing abrasivity to dentin. J Dent Res 1984;63:1176–1179.

33 Dörfer CE, Hefferren JJ, González-Cabezas C, Imfeld T, Addy M: Methods to determine dentifrice abrasiveness. J Clin Dent 2010;21(suppl):S14.

Carlos González-Cabezas, DDS, MSD, PhD
Department of Cariology, Restorative Sciences and Endodontics
School of Dentistry, University of Michigan
1011 N. University Room 2395, Ann Arbor, MI 48109-1078 (USA)
E-Mail carlosgc@umich.edu

van Loveren C (ed): Toothpastes. Monogr Oral Sci. Basel, Karger, 2013, vol 23, pp 108–124
DOI: 10.1159/000350479

Laboratory and Human Studies to Estimate Anticaries Efficacy of Fluoride Toothpastes

Livia M.A. Tenuta · Jaime A. Cury

Piracicaba Dental School, University of Campinas, Piracicaba, Brazil

Abstract

Much more than mechanical biofilm removal, tooth-brushing with fluoride toothpastes is an effective way of increasing the availability of fluoride in the oral cavity to reduce demineralization and enhance remineralization of enamel and dentine. These effects of fluoride toothpastes have been estimated by a wide range of laboratory and human studies, which have helped to develop anticaries effective formulations and understand their mechanism of action. These studies have focused on the availability of fluoride in the toothpaste formulations, its bioavailability in saliva and remnants of disturbed biofilm, its reaction with the dental substrate to form loosely bound reservoirs as well as the ultimate reduction of mineral loss and increase in mineral and fluoride content of caries lesions. The specifics of these modes of action and their application in in vitro, in situ and in vivo preclinical tests is presented and discussed.

Fluoride toothpastes have played a major role in the pronounced caries decline observed worldwide since their widespread availability [1]. In fact, fluoride toothpaste was pointed out, by a panel of experts, as the main responsible for the decline in caries in the last century [2]. Nevertheless, as detailed elsewhere [3], the pioneer fluoride toothpaste formulations, prepared using highly soluble fluoride salts and calcium-based abrasives, were unable to demonstrate a significant anticaries effect in clinical trials [4–6] due to the reaction between calcium and fluoride and the reduced concentration of soluble fluoride to interfere with the caries process. Therefore, the history of toothpaste development is a good example of the importance of scrutinized evaluation of their anticaries efficacy in order to produce effective formulations.

The efficacy of toothpastes has been estimated using distinct types of models, either in vitro, in situ or in vivo. In in vitro studies, the clinical efficacy of toothpastes is usually predicted from distinct outcomes that intend to simulate the intraoral effect of the formulation. In situ studies are designed to overcome the limitations of laboratory models regarding the pharmacokinetics of the formulations in the oral cavity. They usually use either extensively demineralized samples or highly cariogenic in situ conditions aiming at reduction of the time for estimating the anticaries effect of the formulations, which is also accomplished by using highly sensitive tools for evaluation of enamel or dentine de- or remineralization. Short-term in vivo studies assessing the bioavailability of fluoride from toothpastes provide important information on the expected clinical effect. All these models, in vitro, in situ and in vivo, when adequately used, can function as good predictors of the anticaries efficacy of a toothpaste formulation giving support for a clinical trial to be conducted. Also, they can be used as preliminary tests of equivalence between a new formulation and a clinically proven one and/or to explain the mechanism of action [7]. Nevertheless, the many distinct types of models and outcomes measured in such studies advise a scrutinized review of their strengths and limitations [8]. It is also of utmost importance that the factors being modeled are adequately understood in order to mirror the clinical outcome as precisely as possible. Therefore, it is the aim of this chapter to present strengths and limitations of laboratory and human studies to estimate the efficacy of toothpastes, discussing the models' details against the proposed mode of action of the formulations.

Fluoride Toothpastes: Mechanism of Action

Brushing teeth is a routine task with two resulting effects: (1) the mechanical removal of remnants of food and dental biofilm by the toothbrush, and (2) the chemical effect of the anticaries active ingredient in the toothpaste formulation (in this case, fluoride). The importance of 2 to the overall clinical performance of a formulation is exemplified by the results of a systematic review of clinical trials testing fluoride toothpastes against no fluoride toothpaste controls [1].

During toothbrushing with fluoride toothpastes, fluoride diffuses to saliva, teeth, remaining biofilm not removed by brushing and the oral mucosa, an important reservoir of fluoride in the mouth [9]. However, since the oral cavity is an open system, fluoride concentration in saliva will decrease sharply after the use of fluoride toothpastes [10]. Nevertheless, fluoride concentration in saliva can be maintained at levels higher than baseline for longer periods of time, mainly from fluoride released from the oral mucosa [11]. Also, fluoride in the remaining biofilm and tooth surface will be important to interfere with the caries process at these sites. Therefore, the transient high fluoride concentration in the oral cavity after toothpaste use, as well as the prolonged slightly elevated fluoride concentration maintained in certain sites, will be responsible to positively affect the balance of enamel and dentine demineralization towards remineralization [12]. This mode of action is depicted in figure 1. Shortly after brushing, fluoride will be able to enhance the remineralizing potential of saliva and plaque fluid; when a cariogenic challenge is performed hours after toothpaste use, fluoride available in biofilm remnants will decrease tooth demineralization [13, 14]. As a result of the reduction of demineralization and enhancement of remineralization by fluoride, the tooth mineral will gain fluoride as firmly bound fluorapatite (FAp), although this uptake should be considered more a consequence of the effect of fluoride on caries process than the reason of the anticaries effect of fluoride. Although the change in mineral composition may play a role decreasing the susceptibility of a remineralized surface to a further caries attack [15], FAp substitution of the tooth mineral is usually around 10% [16], and the limited anticaries effect of high FAp-containing enamel substrate has been demonstrated [17].

The reactivity of fluoride from toothpastes with enamel or dentine can also be listed as a mode of action of fluoride toothpastes, especially for the demineralized tissue which is more reactive. Unlike FAp, loosely bound fluoride reaction products (CaF_2-like minerals) formed on the tooth surface during toothbrushing could function as reservoirs of the ion, releasing it, for example, to a new biofilm formed on the surface to

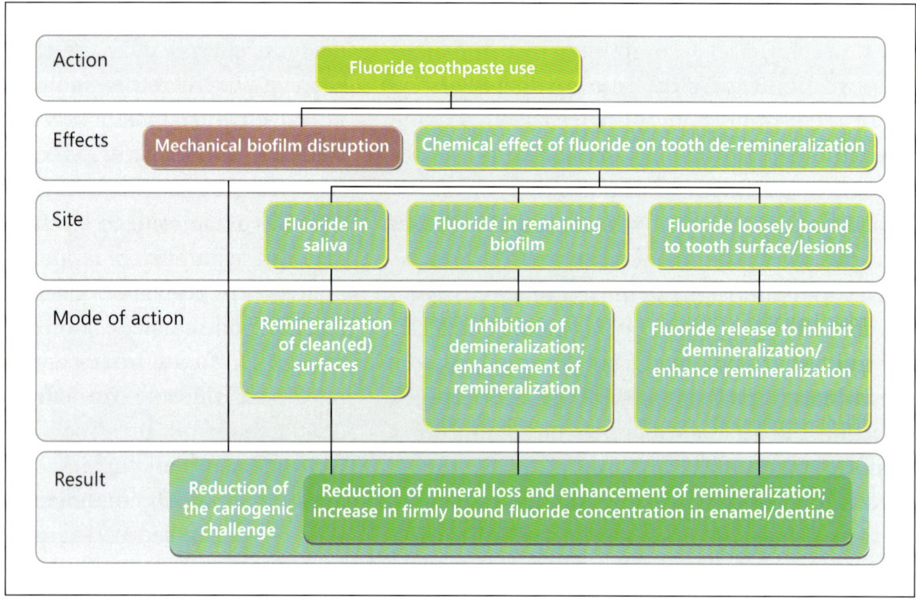

Fig. 1. The effects of fluoride toothpaste use based on the site and mode of action, and the resulting outcome. Effect: Although the main purpose of brushing teeth is the mechanical biofilm removal (reducing the cariogenic challenge by reducing the necessary factor for demineralization which is the presence of biofilm), the main anticaries effect of toothbrushing with fluoride toothpastes is based on the chemical effect of fluoride on tooth de-remineralization. Site: Upon brushing, fluoride is spread through saliva, diffuses to the remaining biofilm and potentially reacts with the tooth surface, especially with preexisting lesions. Mode of action: In each and every site, fluoride will positively affect the balance of de-remineralization towards mineral gain. Result: Fluoride will reduce mineral loss and enhance remineralization, resulting in increasing firmly bound fluoride concentration in the tooth substrate subjected to de-remineralization processes.

subsequently interfere with the caries process [18]. Yet, Tenuta et al. [19] showed experimentally that the effect of these reaction products on reduction of enamel demineralization is significantly lower than that of the fluoride remaining in the biofilm remnants after toothbrushing. Also, the ability of conventional fluoride toothpastes to form significant amounts of CaF_2-like deposits on enamel or dentine in vivo is still debatable.

In addition to the chemical effect of fluoride toothpastes, the biochemical effect of fluoride inhibiting bacterial acidogenesis has been investigated, but given the lack of evidence for a significant effect on the anticaries action of fluoride toothpaste [20–22], it was not included in figure 1.

Fluoride Bioavailability from Toothpastes

To play a role in the de-remineralization process, as well as to react with tooth surface, fluoride must be available in the oral fluids as the F^- ion. It can be delivered from toothpastes as such [formulations containing sodium fluoride (NaF), stannous fluoride (SnF_2) or amine fluoride], or as the monofluorophosphate ion (MFP, FPO_3^{2-}). The latter needs to be hydrolyzed in the oral cavity by phosphatases (mainly in dental biofilm), releasing ionic fluoride [23]. Fluoride ion released from MFP is considered the main responsible for the anticaries effect of this type of fluoride [24].

In terms of anticaries action, all forms of fluoride described above are similarly effective, with minor differences [25–27]. Nevertheless, the type of toothpaste formulation, considering not only the fluoride form used, but also the abrasive system, can significantly affect fluoride bioavailability as well as the type of model that can be used to investigate its efficacy. For example, as of now, there is not an available in vitro model to check for the anticaries effect of MFP-based toothpastes, given that the MFP ion needs to be hydrolyzed to release the active fluoride ion. Thus, the in vitro comparisons with other kinds of fluoride used in toothpastes are not valid because only the effect of free fluoride ion already found in the formulation is evaluated [28, 29], and not that released in the mouth from MFP.

Modeling the Anticaries Effect of Fluoride Toothpastes

The effects briefly described above can be studied using in vitro, in situ or in vivo models. Depending on the level of complexity of the model, more predicting variables can be included. In order to scrutinize the factors that should be considered in the laboratory and/or human studies aiming to assess the efficacy of toothpastes, a detailed description of their rationale is given below:

Fluoride Available in the Toothpaste Formulation – Laboratory Test
The most simple and yet extremely valuable laboratory study to predict the effectiveness of fluoride toothpastes is the determination of the chemical availability of fluoride in the formulation. Chemically available fluoride (also described in this text as 'soluble fluoride') refers to the total amount of soluble, potentially active fluoride in the formulation [as ionic (F^-) and ionizable (FPO_3^{2-}) fluoride]. This type of study is relevant considering that in many fluoride toothpaste formulations, fluoride bioavailability decreases with time due to the un-

desirable reaction of fluoride compounds with calcium-based abrasives, such as dicalcium phosphate dihydrate ($CaH_2PO_4{\cdot}2H_2O$) and calcium carbonate ($CaCO_3$). Formulations containing MFP/$CaCO_3$ are considered affordable choices given that $CaCO_3$ is less expensive than silica to be added as an abrasive to toothpastes [30]. However, the only compatible fluoride salt known at present to be used in such formulations is sodium MFP, although it may hydrolyze over time possibly resulting in less soluble fluoride.

The clinical anticaries effect of toothpaste formulations containing MFP and calcium-based abrasives is well documented [27, 31], and those containing $CaCO_3$ are the most used in developing countries given their lower price of production [30, 32]. Nevertheless, depending on the quality of the formulation or the conditions of storage (since heat accelerates the spontaneous hydrolysis of MFP and the reaction of the ionic fluoride with calcium), a significant reduction in soluble fluoride is expected with time [33–35]. Thus, a preliminary test to assess the anticaries potential of fluoride toothpastes is the determination of their total soluble fluoride concentration in both fresh and aged samples. Aging can be performed under normal conditions or under elevated temperature, which accelerates aging [36, 37].

Concerns on the fluoride availability in toothpastes have been raised recently, since it was shown that in some African and Asiatic countries a significant number of toothpastes present low F availability, potentially impairing their anticaries efficacy [38–40]. In Latin America, this concern is of lesser magnitude because most toothpastes present available fluoride in concentration to control caries [41–45], but it may not be ignored [35].

It is therefore important to discuss the methods for the determination of chemically available fluoride in toothpaste formulations. There are different pools of fluoride in a toothpaste (fig. 2): ionic fluoride, which is readily available in aqueous solutions; ionizable fluoride, such as MFP, which will release ionic fluoride in the mouth upon the action

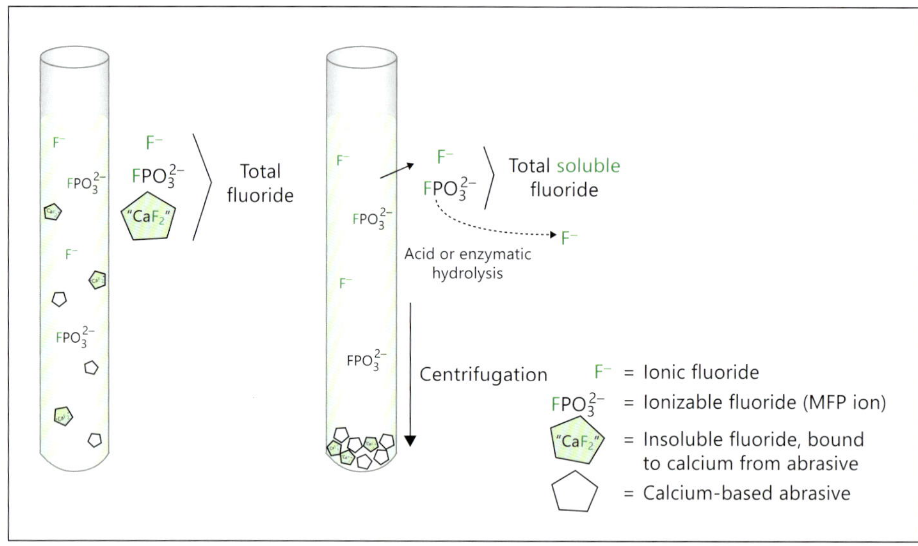

Fig. 2. Schematic representation of toothpaste slurries for determination of fluoride availability in toothpastes. All fluoride forms possible [ionic, ionizable or insoluble (bound to calcium from abrasive)] are represented. The separation of total soluble fluoride from total fluoride can be performed by centrifugation and precipitation of insoluble particles. Total soluble fluoride concentration can be determined using the fluoride electrode after acid or enzymatic hydrolysis of the MFP ion; direct electrode measuring without the hydrolysis step will yield ionic fluoride concentration [28, 43].

of oral phosphatases; and insoluble fluoride, a result of the undesirable reaction of fluoride and calcium from abrasive systems (if present). Ionic + ionizable fluoride can be also referred to as 'total soluble fluoride' and represent the anticaries active fraction from the total fluoride in toothpastes.

For the measurement of total soluble fluoride, a centrifugation can be used to separate insoluble fluoride (precipitated together with abrasive particles) from the soluble forms (fig. 2). Considering the method used for fluoride determination (e.g. fluoride-specific electrode for determination of fluoride ion, or ionic chromatography for determination of the MFP ion), an adequate preparation of the samples should be considered. The fluoride electrode can be used for the determination of both ionic fluoride and MFP ion, once a hydrolysis step, either chemical (by 1 M HCl at 45°C for 1 h) [28, 43] or enzymatic (by acid phos-

phatase) [38], is added to the protocol to ensure the release of fluoride ion from MFP. If one wants to determine the total fluoride concentration in the formulation (soluble + insoluble), the preparation of the samples can either include the acid dissolution of the insoluble fluoride [28, 43], separation of fluoride from the toothpaste slurry by microdiffusion techniques [37, 46] or a direct measurement using gas chromatography [38]. Given the cost effectiveness of the method, the standardized protocol to determine all fluoride forms in toothpastes using the fluoride electrode [43–45, 47] seems a straightforward option.

Another test to estimate the bioavailability of fluoride in toothpastes during toothbrushing is the 'one minute fluoride release rate' test described in the Guidelines for Fluoride-Containing Dentifrices of the American Dental Association [37]. In this test, a 1:3 toothpaste slurry is created in water or saliva (artificial or natural) and after 1-min mixing, soluble fluoride concentration (either as ion, determined with the fluoride electrode, or as the MFP ion, determined by ion chromatography) is quantified in the supernatant. Correlation studies between this test and salivary fluoride pharmacokinetics should be conducted to validate this methodology, but it has shown to be able to differentiate fluoride toothpastes with distinct anti-erosion potentials [48].

Fluoride Bioavailable in Saliva and the Remaining Biofilm by Toothpaste Use

As detailed elsewhere [9], the pharmacokinetics of fluoride in the oral cavity after the use of toothpastes is well known and certainly plays a role in its anticaries efficacy. For example, there is evidence in the literature that higher daily brushing frequencies are significantly correlated with lower caries increment [1, 49, 50], and also that more thorough rinse with water accelerates elimination of fluoride from saliva [51–53] and reduces the anticaries benefit [49, 50, 54]. Therefore, fluoride concentration in saliva has been used to indicate its bioavailability from toothpaste formulations and consequently their anticaries effect.

Although the hypothetical mode of action of fluoride in saliva after fluoride toothpaste use may be to promote the remineralization of demineralized clean(ed) tooth surfaces (fig. 1), saliva can also be regarded as the exchange fluid from which fluoride reaches other oral reservoirs (remaining biofilm, tooth surfaces and oral mucosa). This exchange will be a function of fluoride concentration in saliva or the thin salivary film covering oral tissues and teeth [11, 55], given that this concentration limits fluoride ability to react with tooth surface or to diffuse into the biofilm.

Because of the ease of collection and the straightforward response on fluoride clearance in the oral cavity after fluoride toothpaste use, fluoride availability in saliva has been used in a significant number of studies to estimate the anticaries potential of different fluoride formulations or the potential mechanism of action of different toothpastes or brushing protocols (table 1).

Fluoride available in the biofilm can also be regarded as an important outcome in studies assessing the anticaries effect of fluoride toothpastes given the role of the biofilm in the caries process. When the inhibition of enamel demineralization was assessed using a short-term in situ model, the fluoride held up by the fluid phase of a test plaque after use of a fluoride toothpaste has demonstrated a greater anticaries effect when compared to fluoride loosely bound to the cleaned enamel surface, mainly due to the significantly higher capacity of the biofilm to retain fluoride when compared to sound enamel [19]. This effect studied in this in situ model emphasizes that fluoride toothpaste is indispensable to enrich biofilm remnants with fluoride and explain why toothbrushing with fluoride toothpastes is an effective strategy for oral health promotion [76].

In fact, fluoride availability in fasting dental biofilm has been shown to be a reflection of the fluoride concentration in the toothpaste use, even 18 h after brushing [10, 77]. Also, a higher biofilm fluoride concentration was related to lower caries rates in a dose-response 3-year clinical study [78].

It should be emphasized, however, that measurements of total fluoride concentration in dental biofilm may result in biased interpretations of its potential as a fluoride reservoir. Although total biofilm fluoride has been shown to reflect fluoride toothpaste use [10], it is not a good predictor of fluoride that is available in the biofilm fluid, since the correlation between total fluoride and biofilm fluid fluoride is only poor, even after the use of fluoride products [79]. This may be partially explained by the great effect that the condition of biofilm accumulation has on the concentration of fluoride and other inorganic ions in whole biofilm. It has been consistently shown in situ [80–86] and in vivo [87] that the frequent exposure to fermentable carbohydrates reduces the concentration of mineral ions, including fluoride, in the biofilm. Therefore, whole biofilm fluoride concentration is affected not only

Table 1. In vivo estimation of anticaries efficacy and mechanism of action of fluoride toothpastes

Test	References	Outcomes and/or conclusions
Salivary and biofilm fluoride clearance after one exposure to fluoride toothpastes	Zero et al. [56] Serra and Cury [57] Sjögren and Birkhed [52] Sjögren et al. [58] Sjögren and Melin [59] Issa and Toumba [53] Heijnsbroek et al. [60] Zamataro et al. [61]	Rinsing with water significantly reduces salivary fluoride retention after toothpaste use; a fluoride rinse after fluoride toothpaste use enhances salivary fluoride retention
	Zero et al. [56] Zero et al. [62]	Fluoride use before bedtime prolongs oral fluoride retention
	Zero et al. [62] Heijnsbroek et al. [60]	Saliva and plaque present dissimilar fluoride clearances after the use of fluoride toothpastes/rinses
	Raven et al. [63] Duckworth et al. [64]	Salivary and biofilm fluoride concentration for fluoride-containing toothpastes inversely associated with 3-year caries increments in a clinical trial
	Afflitto et al. [65]	Correlation between salivary fluoride availability after fluoride toothpaste use and cariostatic efficacy (in a rat model)
	Sjögren et al. [66]	Rinsing with water significantly reduces saliva and biofilm interdental fluoride concentration after toothpaste use; a fluoride rinse enhances interdental fluoride retention
	Whitford et al. [67, 68] Pessan et al. [69, 70]	The effect of fluoridated water and fluoride toothpaste on salivary and biofilm fluoride assessed
	Vogel et al. [71] Pessan et al. [72]	A calcium pre-rinse may enhance oral fluoride retention after fluoride toothpaste use
	Zero et al. [73]	Higher brushing times and toothpaste amounts increase fluoride retention in saliva and enhance enamel fluoride uptake and rehardening of demineralized enamel blocks used in situ
Residual salivary and biofilm fluoride concentration due to continuous fluoride toothpaste use	Duckworth et al. [64]	Salivary and biofilm fluoride concentration for fluoride-containing toothpastes inversely associated with 3-year caries increments in a clinical trial
Fluoride incorporation into enamel due to fluoride toothpaste use	Mushanoff et al. [74] Barbakow et al. [75]	In vivo enamel acid biopsies taken to evaluate fluoride incorporation from amine fluoride toothpaste use

by fluoride exposure from toothpastes or rinses, but also by the condition of biofilm formation. More importantly, little is known about the capacity of distinct biofilm reservoirs to release fluoride to the biofilm fluid to interfere with de/remineralization, as it seems that biofilms with dissimilar fluoride concentrations release fluoride to the fluid at a similar extent during a cariogenic challenge [84].

Given that fluoride concentration in whole biofilm is not only a function of exposure from toothpastes or rinses, and that release from its reservoirs is not directly related to total fluoride concentration, the use of biofilm fluid fluoride measurements should be preferred in order to avoid biased interpretations of the role of biofilm fluoride on caries.

Another debatable issue is the difference in fluoride bioavailability from NaF and MFP. It is not expected that the amount of total fluoride in the mouth from both compounds would differ, but the amount of ionic fluoride will be considerably lower for the MFP toothpastes [88]. Using NaF and MFP rinses, Vogel et al. [89] showed that NaF promoted a higher fluoride bioavailability in saliva and in the biofilm fluid when compared to MFP. Since little is known about the parameters involved in the MFP hydrolysis in the biofilm, such as its diffusion and concomitant conversion to ionic fluoride, and the effect of toothpaste pH, which can affect the activity of phosphatases in vivo, models to further study the ionic fluoride bioavailability from MFP should be investigated, as proposed by Pearce and Dibdin [23].

Fluoride Reactivity with Dental Enamel and Dentine

If fluoride is chemically available in the toothpaste formulation, it would be expected that it forms products on enamel and dentine. However, the capacity of fluoride from toothpastes to react with the tooth structure is limited by the fluoride concentration in the toothpaste-saliva slurry, as well as by interfering ingredients, such as soap [90, 91], which competes with fluoride for calcium on the tooth surface. Nevertheless, fluoride incorporation as loosely bound reaction products on enamel or dentine can be used as a predictive tool of a formulation's anticaries efficacy. In fact, the capacity of fluoride in the formulation to react with demineralized enamel has been used, besides fluoride availability in the formulation, as a qualifying test to sustain caries control claims of fluoride toothpastes [7, 37, 63].

A distinction needs to be made regarding the two main pools of fluoride in the tooth structure: (1) the loosely bound fluoride, which will be released and affect tooth de- and remineralization [18], and (2) the firmly bound fluoride, which can also be formed, to a small extent, during toothpaste use (table 1) but considered mainly as the result of the caries process in the presence of fluoride. The latter will be discussed further in the section 'Fluoride Uptake by Enamel/Dentine as a Result of De-Remineralization in the Presence of Fluoride'. Although both can be regarded as screening tools for the anticaries effect of fluoride toothpastes, they are representing distinct aspects of the caries process and the effect of fluoride to control it (fig. 1, mode of action versus result). It is therefore important that the method of fluoride determination clearly differentiates both. For instance, potassium hydroxide has been used to selectively extract loosely bound fluoride [92] prior to the extraction of firmly bound fluoride by acid dissolution. The extraction of total fluoride from the tooth surface may impair the distinction of both fluoride sources.

Also, it should be considered that the clinical relevance of fluoride reactivity results obtained in vitro and in situ may be different. In in vitro studies, the fluoride reactivity is directly related to the ionic, reactive fluoride available in the formulation. Since the in vitro reactivity of MFP-containing toothpastes with enamel is a result of ionic fluoride present in the formulation [93], it is a poor predictor of its clinical anticaries effect. In in situ studies, on the other hand, fluoride uptake is directly related to fluoride bioavailability, i.e. fluoride ion reaching the tooth samples. Nevertheless, in vitro models usually favor fluoride reactivity with tooth minerals, whereas in situ the reactivity may be impaired by biological coatings such as the pellicle, or by a lower contact of the toothpaste slurry with the enamel/dentine specimens. However, the latter would represent better the clinical situation.

Another important issue to be considered is that demineralized enamel, especially artificial caries lesions formed in vitro, can take up much more fluoride than a sound surface. This is particularly useful to differentiate formulations in terms of fluoride reactivity, but the clinical significance of the high uptake of loosely bound fluoride by highly porous, artificial enamel lesions used in vitro tests, considering the type of lesions available in the mouth, is yet to be determined.

Another point that requires further studies is the reactivity of fluoride toothpastes with dentine, which has been underexplored in the literature. Although dentine is more reactive with fluoride than enamel, the relevance of this test to predict the anticaries effect of a toothpaste formulation is limited by the same reason described above for carious enamel.

Inhibition of Enamel/Dentine Demineralization in Protocols Simulating Clinical Use

Although the parameters described above can be successfully used as indicators of the anticaries effect of fluoride toothpastes, the actual reduction of demineralization or enhancement of remineralization of tooth substrates is the main outcome to be considered. The inhibition of mineral loss or the net remineralization of tooth substrates should be estimated under conditions that more closely resemble the clinical use of toothpastes and the caries process. Given the nature of the caries process as the result of cycles of demineralization and remineralization, it is advisable that the anticaries effect of toothpastes be studied under such conditions. Many in vitro pH-cycling models have been developed with this aim and can be successfully used to test the anticaries efficacy of toothpastes. Also, in situ protocols favoring demineralization of sound substrates or remineralization of demineralized ones (according to the cariogenic challenge used) are widely available. These models will be discussed in more detail in the section 'Particularities of Laboratory and Human Models to Estimate the Anticaries Efficacy of Fluoride Toothpastes'.

Also, in in vitro and in situ studies, sensitive methods can be used to assess a change in mineral content of enamel or dentine (demineralization or remineralization). This is a main advantage of these types of studies over clinical trials because toothpaste effect can be assessed using shorter experimental times. Nevertheless, they must present dose-response to fluoride in order to be valid [94], as will be discussed later.

Fluoride Uptake by Enamel/Dentine as a Result of De-Remineralization in the Presence of Fluoride

As ten Cate and Mundorff-Shrestha [95] stated, it is acknowledged by the scientific community that fluoride uptake by enamel may no longer be accepted as a critical indicator of the mechanism of action of fluoride; however, it can be accepted as an excellent pre-screening tool. As described above, firmly-bound fluoride is supposed to increase as a result of the de- and remineralization process in the presence of fluoride, and can therefore be used as a surrogate of the de-remineralization analyses on the tooth substrate [96]. It has been conventionally extracted from enamel by acid-etching or abrading the surface and measuring the fluoride concentration in the extracted tissue using an ion-selective electrode [97].

Particularities of Laboratory and Human Models to Estimate the Anticaries Efficacy of Fluoride Toothpastes

A short description of type of models described in the literature to assess the efficacy of fluoride toothpastes is presented. By no means is this list intended to describe all the available literature; it is intended to present and further discuss some important particularities of the models.

pH-Cycling Models

Since the caries process is a continuum of de- and remineralization cycles, pH-cycling models [98]

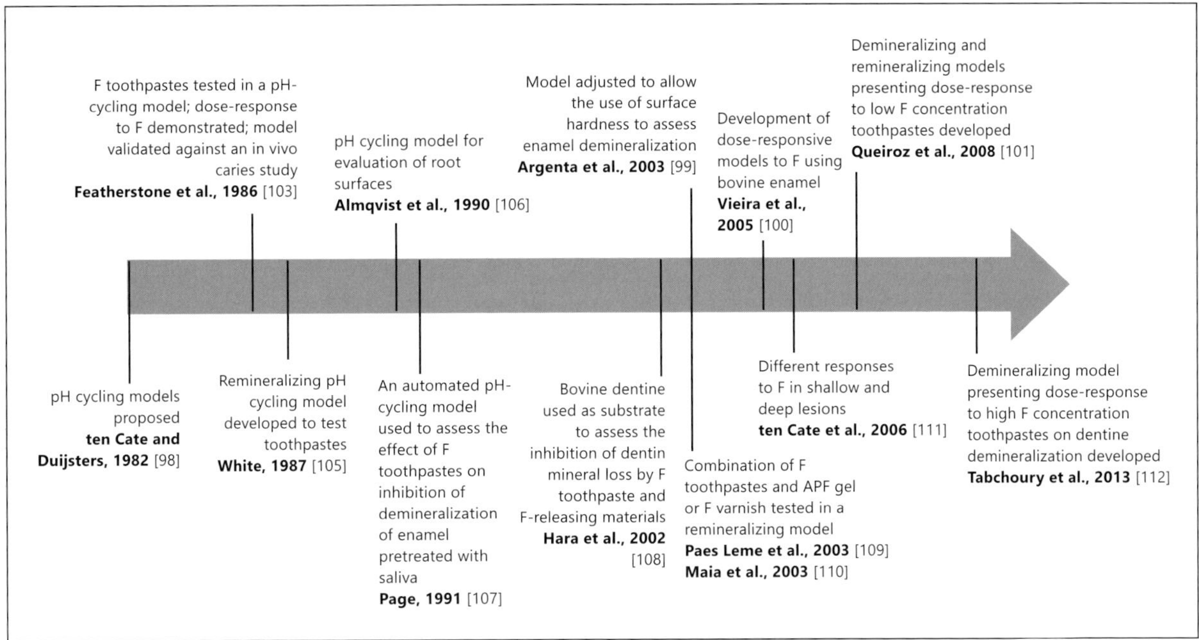

Fig. 3. Development of pH-cycling models and their use to estimate the anticaries efficacy of fluoride toothpastes.

seem to be the most suitable to study the effect of anticaries agents, with emphasis on fluoride toothpaste. An important prerequisite of these models is that they present a dose response to fluoride [99–102]. This might be tested using solutions with increasing fluoride concentrations, prior to the test of the toothpaste formulations of interest. The failure to fulfill this requirement will end up in biased models since the comparison of toothpaste efficacies, especially when proof of equivalence to a gold-standard toothpaste is intended, will be compromised by the lack of response to fluoride doses. Also, a good correspondence between data obtained from pH-cycling studies and clinical studies is aimed at and has been demonstrated before [103, 104].

Given the dual role of fluoride in the inhibition of demineralization and enhancement of remineralization, the possibility of evaluating these two effects separately has been explored in pH cycling models using two different types of protocols:

a De > Re models, used to assess the effect of fluoride on the reduction of dental demineralization. In these models, either sound or carious substrates are used, but the model is built to induce further mineral loss, and the effect of fluoride to reduce it is tested.

b Re > De models, used to assess the effect of fluoride on the enhancement of remineralization. Pre-demineralized substrates are needed, and although a demineralization cycle is included, the overall model induces remineralization, which may be enhanced by fluoride.

Although many types of models with distinct protocols were developed (fig. 3), their main feature is at least one daily demineralization-remineralization cycle, interspersed by short-term (1–5 min) exposure of the tooth specimens to the fluoride toothpaste prepared in a slurry (simulating in vivo salivary dilution). Therefore, the mechanism of action being modeled in such studies is the reactivity of fluoride with the substrates during each exposure and the subsequent release of fluoride to the de- and remineralizing solutions. For this reason, only ionic fluoride will be effective. The inhibition of demineralization is assessed after 1 or 2 weeks of cycling, as a result of the added effects of the individual exposures.

Although these models present a straightforward and relatively simple design, there are many factors interfering with the ultimate response. These include: substrate preparation (with either natural or polished surface, according to the requirements of the mineral content evaluation method), cycling regimen, ratio of de/remineralizing solution volume to area of enamel/dentine exposed to it, pH of the de/remineralizing solutions and sources of salts used to prepare these solutions. Different salts used to prepare the de- and remineralizing solutions have resulted in remarkable differences in the model response [Cury, unpubl. data], probably due to different background contamination with fluoride. These interfering factors must be kept in mind when developing and using pH-cycling models. Figure 3 presents an overview of the development and evolution of pH cycling models to assess the anticaries effect of fluoride toothpastes on distinct substrates (human permanent and deciduous enamel, bovine enamel, human and bovine dentine) and under distinct conditions (De > Re or Re > De).

In situ Studies
Since they were proposed [113], in situ models have been widely used in cariology due to their advantages over in vitro studies, and the reduced concerns on ethical issues when compared to a clinical trial. Also, the use of highly sensitive methods to assess mineral gain or loss by tooth substrates reduces the experimental time when compared to clinical studies [114].

As with in vitro models, in situ studies are also subjected to the scrutiny of presenting validity, reliability and sensitivity [94] to assess and compare toothpaste formulations. Moreover, it should be noted that controlled in situ models are designed to test the efficacy of toothpastes, and therefore the ultimate clinical effectiveness will be attested by proper clinical trials or systematic reviews of clinical trials. In this regard, the results of controlled in situ studies testing toothpastes with distinct fluoride concentrations [77, 115] or the combination of fluoride toothpaste use and professionally applied topical fluoride [116] are according to clinical studies or systematic reviews of the literature on these subjects [78, 117–119].

Although the particularities of each in situ model prevents their straightforward classification into distinct types, a clear distinction has been made based on the length (and type of cariogenic challenge) between long-term models – based on a biofilm forming during the intraoral test and/or by the effect of the volunteer's diet – and short-term models – based on a test plaque used to standardize the biofilm and therefore allow the study of specifics of the mechanism of action. Both types of models have been used to assess the efficacy of fluoride toothpastes, with strengths and limitations discussed in detail elsewhere [114]. Many aspects of the model should be considered, especially those related to the intraoral exposure to the formulations. Aspects that have a clear interference with that are the positioning of specimens in the mouth (either palatal or mandibular, in removable devices or fixed in the dentition, etc.), the type of exposure to the formulation to be tested (brushing, exposure to a slurry, etc.), the type of substrate being evaluated (sound or demineralized and the characteristics of the lesion) and the condition of biofilm accumulation and cariogenic challenge, among many others. These many features of the in situ models that might interfere with the study outcome have been reviewed before [120, 121]. Figure 4 presents the development and use of in situ models to test toothpastes' efficacy and mode of action.

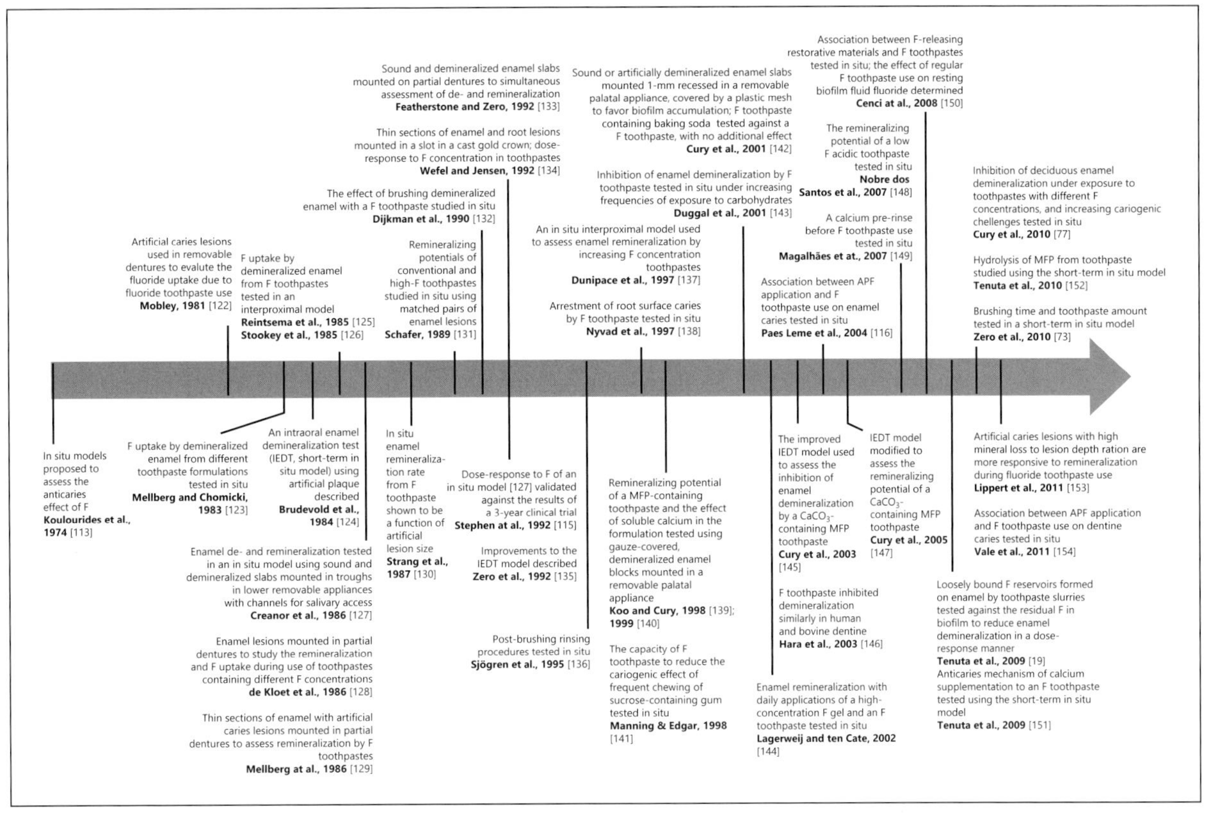

Fig. 4. Development of in situ models and their use to estimate the anticaries efficacy and mechanism of action of fluoride toothpastes.

In vivo Studies

Although clinical studies are necessary to prove the anticaries effectiveness of toothpaste formulations, some in vivo short-term tests can provide information on their efficacy in shorter periods of time. This is the case of the saliva and biofilm fluoride tests performed during the use of fluoride toothpastes. The value of these measurements, their strengths and limitations, have been discussed earlier in this chapter. Some examples of studies using saliva and biofilm fluoride concentration as estimates of the efficacy of fluoride toothpastes are presented in table 1.

Conclusions

The success of fluoride toothpaste use to control dental caries worldwide is broadly recognized, and has evolved from the development of effective formulations which have been continuously tested in a range of in vitro, in situ and in vivo tests before being widely used by the general population. Understanding the specifics of each of these models and the mechanism(s) of action being assessed by them is necessary to continue the translation of scientific development of new fluoride toothpaste formulations to highly effective clinical use.

References

1 Marinho VCC, Higgins JPT, Logan S, Sheiham A: Fluoride toothpastes for preventing dental caries in children and adolescents. Cochrane Database Syst Rev 2003;CD002278.

2 Bratthall D, Hänsel-Petersonn G, Sundberg H: Reasons for the caries decline: what do experts believe? Eur J Oral Sci 1996;104:416–422.

3 Lippert F: An Introduction to Toothpaste - Its Purpose, History and Ingredients; in van Loveren C (ed): Toothpastes. Monogr Oral Sci. Basel, Karger, 2013, vol 23, pp 1–14.

4 Bibby BG: A test of the effect of fluoride-containing dentifrices on dental caries. J Dent Res 1945;24:297–303.

5 Muhler JC: Effect on dental caries of a dentifrice containing stannous fluoride and dicalcium phosphate. J Dent Res 1957;36:399–402.

6 Winkler KC, Backer-Dirks O, van Amerongen J: A reproducible method for caries evaluation. Test in a therapeutic experiment with a fluorinated dentifrice. Br Dent J 1953;95:119–124.

7 Zero DT: Dentifrices, mouthwashes, and remineralization/caries arrestment strategies. BMC Oral Health 2006;6(suppl 1):S9.

8 White DJ: The comparative sensitivity of intra-oral, in vitro, and animal models in the 'profile' evaluation of topical fluorides. J Dent Res 1992;71:884–894.

9 Duckworth R: Pharmokinetics in the oral cavity: Fluoride and other active Ingredients; in van Loveren C (ed): Toothpastes. Monogr Oral Sci. Basel, Karger, 2013, vol 23, pp 121–1353.

10 Duckworth RM, Morgan SN: Oral fluoride retention after use of fluoride dentifrices. Caries Res 1991;25:123–129.

11 Zero DT, Raubertas RF, Pedersen AM, Fu J, Hayes AL, Featherstone JD: Studies of fluoride retention by oral soft tissues after the application of home-use topical fluorides. J Dent Res 1992;71:1546–1552.

12 ten Cate JM: Mechanistic interactions of dentifrices with de- and remineralization; in Embery G, Rölla G (eds): Clinical and Biological Aspects of Dentifrices. Oxford, Oxford University Press, 1992, pp 51–60.

13 ten Cate JM: Review on fluoride, with special emphasis on calcium fluoride mechanisms in caries prevention. Eur J Oral Sci 1997;105:461–465.

14 Cury JA, Tenuta LMA: How to maintain a cariostatic fluoride concentration in the oral environment. Adv Dent Res 2008;20:13–16.

15 Koulourides T, Cameron B: Enamel remineralization as a factor in the pathogenesis of dental caries. J Oral Pathol 1980;9:255–269.

16 Weatherell JA, Robinson C, Schaper R, Künzel W: Distribution of fluoride in clinically sound enamel surfaces of permanent upper incisors. Caries Res 1983;17:118–124.

17 Ögaard B, Rölla G, Ruben J, Dijkman T, Arends J: Microradiographic study of demineralization of shark enamel in a human caries model. Scand J Dent Res 1988;96:209–211.

18 Rølla G, Saxegaard E: Critical evaluation of the composition and use of topical fluorides, with emphasis on the role of calcium fluoride in caries inhibition. J Dent Res 1990;69:780–785.

19 Tenuta LM, Zamataro CB, Del Bel Cury AA, Tabchoury CP, Cury JA: Mechanism of fluoride dentifrice effect on enamel demineralization. Caries Res 2009;43:278–285.

20 Simone AJ, Gulya M, Mukerjee C, Kashuba A, Polefka TG: Assessment of the effects of dentifrices on plaque acidogenesis via intra-oral measurement of plaque acids. J Dent Res 1992;71:864–866.

21 van Loveren C, Buijs JF, Kippuw N, ten Cate JM: Plaque composition, fluoride tolerance and acid production of mutans streptococci before and after the suspension of the use of fluoride toothpastes. Caries Res 1995;29:442–448.

22 van Loveren C: Antimicrobial activity of fluoride and its in vivo importance: identification of research questions. Caries Res 2001;35(suppl 1):65–70.

23 Pearce EI, Dibdin GH: The diffusion and enzymic hydrolysis of monofluorophosphate in dental plaque. J Dent Res 1995;74:691–697.

24 Shellis RP, Duckworth RM: Studies on the cariostatic mechanisms of fluoride. Int Dent J 1994;44(suppl 1):263–273.

25 Mellberg JR: Fluoride dentifrices: current status and prospects. Int Dent J 1991;41:9–16.

26 DePaola PF, Soparkar PM, Triol C, Volpe AR, Garcia L, Duffy J, Vaughan B: The relative anticaries effectiveness of sodium monofluorophosphate and sodium fluoride as contained in currently available dentifrice formulations. Am J Dent 1993;6:S7–S12.

27 Volpe AR, Petrone ME, Davies RM: A critical review of the 10 pivotal caries clinical studies used in a recent meta-analysis comparing the anticaries efficacy of sodium fluoride and sodium monofluorophosphate dentifrices. Am J Dent 1993;6:S13–S42.

28 Pearce EI: A laboratory evaluation of New Zealand fluoride toothpastes. N Z Dent J 1974;70:98–108.

29 Toda S, Featherstone JD: Effects of fluoride dentifrices on enamel lesion formation. J Dent Res 2008;87:224–227.

30 Petersen PE, Lennon MA: Effective use of fluorides for the prevention of dental caries in the 21st century: the WHO approach. Community Dent Oral Epidemiol 2004;32:319–321.

31 Lynch RJ, ten Cate JM: The anti-caries efficacy of calcium carbonate-based fluoride toothpastes. Int Dent J 2005;55(suppl 1):175–178.

32 Cury JA, Tenuta LM, Ribeiro CC, Paes Leme AF: The importance of fluoride dentifrices to the current dental caries prevalence in Brazil. Braz Dent J 2004;15:167–174.

33 Conde NC, Rebelo MA, Cury JA: Evaluation of the fluoride stability of dentifrices sold in Manaus, AM, Brazil. Pesqui Odontol Bras 2003;17:247–253.

34 Hashizume LN, Lima YB, Kawaguchi Y, CuryJA: Fluoride availability and stability of Japanese dentifrices. J Oral Sci 2003;45:193–199.

35 Ricomini Filho AP, Tenuta LMA, Cury JA: Author's reply – Comments by Dr. Benzian et al. (2012) on the paper 'Fluoride concentration in the top-selling Brazilian toothpastes purchased at different regions'. Braz Dent J 2012;23:312–314.

36 Tabchoury CPM, Cury JA: Study of toothpastes aging conditions to predict fluoride behavior in environmental conditions (in Portuguese). Rev Bras Farm 1994;75:67–71.

37 American Dental Association, Council on Scientific Affairs. Fluoride-containing dentifrices. Chicago, American Dental Association, 2005.

38 van Loveren C, Moorer WR, Buijs MJ, van Palenstein Helderman WH: Total and free fluoride in toothpastes from some non-established market economy countries. Caries Res 2005;39:224–230.

39 Kikwilu EN, Frencken JE, Mulder J: Utilization of toothpaste and fluoride content in toothpaste manufactured in Tanzania. Acta Odontol Scand 2008;66: 293–299.

40 Benzian H, Holmgren C, Buijs M, van Loveren C, van der Weijden F, van Palenstein Helderman W: Total and free available fluoride in toothpastes in Brunei, Cambodia, Laos, the Netherlands and Suriname. Int Dent J 2012;62:213–221.

41 Villena RS, Cury JA, Issao M: A study on the availability and stability of fluoride dentifrices commercialized in Peru (in Spanish). Rev Estomatol Herediana 1994;4:12–20.

42 Cury JA, Tabchoury CPM, Piovano S: Concentración y estabilidad del fluoruro en dentífricos en venta en la Ciudad Autónoma de Buenos Aires (in Spanish). Bol Asociac Argent Odontol Niños 2006;35:4–8.

43 Cury JA, Oliveira MJL, Martins CC, Tenuta LMA, Paiva SM: Available fluoride in toothpastes used by Brazilian children. Braz Dent J 2010;21:396–400.

44 Ricomini Filho AP, Tenuta LMA, Fernandes FSF, Calvo AFB, Kusano SC, Cury JA: Fluoride concentration in the top-selling Brazilian toothpastes purchased at different regions. Braz Dent J 2012;23:45–48.

45 Carrera CA, Giacaman RA, Muñoz-Sandoval C, Cury JA: Total and soluble fluoride content in commercial dentifrices in Chile. Acta Odontol Scand 2012;70: 583–588.

46 Taves DR: Separation of fluoride by rapid diffusion using hexamethyldisiloxane. Talanta 1968;15:969–974.

47 Giacaman RA, Carrera CA, Muñoz-Sandoval C, Fernandez C, Cury JA: Fluoride content in toothpastes commercialized for children in Chile and discussion on professional recommendations of use. Int J Paediatr Dent 2013;23:77–83.

48 Hara AT, Kelly SA, González-Cabezas C, Eckert GJ, Barlow AP, Mason SC, Zero DT: Influence of fluoride availability of dentifrices on eroded enamel remineralization in situ. Caries Res 2009;43:57–63.

49 Chesters RK, Huntington E, Burchell CK, Stephen KW: Effect of oral care habits on caries in adolescents. Caries Res 1992;26:299–304.

50 Chestnutt IG, Schäfer F, Jacobson AP, Stephen KW: The influence of toothbrushing frequency and post-brushing rinsing on caries experience in a caries clinical trial. Community Dent Oral Epidemiol 1998;26:406–411.

51 Duckworth RM, Knoop DT, Stephen KW: Effect of mouthrinsing after toothbrushing with a fluoride dentifrice on human salivary fluoride levels. Caries Res 1991;25:287–291.

52 Sjögren K, Birkhed D: Effect of various post-brushing activities on salivary fluoride concentration after toothbrushing with a sodium fluoride dentifrice. Caries Res 1994;28:127–131.

53 Issa AI, Toumba KJ: Oral fluoride retention in saliva following toothbrushing with child and adult dentifrices with and without water rinsing. Caries Res 2004; 38:15–19.

54 Sjögren K, Birkhed D: Factors related to fluoride retention after toothbrushing and possible connection to caries activity. Caries Res 1993;27:474–477.

55 Weatherell JA, Strong M, Robinson C, Ralph JP: Fluoride distribution in the mouth after fluoride rinsing. Caries Res 1986;20:111–119.

56 Zero DT, Fu J, Espeland MA, Featherstone JD: Comparison of fluoride concentrations in unstimulated whole saliva following the use of a fluoride dentifrice and a fluoride rinse. J Dent Res 1988;67: 1257–1262.

57 Serra MC, Cury JA: Kinetics of fluoride in saliva after use of fluoride dentifrices and rinses (in Portuguese). Rev Assoc Paul Cirurg Dent 1992;46:875–888.

58 Sjögren K, Birkhed D, Rangmar B: Effect of a modified toothpaste technique on approximal caries in preschool children. Caries Res 1995;29:435–441.

59 Sjögren K, Melin NH: The influence of rinsing routines on fluoride retention after toothbrushing. Gerodontology 2001;18:15–20.

60 Heijnsbroek M, Gerardu VA, Buijs MJ, van Loveren C, ten Cate JM, Timmerman MF, van der Weijden GA: Increased salivary fluoride concentrations after post-brush fluoride rinsing not reflected in dental plaque. Caries Res 2006;40:444–448.

61 Zamataro CB, Tenuta LM, Cury JA: Low-fluoride dentifrice and the effect of postbrushing rinsing on fluoride availability in saliva. Eur Arch Paediatr Dent 2008;9:90–93.

62 Zero DT, Raubertas RF, Fu J, Pedersen AM, Hayes AL, Featherstone JD: Fluoride concentrations in plaque, whole saliva, and ductal saliva after application of home-use topical fluorides. J Dent Res 1992;71:1768–1775.

63 Raven SJ, Schäfer F, Duckworth RM, Gilbert RJ, Parr TA: Comparison between evaluation methods for the anticaries efficacy of monofluorophosphate-containing dentifrices. Caries Res 1991; 25:130–137.

64 Duckworth RM, Morgan SN, Gilbert RJ: Oral fluoride measurements for estimation of the anti-caries efficacy of fluoride treatments. J Dent Res 1992;71: 836–840.

65 Afflitto J, Schmid R, Esposito A, Toddywala R, Gaffar A: Fluoride availability in human saliva after dentifrice use: correlation with anticaries effects in rats. J Dent Res 1992;71:841–845.

66 Sjögren K, Birkhed D, Rangmar S, Reinhold AC: Fluoride in the interdental area after two different post-brushing water rinsing procedures. Caries Res 1996;30: 194–199.

67 Whitford GM, Wasdin JL, Schafer TE, Adair SM: Plaque fluoride concentrations are dependent on plaque calcium concentrations. Caries Res 2002;36:256–265.

68 Whitford GM, Buzalaf MA, Bijella MF, Waller JL: Plaque fluoride concentrations in a community without water fluoridation: effects of calcium and use of a fluoride or placebo dentifrice. Caries Res 2005;39:100–107.

69 Pessan JP, Silva SM, Lauris JR, Sampaio FC, Whitford GM, Buzalaf MA: Fluoride uptake by plaque from water and from dentifrice. J Dent Res 2008;87: 461–465.

70 Pessan JP, Alves KM, Ramires I, Taga MF, Sampaio FC, Whitford GM, Buzalaf MA: Effects of regular and low-fluoride dentifrices on plaque fluoride. J Dent Res 2010;89:1106–1110.

71 Vogel GL, Shim D, Schumacher GE, Carey CM, Chow LC, Takagi S: Salivary fluoride from fluoride dentifrices or rinses after use of a calcium pre-rinse or calcium dentifrice. Caries Res 2006;40: 449–454.

72 Pessan JP, Sicca CM, de Souza TS, da Silva SM, Whitford GM, Buzalaf MA: Fluoride concentrations in dental plaque and saliva after the use of a fluoride dentifrice preceded by a calcium lactate rinse. Eur J Oral Sci 2006;114:489–493.

73 Zero DT, Creeth JE, Bosma ML, Butler A, Guibert RG, Karwal R, Lynch RJ, Martinez-Mier EA, González-Cabezas C, Kelly SA: The effect of brushing time and dentifrice quantity on fluoride delivery in vivo and enamel surface microhardness in situ. Caries Res 2010;44: 90–100.

74 Mushanoff O, Gedalia I, Daphni L: Fluoride acquisition by surface enamel of human teeth in vivo following toothbrushing with an amine-fluoride toothpaste. J Dent 1981;9:144–149.

75 Barbakow F, Cornec S, Rozencweig D, Vadot J: Enamel fluoride content after using amine fluoride- or monofluorophosphate-sodium fluoride-dentifrices. J Dent Child 1983;50:186–191.

76 Kay E, Locker D: A systematic review of the effectiveness of health promotion aimed at improving oral health. Community Dent Health 1998;15:132–144.

77 Cury JA, do Amaral RC, Tenuta LM, Del Bel Cury AA, Tabchoury CP: Low-fluoride toothpaste and deciduous enamel demineralization under biofilm accumulation and sucrose exposure. Eur J Oral Sci 2010;118:370–375.

78 Stephen KW, Creanor SL, Russell JI, Burchell CK, Huntington E, Downie CF: A 3-year oral health dose-response study of sodium monofluorophosphate dentifrices with and without zinc citrate: anti-caries results. Community Dent Oral Epidemiol 1988;16:321–325.

79 Vogel GL: Oral fluoride reservoirs and the prevention of dental caries. Monog Oral Sci 2011;22:146–157.

80 Cury JA, Rebello MA, Del Bel Cury AA: In situ relationship between sucrose exposure and the composition of dental plaque. Caries Res 1997;31:356–360.

81 Cury JA, Rebelo MA, Del BelCury AA, Derbyshire MT, Tabchoury CP: Biochemical composition and cariogenicity of dental plaque formed in the presence of sucrose or glucose and fructose. Caries Res 2000;34:491–497.

82 Ribeiro CCC, Tabchoury CPM, Del Bel Cury AA, Tenuta LMA, Rosalen PL, Cury JA: Composition and cariogenicity of dental biofilm formed in situ in the presence of starch and sucrose. Br J Nutr 2005;94:44–50.

83 Aires CP, Tabchoury CP, Del Bel Cury AA, Koo H, Cury JA: Effect of sucrose concentration on dental biofilm formed in situ and on enamel demineralization. Caries Res 2006;40:28–32.

84 Tenuta LM, Del Bel Cury AA, Bortolin MC, Vogel GL, Cury JA: Ca, Pi, and F in the fluid of biofilm formed under sucrose. J Dent Res 2006;85:834–838.

85 Ccahuana-Vásquez RA, Vale GC, Tenuta LMA, Del Bel Cury AA, Vale GC, Cury JA: Effect of frequency of sucrose exposure on dental biofilm composition and enamel demineralization in the presence of fluoride. Caries Res 2007;41:9–15.

86 Vale GC, Tabchoury CP, Arthur RA, Del Bel Cury AA, Paes Leme AF, Cury JA: Temporal relationship between sucrose-associated changes in dental biofilm composition and enamel demineralization. Caries Res 2007;41:406–412.

87 Nobre dos Santos M, Melo dos Santos L, Francisco SB, Cury JA: Relationship among dental plaque composition, daily sugar exposure and caries in the primary dentition. Caries Res 2002;36:347–352.

88 Bruun C, Givskov H, Thylstrup A: Whole saliva fluoride after toothbrushing with NaF and MFP dentifrices with different F concentrations. Caries Res 1984;18:282–288.

89 Vogel GL, Mao Y, Chow LC, Proskin HM: Fluoride in plaque fluid, plaque, and saliva measured for 2 h after a sodium fluoride monofluorophosphate rinse. Caries Res 2000;34:404–411.

90 Barkvoll P, Rölla G, Lagerlöf F: Effect of sodium lauryl sulfate on the deposition of alkali-soluble fluoride on enamel in vitro. Caries Res 1988;22:139–144.

91 Franco EM, Cury JA: Effect of Plax prebrushing rinse on enamel fluoride deposition. Am J Dent 1994;7:119–121.

92 Caslavska V, Moreno EC, Brudevold F: Determination of the calcium fluoride formed from in vitro exposure of human enamel to fluoride solutions. Arch Oral Biol 1975;20:333–339.

93 Pearce EI, More RD: Uptake of fluoride by enamel from monofluorophosphate dentifrices. Caries Res 1975;9:459–474.

94 Stephen KW: Technical advances in intra-oral model systems used to assess cariogenicity: experimental design and analysis (reactor paper). J Dent Res 1992;71:905–907.

95 ten Cate JM, Mundorff-Shrestha SA: Working Group Report 1: Laboratory models for caries (in vitro and animal models). Adv Dent Res 1995;9:332–334.

96 White DJ: The application of in vitro models to research on demineralization and remineralization of the teeth. Adv Dent Res 1995;9:175–193.

97 Duckworth RM, Gilbert RJ: Intra-oral models to assess cariogenicity: evaluation of oral fluoride and pH. J Dent Res 1992;71:934–944.

98 ten Cate JM, Duijsters PP: Alternating demineralization and remineralization of artificial enamel lesions. Caries Res 1982;16:201–210.

99 Argenta RM, Tabchoury CP, Cury JA: A modified pH-cycling model to evaluate fluoride effect on enamel demineralization. Pesqui Odontol Bras 2003; 17:241–246.

100 Vieira AE, Delbem AC, Sassaki KT, Rodrigues E, Cury JA, Cunha RF: Fluoride dose response in pH-cycling models using bovine enamel. Caries Res 2005;39:514–520.

101 Queiroz CS, Hara AT, PaesLeme AF, Cury JA: pH-cycling models to evaluate the effect of low fluoride dentifrice on enamel de- and remineralization. Braz Dent J 2008;19:21–27.

102 Stookey GK, Featherstone JD, Rapozo-Hilo M, Schemehorn BR, Williams RA, Baker RA, Barker ML, Kaminski MA, McQueen CM, Amburgey JS, Casey K, Faller RV: The Featherstone laboratory pH cycling model: a prospective, multi-site validation exercise. Am J Dent 2011;24:322–328.

103 Featherstone JDB, O'Reilly MM, Shariati M, Brugler S: Enhancement of remineralisation in vitro and in vivo; in Leach SA (ed): Factors Relating to Demineralisation and Remineralisation of the Teeth. Oxford, IRL Press, 1986, pp 23–34.

104 O'Reilly MM, Featherstone JD: Demineralization and remineralization around orthodontic appliances: an in vivo study. Am J Orthod Dentofacial Orthop 1987;92:33–40.

105 White DJ: Reactivity of fluoride dentifrices with artificial caries. I. Effects on early lesions: F uptake, surface hardening and remineralization. Caries Res 1987;21:126–140.

106 Almqvist H, Lagerlöf F, Angmar-Månsson B: Automatic pH-cycling caries model applied on root hard tissue. Caries Res 1990;24:1–5.

107 Page DJ: A study of the effect of fluoride delivered from solution and dentifrices on enamel demineralization. Caries Res 1991;25:251–255.

108 Hara AT, Magalhães CS, Serra MC, Rodrigues AL Jr: Cariostatic effect of fluoride-containing restorative systems associated with dentifrices on root dentin. J Dent 2002;30:205–212.

109 Paes Leme AF, Tabchoury CP, Zero DT, Cury JA: Effect of fluoridated dentifrice and acidulated phosphate fluoride application on early artificial carious lesions. Am J Dent 2003;16:91–95.

110 Maia LC, de Souza IP, Cury JA: Effect of a combination of fluoride dentifrice and varnish on enamel surface rehardening and fluoride uptake in vitro. Eur J Oral Sci 2003;111:68–72.

111 ten Cate JM, Exterkate RA, Buijs MJ: The relative efficacy of fluoride toothpastes assessed with pH cycling. Caries Res 2006;40:136–141.

112 Tabchoury CPM, Ratti A, Cook KE, Cury JA: pH-cycling model for evaluation of high-fluoride toothpaste in root dentine (abstract 1536). J Dent Res 2013;92(Spec Iss A).

113 Koulourides T, Phantumvanit P, Munksgaard EC, Housch T: An intraoral model used for studies of fluoride incorporation in enamel. J Oral Pathol 1974;3:185–196.

114 Zero DT: In situ caries models. Adv Dent Res 1995;3:214–230.

115 Stephen KW, Damato FA, Strang R: An in situ enamel section model for assessment of enamel re/demineralization potential. J Dent Res 1992;71:856–859.

116 Paes Leme AF, Dalcico R, Tabchoury CPM, Del BelCury AA, Rosalen PL, Cury JA: In situ effect of frequent sucrose exposure on enamel demineralization and on plaque composition after APF application and F dentifrice use. J Dent Res 2004;83:71–75.

117 Marinho VC, Higgins JP, Sheiham A, Logan S: Combinations of topical fluoride (toothpastes, mouthrinses, gels, varnishes) versus single topical fluoride for preventing dental caries in children and adolescents. Cochrane Database Syst Rev 2004;CD002781.

118 Lima TJ, Ribeiro CCC, Tenuta LMA, Cury JA: Low-fluoride dentifrice and caries lesions control in children with different caries experience: a randomized clinical trial. Caries Res 2008;42:46–50.

119 Walsh T, Worthington HV, Glenny A-M, Appelbe P, Marinho VC, Shi X: Fluoride toothpastes of different concentrations for preventing dental caries in children and adolescents. Cochrane Database Syst Rev 2010;CD007868.

120 American Dental Association, Council on Dental Therapeutics. Proceedings of the meeting 'Technological advances in intra-oral model systems used to assess cariogenicity'. J Dent Res 1992;71:801–956.

121 Featherstone JDB (ed): Clinical aspects of de/remineralization of teeth. Proceedings of Models Conference, 1994. Adv Dent Res 1995;9:169–340.

122 Mobley MJ: Fluoride uptake from in situ brushing with a SnF_2 and a NaF dentifrice. J Dent Res 1981;60:1943–1948.

123 Mellberg JR, Chomicki WG: Fluoride uptake by artificial caries lesions from fluoride dentifrices in vivo. J Dent Res 1983;62:540–542.

124 Brudevold F, Attarzadeh F, Tehrani A, van Houte J, Russo J: Development of anew intraoral demineralization test. Caries Res 1984;18:421–429.

125 Reintsema H, Schuthof J, Arends J: An in vivo investigation of the fluoride uptake in partially demineralized human enamel from several different dentifrices. J Dent Res 1985;64:19–23.

126 Stookey GK, Schemehorn BR, Cheetham BL, Wood GD, Walton GV: In situ fluoride uptake from fluoride dentifrices by carious enamel. J Dent Res 1985;64:900–903.

127 Creanor SL, Strang R, Telfer S, MacDonald I, Smith MJ, Stephen KW: In situ appliance for the investigation of enamel de- and remineralization. A pilot study. Caries Res 1986;20:385–391.

128 De Kloet HJ, Exterkate RA, Rempt HE, ten Cate JM: In vivo bovine enamel remineralization and fluoride uptake from two dentifrices containing different fluoride concentrations. J Dent Res 1986;65:1410–1414.

129 Mellberg JR, Castrovince LA, Rotsides ID: In vivo remineralization by a monofluorophosphate dentifrice as determined with a thin-section sandwich method. J Dent Res 1986;65:1078–1083.

130 Strang R, Damato FA, Creanor SL, Stephen KW: The effect of baseline lesion mineral loss on in situ remineralization. J Dent Res 1987;66:1644–1646.

131 Schäfer F: Evaluation of the anticaries benefit of fluoride toothpastes using an enamel insert model. Caries Res 1989;23:81–86.

132 Dijkman A, Huizinga E, Ruben J, Arends J: Remineralization of human enamel in situ after 3 months: the effect of not brushing versus the effect of an F dentifrice and an F-free dentifrice. Caries Res 1990;24:263–266.

133 Featherstone JDB, Zero DT: An in situ model for simultaneous assessment of inhibition of demineralization and enhancement of remineralization. J Dent Res 1992;71:804–810.

134 Wefel JS, Jensen ME: An intra-oral single-section demineralization/remineralization model. J Dent Res 1992;71:860–863.

135 Zero DT, Fu J, Anne KM, Cassata S, McCormack SM, Gwinner LM: An improved intra-oral enamel demineralization test model for the study of dental caries. J Dent Res 1992;71:871–878.

136 Sjögren K, Birkhed D, Ruben J, Arends J: Effect of post-brushing water rinsing on caries-like lesions at approximal and buccal sites. Caries Res 1995;29:337–342.

137 Dunipace AJ, Hall AF, Kelly SA, Beiswanger AJ, Fischer GM, Lukantsova LL, Eckert GJ, Stookey GK: An in situ interproximal model for studying the effect of fluoride on enamel. Caries Res 1997;31:60–70.

138 Nyvad B, ten Cate JM, Fejerskov O: Arrest of root surface caries in situ. J Dent Res 1997;76:1845–1853.

139 Koo RH, Cury JA: Soluble calcium/SMFP dentifrice: effect on enamel fluoride uptake and remineralization. Am J Dent 1998;11:173–176.

140 Koo H, Cury JA: In situ evaluation of a dentifrice containing MFP/DCPD on fluoride uptake and human dental enamel remineralization (in Portuguese). Rev Odontol USP 1999;13:245–249.

141 Manning RH, Edgar WM: In situ de- and remineralisation of enamel in response to sucrose chewing gum with fluoride or non-fluoride dentifrices. J Dent 1998;26:665–668.

142 Cury JA, Hashizume LN, Del BelCury AA, Tabchoury CP: Effect of dentifrice containing fluoride and/or baking soda on enamel demineralization/remineralization: an in situ study. Caries Res 2001;35:106–110.

143 Duggal MS, Toumba KJ, Amaechi BT, Kowash MB, Higham SM: Enamel demineralization in situ with various frequencies of carbohydrate consumption with and without fluoride toothpaste. J Dent Res 2001;80:1721–1724.

144 Lagerweij MD, ten Cate JM: Remineralisation of enamel lesions with daily applications of a high-concentration fluoride gel and a fluoridated toothpaste: an in situ study. Caries Res 2002;36:270–274.

145 Cury JA, Francisco SB, Simões GS, Del BelCury AA, Tabchoury CP: Effect of a calcium carbonate-based dentifrice on enamel demineralization in situ. Caries Res 2003;37:194–199.

146 Hara AT, Queiroz CS, Paes Leme AF, Serra MC, Cury JA: Caries progression and inhibition in human and bovine root dentine in situ. Caries Res 2003;37:339–344.

147 Cury JA, Simões GS, Del BelCury AA, Gonçalves NC, Tabchoury CP: Effect of a calcium carbonate-based dentifrice on in situ enamel remineralization. Caries Res 2005;39:255–257.

148 Nobre dos Santos M, Rodrigues LK, Del Bel Cury AA, Cury JA: In situ effect of a dentifrice with low fluoride concentration and low pH on enamel remineralization and fluoride uptake. J Oral Sci 2007;49:147–154.

149 Magalhães AC, Furlani Tde A, Italiani F de M, Iano FG, Delbem AC, Buzalaf MA: Effect of calcium pre-rinse and fluoride dentifrice on remineralisation of artificially demineralised enamel and on the composition of the dental biofilm formed in situ. Arch Oral Biol 2007;52:1155–1160.

150 Cenci MS, Tenuta LM, Pereira-Cenci T, Del BelCury AA, ten Cate JM, Cury JA: Effect of microleakage and fluoride on enamel-dentine demineralization around restorations. Caries Res 2008;42:369–379.

151 Tenuta LM, Cenci MS, Cury AA, Pereira-Cenci T, Tabchoury CP, Moi GP, Cury JA: Effect of a calcium glycerophosphate fluoride dentifrice formulation on enamel demineralization in situ. Am J Dent 2009;22:278–282.

152 Tenuta LM, Del Bel Cury AA, Tabchoury CP, Moi GP, Silva WJ, Cury JA: Kinetics of monofluorophosphate hydrolysis in a bacterial test plaque in situ. Caries Res 2010;44:55–59.

153 Lippert F, Lynch RJ, Eckert GJ, Kelly SA, Hara AT, Zero DT: In situ fluoride response of caries lesions with different mineral distributions at baseline. Caries Res 2011;45:47–55.

154 Vale GC, Tabchoury CP, Del Bel Cury AA, Tenuta LM, ten Cate JM, Cury JA: APFand dentifrice effect on root dentin demineralization and biofilm. J Dent Res 2011;90:77–81.

Livia Maria Andaló Tenuta
Faculdade de Odontologia de Piracicaba, UNICAMP
PO Box 52, Av. Limeira, 901
CEP 13414-903 Piracicaba, SP (Brazil)
E-Mail litenuta@fop.unicamp.br

van Loveren C (ed): Toothpastes. Monogr Oral Sci. Basel, Karger, 2013, vol 23, pp 125–139
DOI: 10.1159/000350590

Pharmacokinetics in the Oral Cavity: Fluoride and Other Active Ingredients

Ralph M. Duckworth

Centre for Oral Health Research, School of Dental Sciences, Newcastle University, Newcastle upon Tyne, UK

Abstract

Modern commercial toothpastes contain therapeutic ingredients to combat various oral conditions, for example, caries, gingivitis, calculus and tooth stain. The efficient delivery and retention of such ingredients in the mouth is essential for good performance. The aim of this chapter is to review the literature on the oral pharmacokinetics of, primarily, fluoride but also other active ingredients, mainly anti-plaque agents. Elevated levels of fluoride have been found in saliva, plaque and the oral soft tissues after use of fluoridated toothpaste, which persist at potentially active concentrations for hours. Both experiment and mathematical modelling suggest that the soft tissues are the main oral reservoir for fluoride. Qualitatively similar observations have been made for anti-plaque agents such as triclosan and metal cations, though their oral substantivity is generally greater. Scope for improved retention and subsequent efficacy exists.

The first clinically proven fluoridated toothpaste appeared in the 1950s. Since then, developments have led to the incorporation of many different ingredients of potential activity against a variety of oral conditions. Modern commercial toothpaste formulations contain therapeutic ingredients that purport to be active against, for example, caries, gingivitis, calculus, dentine hypersensitivity, halitosis and tooth stain. Such formulations and their benefits are discussed in detail in earlier chapters.

To be effective, any potential active ingredient needs to be delivered to the mouth and ideally be retained at target sites for as long as possible. The delivery and retention of fluoride (oral fluoride pharmacokinetics) has been studied for many years, and a number of retention sites have been identified. Various factors involved in these processes have been studied, some of which have been modelled mathematically. This chapter primarily reviews the current research position concerning fluoride. A second aim is to review the literature that concerns other active ingredients, mainly those included in toothpastes as so-called anti-plaque agents.

Modes of Action of Fluoride

The success of fluoride in controlling dental caries has been well documented. Fluoride exhibits a number of diverse modes of action [1–3] that confer advantages compared with other potential anti-caries agents. These are: lowering of enamel solubility, inhibition of acid production by plaque bacteria, inhibition of demineralisation and promotion of remineralisation. The most important effects are believed to be the last two, with emphasis on the former.

The delivery and retention of fluoride (F) at, or close to, the site of action is regarded as an important feature of the successful application of the agent [4, 5]. In particular, the maintenance of an elevated, even if low, F ion concentration adjacent to the tooth surface has long been believed to be the key to achieve optimal caries control [6].

Fluoride in Saliva

Application of a topical fluoride product brings the fluoride into contact with the oral environment in general but primarily with the saliva. To the author's knowledge, Aasenden et al. [7] were the first authors to monitor the salivary clearance of fluoride over a number of hours after the application of topical fluoride, in their case a NaF solution. Of significance with respect to potential anti-caries action, salivary F concentration tended to fall rapidly to below 1 ppm (53 µmol/l) within 30–60 min after treatment application. Heintze and Petersson [8] and Bruun et al. [9] also studied salivary clearance after use of NaF mouthwashes. These authors further demonstrated that clearance profiles were qualitatively similar after application of a fluoridated dentifrice, a varnish, a tablet and gums. Such measurements indicated that salivary fluoride concentration tended to increase with increasing F concentration of the applied treatment, a finding also reported specifically for toothpastes by Finidori and Lamendin [10] and by Bruun et al. [11].

Only Aasenden et al. [7] of the above authors attempted to analyse the clearance profile itself, and they found a linear relationship between log (F⁻) and log (time). Later, Bruun et al. [12] used the Weibull function [13] to fit similar clearance

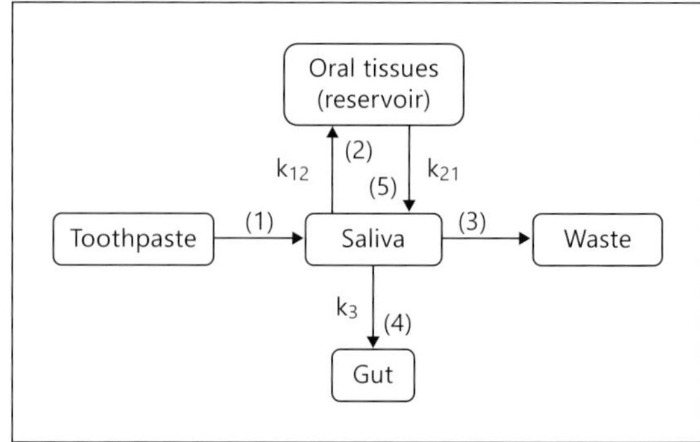

Fig. 1. The fate of fluoride during and after toothpaste application, adapted from Duckworth and Morgan [14]. For further explanation see text.

curves during the first 30 min after application of various fluoridated toothpastes. However, although that function fitted the data well, Duckworth and Morgan [14] believed that their application of conventional pharmacokinetic principles was more informative about the mechanisms involved in oral F retention. The various processes involved in the delivery and retention of F from toothpaste are represented schematically in figure 1. Five stages are depicted: (1) during brushing the toothpaste becomes mixed with saliva in the mouth; (2) fluoride species are taken up by the oral tissues; (3) after ca. 1 min, a major fraction of the applied fluoride is lost from the mouth – the bulk of the saliva/toothpaste slurry is spat out, some paste is retained on the toothbrush and the mouth is rinsed with water; (4) the remaining fluoride is mostly cleared from the mouth by swallowing, or is taken up by the oral tissues, and (5) as the salivary fluoride concentration decreases with time, the concentration gradient between the oral tissues and saliva increases, thus favouring the release of fluoride from the tissues.

Figure 2 shows a typical salivary F clearance curve, where mean saliva F concentrations are plotted on a logarithmic scale against time after application of a conventional 1,500 µg F/g tooth-

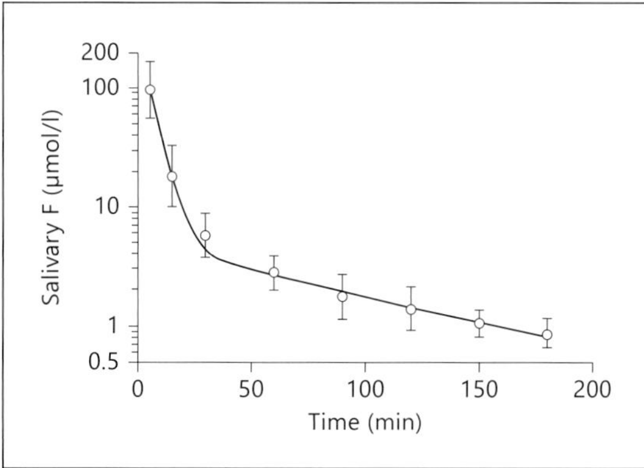

Fig. 2. Mean salivary fluoride clearance curve after use of a 1,500 µg F/g Na$_2$FPO$_3$ toothpaste (n = 10). Open circles = experimental data (bars = SD); solid line = computer-fitted model curve. From Duckworth and Morgan [14].

This leads to a solution for the concentration of fluoride in saliva as a function of time of the form:

$$F_S(t) = A \exp(-\alpha t) + B \exp(-\beta t) \qquad (1)$$

where A and B are arbitrary constants and α and β are functions of the three rate constants.

Figure 2 shows that a computer-generated curve, calculated using equation 1, fits the experimental data very well (r^2 = 0.999). Indeed, in this study, values of r^2 >0.99 were recorded for the individual clearance data. Similar curve fits have been obtained for both NaF- and Na$_2$FPO$_3$-containing toothpastes [14, 18]. The fact that the two phases of such curves are clearly distinct implies that, in approximation, α and β are the slopes and A and B the intercepts at t = 0 of the first and second clearance phases, respectively.

The initial, relatively rapid, clearance phase is determined by salivary flow rate, as predicted, e.g. by the theoretical model of Lagerlöf and Oliveby [19]. Zero et al. [20] reported that lower saliva F concentrations were associated with higher saliva flow rates. Of potentially greater relevance for toothpaste, Bruun et al. [12] found that fluoridated toothpastes without the usual flavouring agents yielded higher salivary F concentrations after brushing than corresponding standard formulations, which they attributed to stimulation of saliva flow caused by the flavour. This effect was demonstrated clearly in a study by Duckworth and Jones [21], who found that salivary F concentrations were significantly lower after application of NaF mouthrinses that contained either sucrose or sodium chloride, both of which compounds markedly enhanced saliva flow, than after use of corresponding mouthrinses without any additive.

Other influences on oral fluoride retention and clearance from toothpastes have been studied. Duckworth et al. [22] reported the effects of mouthrinsing with water after toothbrushing with a fluoridated toothpaste. They showed that salivary fluoride concentrations decreased with increasing thoroughness of rinsing caused by increasing rinse

paste [14]. The curve shows two distinct clearance phases over 3 h: a relatively rapid initial phase, which lasted from 40 to 80 min depending on the individual, and a relatively slow second phase. Duckworth and Morgan [14] fitted such biphasic clearance curves using a so-called two-compartment open pharmacokinetic model [15], as applied earlier by Ekstrand et al. [16] and Ekstrand [17] to the analysis of fluoride clearance from blood following ingestion. The model is, in essence, the core of figure 1, where saliva is one compartment and the oral tissues (or oral reservoir) are the second compartment. The concentrations of fluoride as a function of time t in saliva, $F_S(t)$, and in the oral reservoir, $F_R(t)$, are controlled by rate constants for uptake of fluoride by the reservoir, k_{12} (process 2), release of fluoride from the reservoir, k_{21} (process 5), and elimination of fluoride from the mouth by swallowing, k_3 (process 4).

The overall rate of change of F concentration in saliva is given by:

rate of change in saliva = rate of gain from reservoir – rate of uptake by reservoir – rate of elimination, i.e.:

$$dF_S(t)/dt = k_{21} F_R(t) - k_{12} F_S(t) - k_3 F_S(t)$$

volume, rinse duration and rinse frequency. Sjögren and Birkhed [23, 24] confirmed such findings and developed the so-called slurry-rinse procedure, whereby no actual water rinse is undertaken after brushing: instead subjects were required to mix a small amount of water with the existing toothpaste slurry and use the resultant mixture as an extended rinse before finally spitting it out. Salivary F concentrations were markedly elevated after use of the slurry-rinse compared with corresponding values after a conventional water rinse. Furthermore, Sjögren et al. [25] were able to demonstrate reduced demineralisation of enamel and dentine positioned approximately in an in situ model as a result of the new procedure. Duckworth et al. [26] showed that the loss of F delivered from a 1,450 µg F/g NaF toothpaste by water rinsing could be offset by subsequently rinsing with a 100 µg F/g (5.3 mmol/l) NaF mouthwash. In a related study, a post-brush rinse with a 226 µg F/g (11.9 mmol/l) NaF mouthwash yielded significantly elevated salivary F concentrations compared to brushing with fluoridated paste alone [27].

Recently, Zero et al. [28] demonstrated that salivary fluoride concentrations measured up to 2 h after brushing with a 1,100 µg F/g NaF toothpaste increased when the brushing time was increased from 30 to 180 s. The authors inferred that the longer brushing time allowed more fluoride to be retained in oral reservoirs, in contrast to thorough water rinsing which allows less fluoride to be retained. The last-mentioned study also showed that salivary F concentrations increased when the amount of applied paste increased from 0.5 to 1.5 g. Although this is an intuitively reasonable observation, the authors noted that the findings of related studies have been contradictory [28].

Two measures have been used to assess oral retention of fluoride: so-called total oral retention, measured by difference between applied amount and amount recovered after brushing (amount spat out as foam and in rinse water plus toothbrush washings), and AUC, area under the salivary clearance curve, estimated either empirically by procedures such as the trapezoidal rule or by computer-fitting to a pharmacokinetic model. For the case of the two-compartment model discussed earlier, integration of equation 1 between the limits t = 0 and t = ∞ gives: AUC = A/α + B/β. In general, total oral retention values of active ingredients are regarded as overestimates because of unmeasured losses [29]. In contrast, the AUC value may be an underestimate of retention because only relatively loosely bound material is accounted for in the time scale of measurement. However, the latter parameter may be a better measure of potential efficacy for that same reason: to be active an agent should be free to be transported to the site of action over as long a period as possible.

Table 1 lists published findings for studies of fluoridated toothpastes that involved adults. Total retention values range from 7 to 32% of the applied amount. As expected, such values are

Table 1. Oral retention of fluoride delivered from toothpaste (mean values)

Formulation	Total retention (% applied amount)	AUC[a] (% applied amount)	Reference
1,000 µg F/g Na$_2$FPO$_3$	14.7[b]	3.9	[12]
1,000 µg F/g NaF	9.0[b]	3.0	
1,000 µg F/g Na$_2$FPO$_3$		1.2	[14]
1,500 µg F/g Na$_2$FPO$_3$		0.9	
2,500 µg F/g Na$_2$FPO$_3$		1.0	
1,000 µg F/g NaF		1.8	[18]
1,500 µg F/g NaF		2.1	
2,500 µg F/g NaF		2.1	
4,000 µg F/g NaF	7, 14[c]		[35]
1,100 µg F/g NaF	10–14	1.8	[20]
1,100 µg F/g NaF	32	2.1	[28]

[a] Values calculated from original data assuming a saliva flow rate of 0.5 ml/min, as used for anti-plaque agents [29] and adopted for table 2.
[b] Toothpaste foam only.
[c] Thorough rinse and slurry rinse, respectively.

lower than the more extensively reported values for young children that are usually in the range 40–60% [30–32] because of less effective rinsing and spitting. Of more importance, AUC values are roughly 10 times lower than the total retention values, reflecting the relatively low substantivity of the negatively charged fluoride species and the relative inefficiency of toothpaste as a delivery vehicle. Fortunately, fluoride ions have been shown to inhibit demineralisation and promote remineralisation of enamel and dentine at surprisingly low concentrations [33, 34].

Oral Fluoride Reservoirs

A key requirement of the two-compartment pharmacokinetic model discussed above is the presence of an oral reservoir that is able to exchange F with saliva. One obvious candidate for such a reservoir is dental plaque, which is known to contain fluoride and is discussed in a separate section below. A second candidate is systemic saliva. However, the amounts of fluoride associated with both plaque [36] and systemic saliva [17, 37] are too small to account for the observed saliva F concentrations. A third candidate is tooth enamel and dentine, both of which have been associated with relatively high F content. However, this fluoridated apatite is highly insoluble, and such fluoride is not readily exchanged with adjacent fluid. A fourth candidate for an oral F reservoir is the oral soft tissues of the gums, tongue and oral mucosa. These tissues have a high surface area, ca. 200 cm^2 [38], relative to other potential reservoir sites, and are discussed in more detail in a separate section below. Fifth reservoir candidates are various stagnation zones around the mouth, e.g. the buccal sulcus and interproximal tooth sites. However, fluoride in toothpaste retained at such locations immediately after brushing will be free to diffuse into the continuous flow of saliva and hence is most likely to contribute only to the initial, rapid phase of salivary F clearance.

It is reasonable to conclude from the above list that the oral soft tissues are the most probable candidate for the oral reservoir responsible for the second phase of salivary F clearance observed in figure 2.

Despite the apparent goodness of fit, the two-compartment open model does not tell the whole story. Further work recorded changes in so-called equilibrium salivary F concentration during continuous daily use over months of a series of fluoridated toothpastes [14]. Subjects brushed with their test paste once per day, and samples of saliva were collected at least 18 h after brushing. Salivary F concentration increased steadily from baseline (achieved during at least 1 month's use of a non-fluoridated control toothpaste) to reach a plateau value after about 2 weeks, during use of a 1,000 µg F/g paste. Further, though smaller, increases occurred during the successive use of 1,500 and 2,500 µg F/g pastes, respectively. When brushing with the latter toothpaste stopped and subjects switched to using the non-fluoridated control paste, salivary F concentration returned to the original baseline value over a further 2 weeks or so. This behaviour was also found, and more clearly illustrated, during regular use of NaF mouthrinses [39]. These observations suggest that at least one further pharmacokinetic compartment must be present, which exchanges F with saliva on a much slower time scale than the compartment 2 oral reservoir postulated earlier to explain the trends in figure 2.

Of the remaining three reservoir candidates mentioned above, plaque and/or the teeth are possibilities. Fluoride should diffuse from plaque into saliva, based on concentration differences between plaque fluid and whole saliva observed during the period of the second clearance phase of figure 2 [40, 41]. Plaque also contains more strongly bound F (see section on plaque below), which could be a second reservoir.

The teeth are also a possibility. However, 2 independent studies suggest otherwise. Zero et al. [42] reported a salivary fluoride clearance study that involved two groups of subjects: one group was fully dentate and one was edentulous. Both groups applied a variety of F-containing topical treatments (toothpaste, rinse and gel) in a randomised order. After each treatment application, saliva samples were collected for up to 24 h. Elevated saliva F concentrations for all treatments were either the same or higher in the edentulous subjects compared to corresponding values in the dentate subjects. Edgar et al. [43] conducted a small-scale experiment that also involved subjects who possessed no natural teeth. This edentulous group brushed daily for about one month with a non-F paste and rinsed with either water or a 250 µg F/g NaF solution in a crossover design study. Saliva samples were collected at least 18 h after brushing and analysed for F. The elevation in salivary F after regular use of the non-F paste/fluoridated rinse, compared to after use of the non-F paste/non-F rinse, was similar to that recorded by a group of subjects who had all their teeth. Of potential interest, the values recorded for the edentulous subjects were numerically higher (though not statistically significantly different) than those recorded for the dentate subjects, consistent with the findings of Zero et al. [42].

The above experiments notwithstanding, calcium fluoride-like deposits on teeth may be the source of low concentrations of salivary F. Such material could have been present on the surfaces of both the natural teeth and artificial prostheses of the two subject groups. Also, this material may have the slow dissolution characteristics required to generate the observed changes in 'equilibrium' baseline salivary F concentration [44]. However, this author is not aware of any direct evidence for the formation of CaF_2-like material on the teeth or elsewhere in the mouth as a result of the use of a conventional 1,000–1,500 µg F/g toothpaste, despite much discussion on the topic. The required rapid precipitation of such material in the time scale of toothpaste application would require a higher degree of supersaturation than is routinely found in saliva [45], after which time measured F^- ion con-

centrations only decrease. Significantly, Vogel et al. [46] were unable to detect such material in plaque after application of a 228 µg F/g NaF solution.

Finally, the oral soft tissues may be the site of the second oral reservoir as well as the first. There is evidence to support more than one uptake/release mechanism [47, 48], which is discussed in more detail below.

Fluoride in Plaque
Measurements of fluoride in plaque are more difficult than in saliva because of the small amounts of sample collected. In general, two types of measure have been reported: whole plaque fluoride, expressed as F amount per unit wet (or dry) weight of plaque, and plaque fluid F, expressed as F concentration. Zero et al. [20] showed that mean whole plaque F clearance curves followed roughly similar profiles to corresponding saliva F curves up to 2 h after application of F dentifrice, F mouthrinse and F gel, bearing in mind the larger variations observed between subjects for the plaque data. Saliva F concentrations were initially elevated higher relative to baseline than corresponding plaque F values, but the subsequent F clearance rate from plaque appeared to be slower.

The findings of Zero et al. [20] are consistent with those of Vogel et al. [49], who recorded fluoride concentrations in samples of saliva and plaque fluid collected from subjects after use of a 0.048 M NaF mouthrinse. In the latter study, plaque fluid F concentrations at various tooth sites were significantly higher than corresponding saliva F concentrations at baseline and at both 30 and 60 min after F rinse application. These data suggest that plaque is a likely reservoir for fluoride, though the authors noted that the amounts of F in plaque were probably too small to account for the F in saliva. The slower clearance of F from plaque than from saliva probably reflects F binding to specific plaque reservoir sites [50], though restricted diffusion of F^- ions within the plaque matrix may also contribute [51–53].

Vogel et al. [49] found that plaque fluid F and saliva F were correlated, irrespective of tooth collection site. Duckworth et al. [39] also reported an association between mean elevated 'baseline' saliva F concentrations and corresponding mean whole plaque F values after regular daily use of a series of NaF mouthrinses of varying F content. The same group also found a dose-response relationship between applied F amount and mean 'baseline' whole plaque fluoride during regular use of Na_2FPO_3 toothpastes in both a large-scale clinical study and a small-scale crossover laboratory study [54].

Fluoride in Soft Tissue

That oral soft tissue may be a more important source of saliva fluoride than dental plaque was first mentioned by Yao and Gron [55], based on samples collected from a few individuals. The collection and measurement of fluoride in oral soft tissue is difficult. Hence, researchers have tended to measure fluoride adjacent to the soft tissues. Weatherell et al. [56] observed differences in F clearance at different oral sites following a 0.053 mol/l NaF rinse by using small paper points to absorb the salivary film. Essentially, they found higher F concentrations in the upper vestibule of the mouth than in the lower vestibule. Sites where F clearance was relatively rapid were associated with regions where salivary flow was expected to be significant such as close to salivary duct orifices, whereas F retention was most pronounced at sites likely to be regions of salivary stagnation. Zero et al. [42] adopted a similar approach but used paper discs that absorbed the salivary film of a defined area. These authors were also able to show site-to-site differences in local F concentration, though such variations were qualitatively different from those of Weatherell et al. [56], perhaps due to methodological differences. Of most relevance to the present discussion, Zero et al. [42] obtained results for different topical F agents, including a conventional NaF dentifrice, and found that

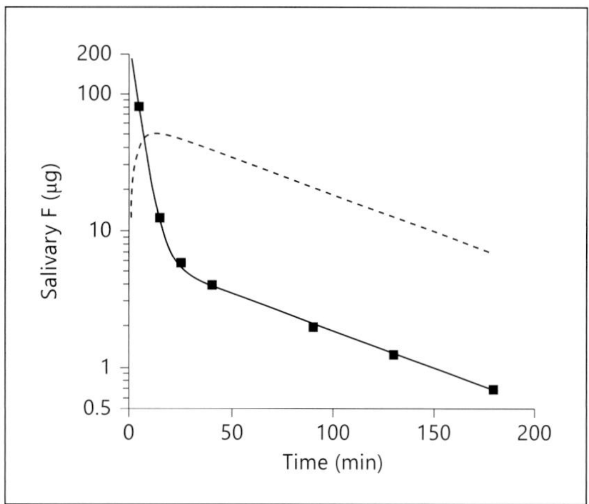

Fig. 3. Application of the two-compartment open pharmacokinetic model to salivary fluoride clearance. ■ = Mean experimental data (0.132 mol/l NaF solution, n = 10), from Duckworth and Stewart [58]; solid line = computer-fitted salivary fluoride clearance curve according to equation 1; dashed line = reservoir fluoride curve calculated using equation 2 and the computer-derived clearance curve parameters. From Duckworth [4].

site-specific F clearance curve profiles were similar to clearance profiles found in whole saliva. Crucially, results for an edentulous panel (i.e. lacking teeth, dental plaque and interproximal spaces) were similar to those for a fully dentate panel, thus highlighting the role of soft tissues as a major oral F reservoir.

To date, the author is only aware of a single study that has been published in which fluoride retention and clearance from oral soft tissue has been measured directly. Jacobson et al. [57] reported elevated amounts of fluoride in buccal mucosal tissue samples collected up to 45 min after application of a 0.2% (0.048 mol/l) NaF mouthrinse. Moreover, both elevated and baseline fluoride concentrations in the tissue were always higher than corresponding values recorded in whole mouth saliva. Figure 3 shows an experimental salivary fluoride clearance curve reported by Duckworth and Stewart [58] for a 0.132 mol/l

NaF rinse, where the mean data points have been expressed in μg F for a salivary volume of 2 ml. This data set was chosen because it was quantitatively similar to that of Jacobson et al. [57] and computer-fitted model clearance parameters were available. Assuming the applicability of the two-compartment open model discussed earlier, the expression for 'reservoir' fluoride as a function of time t, F_R (t), derived from equation 1 is:

$$F_R (t) = \frac{AB (\alpha - \beta) [exp(-\beta t) - exp(-\alpha t)]}{(A\beta - B\alpha)} \qquad (2)$$

The theoretical plot of reservoir fluoride against time, calculated from the above experimental data using equation 2, is markedly higher than the corresponding salivary F clearance curve at all times after F retention attains a maximum value (fig. 3). Of importance, the relative amounts of fluoride associated with the reservoir and in saliva are in qualitative agreement with the data of Jacobson et al. [57]. This suggests once again that the oral soft tissues may indeed be a major F reservoir for salivary F and further confirms the suitability of the two-compartment open model.

Duckworth and Jones [47, 48] conducted a series of in vitro, proof-of-principle experiments that demonstrated fluoride uptake into soft tissue (pig tongue) by both simple diffusion and by association with Ca binding sites. Although these experiments were conducted over time scales of up to 3 h, it is likely that mechanisms involving stronger fluoride binding, such as those found for plaque, will also be present.

Fluoride – Summary and Implications for Anti-Caries Efficacy

Elevated levels of fluoride have been found in saliva, plaque and the oral soft tissues after use of fluoridated topical treatments. Although oral fluoride retention following toothpaste application is low, the rates of subsequent release from oral reservoirs and of salivary clearance from the mouth by swallowing are relatively slow. Moreover, there is evidence for the build-up of retained fluoride during regular use of fluoridated toothpaste over weeks. Significantly, these low but elevated fluoride concentrations have been shown to be able to reduce demineralisation and promote remineralisation of enamel and dentine in mechanistic studies in vitro. The greater our understanding of the pharmacokinetics of fluoride in the mouth, the better able researchers will be to develop new approaches to improving the effectiveness of fluoride to control dental caries. The aim must be to improve the efficiency of fluoride delivery and retention from toothpaste, rather than using the simple expedient of increasing the fluoride content of the formulation with the concomitant concern about fluorosis.

In the context of the potential efficacy of fluoride, ten Cate [59] postulated that salivary calcium was rate limiting for enamel remineralisation. Whitford et al. [60, 61] found that plaque F content after use of a 1,100 μg F/g NaF toothpaste appeared to be limited by plaque Ca. Reservoir binding sites for fluoride most likely predominantly involve some form of Ca bridging mechanism to plaque bacteria and to the oral soft tissues [36, 48, 50]. As mentioned earlier, there is no strong evidence for the formation of CaF_2-like material in the mouth following use of conventional F toothpaste. By implication, a major potential route to improve the anti-caries efficacy of fluoride is to supplement bioavailable calcium and thereby retain a greater proportion of applied fluoride in the mouth. Researchers have sought to do this via Ca ion rinses before brushing with fluoridated toothpaste [for review see 36], or by use of a (preferably sub-micron-sized) particulate source of calcium, e.g. nano calcium carbonate [62], calcium fluoride [63], casein phosphopeptide – amorphous calcium phosphate complex [64]. Soluble calcium offers rapid oral delivery and effective retention at all reservoir sites, whilst particulate calcium offers potentially more achievable product stability and controlled slow release in vivo.

The oral soft tissues are most likely the main oral fluoride reservoir. However, the interaction of fluoride with these tissues has been little studied, probably because of experimental difficulties. In addition, at present there is no theoretical model that adequately describes the mass transfer of fluoride from these tissues to the site of action, the tooth surface, via the intervening medium, saliva. Moreover, the possibility that the oral mucosa is a source of F for plaque cannot be discounted, bearing in mind the relatively high F concentrations detected in the salivary film at certain mucosal sites. Research on these topics could be fruitful.

Other Active Ingredients

The majority of studies of the oral retention and clearance of other active ingredients have involved anti-plaque agents, a topic which was reviewed extensively by Cummins and Creeth [29]. They emphasised that: 'to function effectively as an anti-plaque agent in vivo, an agent must be delivered to its site of action in a biologically active form during the time of application, and it must be retained there for a sufficient period to exert its biological effect'. The most successful agents continue to be broad-spectrum anti-microbials such as chlorhexidine, metal ions and phenolic compounds (primarily triclosan) – see the chapter by Sanz et al. [this vol.]. These agents tend to be multifunctional, not only reducing bacterial metabolism and growth but also bacterial adhesion to oral surfaces. Zinc, in particular, has also long been used as an anti-calculus agent because of its ability to inhibit crystal growth.

The above agents are either positively charged species (chlorhexidine, metal ions) or electrostatically neutral (triclosan) at the pH values normally associated with toothpaste, which means, in contrast to fluoride and monofluorophosphate ions, they are substantive to the largely negatively charged surfaces of oral tissues and bacterial cells. Nevertheless, this advantage can be negated to an extent when compatibility with other toothpaste ingredients is considered. The favoured foaming agent for toothpaste is the negatively charged surfactant sodium lauryl sulphate, which can inactivate positively charged antimicrobials. Furthermore, both surfactants and flavour molecules can solubilise non-ionic antimicrobials and render them inactive. For these reasons, the activity of certain antimicrobial agents, notably chlorhexidine, is more optimal when they are incorporated in less complex delivery vehicles such as mouthrinses and gels.

The general model for delivery and clearance of anti-plaque agents in the mouth is essentially the same as that described earlier for fluoride and illustrated by figure 1. The clearance kinetics of substantive agents has been modelled by both single phase [65–67] and dual phase approaches [68–70]. Data for various active ingredients are listed in table 2.

Both total oral retention and, especially, AUC values are higher than corresponding values summarised for fluoride species in table 1. As expected, the cationic and non-ionic anti-plaque agents are more substantive than anionic fluoride. As for fluoride, AUC values are lower than corresponding total retention values. However, differences tend to be smaller, which suggests that a greater proportion of these anti-plaque agents are actually retained in oral reservoirs, and hence remain available for potential action, rather than be simply swallowed after brushing.

A further measure in the latter context is the half-life of salivary clearance, $t_{1/2}$, values of which are also included in table 2. Values have been derived using the single- and dual-phase models or, in the case of those estimated by Cummins and Creeth [29], using a single-phase model applied (for comparison purposes) only to data collected at 30, 60 and 120 min, as these time

Table 2. Oral substantivity of antibacterial agents delivered from toothpaste (mean values)

Agent (active formulation)	Reference	Total retention, % applied amount	AUC, % applied amount	*$t_{1/2}$ min	Plaque content μg/g
Tin (stannous fluoride)	[70]	5[a]		24	70–60[b]
Tin (stannous fluoride/Na hexametaphosphate)	[71]				33.7[c]
Triclosan (triclosan/zinc citrate)	[65]	25	6[d]	20, 34[d]	
	[68]	36	7[d]	27, 61[d]	120[g]
	[69]	37	7.5	28[e], 42[e]	109[f]
Triclosan (triclosan/copolymer)	[66]		13[d]	26	
	[69]	46	4.8	24[e], 54[e]	78[f]
Triclosan (triclosan/Na pyrophosphate)	[69]	43	4.4	22[e], 69[e]	89[f]
Zinc (zinc citrate)	[72]	38	17[d]	60	
Zinc (triclosan/zinc citrate)	[65]	24	12[d]	47	
	[69]	14	7.7	50[e], 94[e]	153[f]

* $t_{1/2} = \ln2/k_{el}$ and $t_{1/2} = \ln2/\beta$ for single- and dual-phase models, respectively, where k_{el} = rate constant for elimination from single compartment.

[a] Authors' assumption for mathematical model.

[b] 1–6 h after application of 1:3 toothpaste/water slurry.

[c] 12 h after brushing.

[d] Calculated by Cummins and Creeth [29].

[e] 1st, 2nd values from single- and dual-compartment models, respectively.

[f] 10 min after brushing.

[g] 15 min after application of 1:4 toothpaste/water slurry (original value expressed per g protein reduced by factor 10 for consistency with other tabulated data).

points were available for most studies. Both published and calculated half-lives are shorter for the non-ionic agent triclosan than for the cationic ion zinc, reflecting weaker association with its corresponding reservoir sites. Of interest, the half-lives for both agents are shorter than that for anionic fluoride ion (ca. 200 min, [14]). Whereas F ion binding relies on Ca sites, zinc ions may compete with salivary Ca for binding sites [73].

Also worth noting are corresponding values for the half-life of the initial rapid phase of salivary clearance, where a two-compartment model has been applied: 4.6 min, tin [70]; 4.3–4.8 min, triclosan [69]; 5.3 min, zinc [69]. Corresponding values for fluoride are not dissimilar: 6.5–9.1 min for Na_2FPO_3 toothpaste [14] and 2.9–4.1 min for NaF solution [58]. All these data are consistent with values obtained by Sreebny et al. [74] for the 'unstimulated saliva' clearance phase for the non-binding molecules glucose and sucrose of 6.9 and 7.7 min, respectively, reflecting what is a common salivary 'wash-out' phase.

In the case of a variety of toothpastes that contained triclosan, Creeth et al. [69] applied both single- and dual-phase models to experimental clearance curves, and found that the dual phase (i.e. two-compartment open) model fitted the data better for both triclosan and zinc (which was included in one of the tested formulations). These authors believed that the dual-phase model, though more complex mathematically, was also more appropriate as it accounted for both rapid clearance from the mouth and slow clearance from an oral reservoir, rather than just the latter process in the single-phase model. Figure 4 shows that salivary clearance of triclosan was faster than that of zinc during the second phase, which suggests that triclosan was released more easily from an oral reservoir than zinc. However, Creeth et al. [69] noted that total oral retention was higher for triclosan (37–46%, depending on toothpaste formulation) than for zinc (14%), which may indicate that some triclosan was tightly bound at certain oral sites.

The principle oral reservoir for all the antiplaque agents listed in table 2 appears to be the oral soft tissues, as concluded earlier for fluoride. From a safety aspect, antibacterial agents may be required to possess low permeability [29] to avoid penetration into the bloodstream. However, the penetration of triclosan into gingival tissue, for example, is thought to play a role in anti-inflammatory activity [75, 76]. The uptake of triclosan by soft tissue and its subsequent release would be expected to be facilitated by its non-ionic character, whilst the interaction of metal cations such as zinc with soft tissue is expected to be both more specific and stronger. These observations are borne out by the clearance data.

Gilbert and Williams [68] monitored the oral clearance of radiolabelled triclosan delivered from a toothpaste slurry. Their results, plotted in figure 5, showed that clearance from plaque was slower than from saliva or the buccal mucosa, which supports the view that the oral soft tissues are the likely reservoir for triclosan rather than plaque [29]. In this context, the qualitative similarity between these data for triclosan and those discussed earlier for fluoride (cf. fig. 3) is striking.

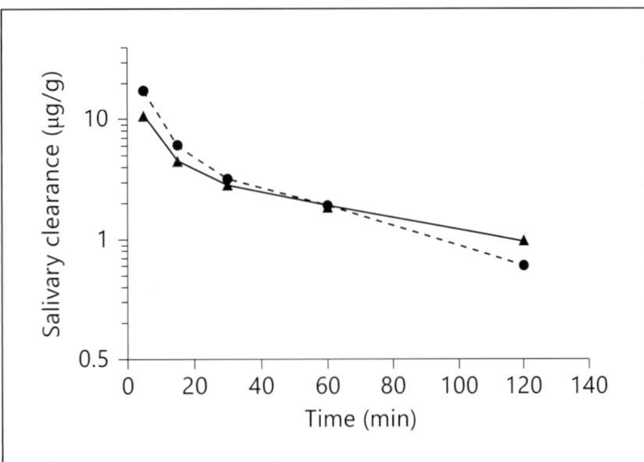

Fig. 4. Salivary clearance curves for triclosan (●, dashed line) and zinc (▲, solid line) after use of a 0.3% triclosan/0.5% zinc citrate toothpaste (mean values, n = 20). Data taken from Creeth et al. [69]. Note: 10 µg/g is equivalent to 34.5 µmol/l for triclosan and 153.0 µmol/l for zinc.

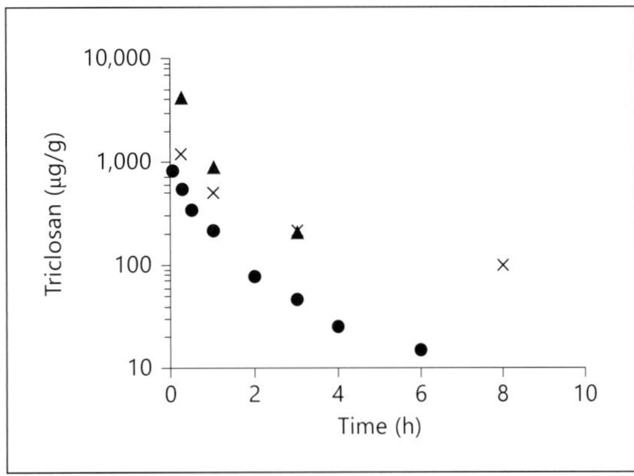

Fig. 5. Clearance of triclosan from saliva (●), plaque (×) and buccal mucosa (▲) after 1-min application of a 1:4 toothpaste (0.2% triclosan/0.5% zinc citrate)/water slurry. Mean values, n = 11–12, saliva values expressed per g saliva ×100, plaque and mucosa values expressed per g protein. Data taken from Gilbert and Williams [68].

Scott et al. [70] used a variation on the two-compartment open model to fit salivary clearance data for tin collected over 6 h following application of a 1:3 stannous fluoride toothpaste/water slurry. Rather than using mean data, they applied a model that utilised the individual data from each of their 20 experimental subjects. In their model, these authors used corresponding plaque tin data as representative of the oral reservoirs. The fit for salivary clearance, which allowed for a variable salivary flow rate over the first several minutes caused by treatment-induced stimulation, was good, whilst that for plaque was unable to simulate an initial accumulation phase that preceded an almost constant elevated level. The authors postulated that smaller than expected model clearance rate constants may have indicated that the retained tin was present as a large complex with salivary protein, rather than as soluble ions or molecules, and that the plaque represented only a small fraction of the oral reservoir.

There is some evidence for a build-up of antibacterial agents in plaque during regular usage, as described earlier for fluoride. This is most marked for zinc. Whilst baseline plaque zinc concentrations have been reported in the range 10–30 µg/g [73], Hall et al. [77] observed a mean value of 149 µg/g 12 h after last brushing with a 0.3% triclosan/2% zinc citrate toothpaste that had been used twice daily for 2 weeks by 43 adults. This value is comparable to the zinc concentration of 153 µg/g recorded by Creeth et al. [69] 10 min after a single brushing with a 0.3% triclosan/0.75% zinc citrate paste.

Hall et al. [77] also observed a small but significantly elevated concentration of triclosan following 2 week's use of the above-mentioned toothpaste, 8.6 µg/g, compared to the baseline control value of <0.1 µg/g.

Anti-Plaque Agents – Summary and Implications

As with fluoride, elevated levels of anti-plaque agents commonly used in toothpaste have been found in saliva, plaque and the oral soft tissues. The importance of the oral substantivity of these agents has been reviewed by, e.g., Marsh [78]. Whilst oral concentrations above traditional MIC values of pathogenic bacteria may persist for a limited period after toothpaste application, bacterial resistance is most often greater in oral biofilms for biological and biochemical as well as pharmacokinetic reasons. Possibly because of this, the effectiveness of anti-plaque agents delivered from toothpaste is probably not optimal despite relatively high retention compared to fluoride. Ironically, another potential issue is the possibility that such agents may be bound too strongly in oral reservoirs and hence never reach the required site of action. For example, the cationic agent sanguinarine exhibits high antimicrobial activity in vitro, yet has poor clinical efficacy [67, 79]. Goodson [67] suggested that sanguinarine was very substantive but was bound too tightly to manifest activity in vivo. Zaura-Arite et al. [80] found that the potent antibacterial chlorhexidine only affected cells in the outer layers of plaque biofilms formed in situ. Notwithstanding the above findings, Marsh [78, 81] has suggested that certain antibacterial agents may act beneficially through selective action against pathogenic organisms that may be more prone than resident microflora to the relatively short contact times experienced in the mouth. This idea is based on the observation that antibacterial agents, even at sub-lethal concentrations, can affect a variety of bacterial metabolic processes implicated in plaque-mediated oral diseases.

Acknowledgements

The author wishes to thank Dr. R.J.M. Lynch (GlaxoSmithKline, Weybridge, UK), Dr. A. Joiner (Unilever, Port Sunlight, UK) and, especially, Dr. V. Zohoori (University of Teesside, UK) for supplying key papers when requested, without which this chapter could not have been written. The author also thanks Prof. P.D. Marsh (University of Leeds, UK) for helpful discussions and Karger Publishers for permission to reproduce figure 2.

References

1 Buzalaf MAR, Pessan JP, Honorio HM, ten Cate JM: Mechanisms of action of fluoride for caries control; in Buzalaf MAR (ed): Fluoride and the Oral Environment. Monogr Oral Sci. Basel, Karger, 2011, vol 22, pp 97–114.
2 Shellis RP, Duckworth RM: Studies on the cariostatic mechanisms of fluoride. Int Dent J 1994;44:263–273.
3 ten Cate JM: Current concepts on the theories of the mechanism of action of fluoride. Acta Odontol Scand 1999;57: 325–329.
4 Duckworth RM: Fluoride in plaque and saliva; thesis, Amsterdam, 1993.
5 Ekstrand J, Oliveby A: Fluoride in the oral environment. Acta Odontol Scand 1999;57:330–333.
6 Fejerskov O, Thylstrup A, Larsen MJ: Rational use of fluorides in caries prevention. A concept based on possible cariostatic mechanisms. Acta Odontol Scand 1981;39:241–249.
7 Aasenden R, Brudevold F, Richardson B: Clearance of fluoride from the mouth after topical treatment or the use of a fluoride mouthrinse. Arch Oral Biol 1968;13:625–636.
8 Heintze U, Petersson LG: Accumulation and clearance of fluoride in human mixed saliva after different topical fluoride treatments. Swed Dent J 1979;3: 141–148.
9 Bruun C, Lambrou D, Larsen MJ, Fejerskov O, Thylstrup A: Fluoride in mixed human saliva after different topical treatments and possible relation to caries inhibition. Community Dent Oral Epidemiol 1982;10:124–129.
10 Finidori C, Lamendin H: Amounts of fluorine in saliva after use of various toothpastes. Chir Dent Fr 1980;50:43–48.
11 Bruun C, Givskov H, Thylstrup A: Whole saliva fluoride after toothbrushing with NaF and MFP dentifrices with different F concentrations. Caries Res 1984;18:282–288.
12 Bruun C, Qvist V, Thylstrup A: Effect of flavour and detergent on fluoride availability in whole saliva after use of NaF and MFP dentifrices. Caries Res 1987; 21:427–434.
13 Weibull W: A statistical distribution function of wide applicability. J Appl Mech 1951;18:293–297.
14 Duckworth RM, Morgan SN: Oral fluoride retention after use of fluoride dentifrices. Caries Res 1991;25:123–129.
15 Wagner JG: Fundamentals of Clinical Pharmacokinetics. Washington, Drug Intelligence Publications, 1975.
16 Ekstrand J, Alván G, Boréus L, Norlin A: Pharmacokinetics of fluoride in man after single and multiple oral doses. Eur J Clin Pharmacol 1977;12: 311–317.
17 Ekstrand J: Fluoride concentrations in saliva after single oral doses and their relation to plasma fluoride. Scand J Dent Res 1979;85:16–17.
18 Duckworth RM, Jones Y, Nicholson J, Jacobson APM, Chestnutt IG: Studies on plaque fluoride after use of F-containing dentifrices. Adv Dent Res 1994;8:202–207.
19 Lagerlöf F, Oliveby A: Computer simulation of oral fluoride clearance. Comput Methods Programs Biomed 1990;31: 97–104.
20 Zero DT, Raubertas RF, Fu J, Pedersen AM, Hayes AL, Featherstone JDB: Fluoride concentrations in plaque, whole saliva and ductal saliva after application of home-use topical fluorides. J Dent Res 1992;71:1768–1775.
21 Duckworth RM, Jones S: On the relationship between salivary fluoride clearance and the rate of salivary flow. Caries Res 1989;23:437.
22 Duckworth RM, Knoop DTM, Stephen KW: Effect of mouthrinsing after toothbrushing with a fluoride dentifrice on human salivary fluoride levels. Caries Res 1991;25:287–291.
23 Sjögren K, Birkhed D: Factors related to fluoride retention after toothbrushing and possible connection to caries activity. Caries Res 1993;27: 474–477.
24 Sjögren K, Birkhed D: Effect of various post-brushing activities on salivary fluoride concentration after toothbrushing with a sodium fluoride dentifrice. Caries Res 1994;28:127–131.
25 Sjögren K, Birkhed D, Ruben J, Arends J: Effect of post-brushing water rinsing on caries-like lesions at approximal and buccal sites. Caries Res 1995;29:337–342.
26 Duckworth RM, Maguire A, Omid N, Steen IN, McCracken GI, Zohoori FV: Effect of rinsing with mouthwashes after brushing with a fluoridated toothpaste on salivary fluoride concentration. Caries Res 2009;43:391–396.
27 Duckworth RM, Horay C, Huntington E, Mehta V: Effects of flossing and rinsing with a fluoridated mouthwash after brushing with a fluoridated toothpaste on salivary fluoride clearance. Caries Res 2009;43:387–390.
28 Zero DT, Creeth JE, Bosma ML, Butler A, Guibert RG, Karwal R, Lynch RJM, Martinez-Mier EA, González-Cabezas C, Kelly SA: The effect of brushing time and dentifrice quantity on fluoride delivery in vivo and enamel surface microhardness in situ. Caries Res 2010;44: 90–100.
29 Cummins D, Creeth JE: Delivery of antiplaque agents from dentifrices, gels, and mouthwashes. J Dent Res 1992;71:1439–1449.
30 Ekstrand J, Smith F: Fluoride in the environment and intake in man; in Ekstrand J, Fejerskov O, Silverstone L (eds): Fluoride in Dentistry. Copenhagen, Munksgaard, 1988, pp 13–27.
31 van Loveren C, Ketley CE, Cochran JA, Duckworth RM, O'Mullane DM: Fluoride ingestion from toothpaste: fluoride recovered from the toothbrush, the expectorate and the after-brush rinses. Community Dent Oral Epidemiol 2004; 32(suppl 1):54–61.
32 Zohoori FV, Duckworth RM, Omid N, O'Hare WT, Maguire A: Fluoridated toothpaste: usage and ingestion of fluoride by 4- to 6-year-old children in England. Eur J Oral Sci 2012;120:415–421.
33 Featherstone JDB: Prevention and reversal of dental caries: role of low level fluoride. Community Dent Oral Epidemiol 1999;27:31–40.
34 Lynch RJM, Navada R, Walia R: Low-levels of fluoride in plaque and saliva and their effects on the demineralisation and remineralisation of enamel; role of fluoride toothpastes. Int Dent J 2004; 54(suppl 1):304–309.
35 Sjögren K, Ekstrand J, Birkhed D: Effect of water rinsing after toothbrushing on fluoride ingestion and absorption. Caries Res 1994;28:455–459.

36 Vogel GL: Oral fluoride reservoirs and the prevention of dental caries; in Buzalaf MAR (ed): Fluoride and the Oral Environment. Monogr Oral Sci. Basel, Karger, 2011, vol 22, pp 146–157.

37 Oliveby A, Lagerlöf F, Ekstrand J, Dawes C: Studies on fluoride excretion in human whole saliva and its relation to flow rate and plasma fluoride levels. Caries Res 1989;23:243–246.

38 Collins LMC, Dawes C: The surface area of the adult human mouth and thickness of the salivary film covering the teeth and oral mucosa. J Dent Res 1987;66:1300–1302.

39 Duckworth RM, Morgan SN, Murray AM: Fluoride in saliva and plaque following use of fluoride-containing mouthrinses. J Dent Res 1987;66:1730–1734.

40 Vogel GL, Mao Y, Chow LC, Proskin HM: Fluoride in plaque fluid, plaque and saliva measured for two hours after a NaF or NaMFP rinse. Caries Res 2000;34:404–411.

41 Vogel GL, Zhang Z, Chow LC, Schumacher GE: Effect of a water rinse on 'labile' fluoride and other ions in plaque and saliva before and after conventional and experimental fluoride rinses. Caries Res 2001;35:116–124.

42 Zero DT, Raubertas RF, Pedersen AM, Fu J, Hayes AL, Featherstone JDB: Studies of fluoride retention by oral soft tissues after the application of home-use topical fluorides. J Dent Res 1992;71:1546–1552.

43 Edgar WM, Ingram GS, Morgan SN: Fluoride in saliva and plaque in relation to fluoride in drinking water and in dentifrice; in Embery G, Rølla G (eds): Clinical and Biological Aspects of Dentifrices. Oxford, Oxford University Press, 1992, pp 157–163.

44 Larsen MJ, Ravnholt G: Dissolution of various calcium fluoride preparations in inorganic solutions and in stimulated human saliva. Caries Res 1994;28:447–454.

45 Larsen MJ, Jensen SJ: Experiments on the initiation of calcium fluoride formation with reference to the solubility of dental enamel and brushite. Arch Oral Biol 1994;39:23–27.

46 Vogel GL, Tenuta LMA, Schumacher GE, Chow LC: No calcium-fluoride-like deposits detected in plaque shortly after a sodium fluoride mouthrinse. Caries Res 2010;44:108–115.

47 Duckworth RM, Jones S: On the interaction between fluorine species and oral soft tissue. Caries Res 1989;68:560.

48 Duckworth RM, Jones S: Involvement of calcium in the interaction between fluoride ions and oral soft tissue. Caries Res 1991;25:223.

49 Vogel GL, Carey CM, Ekstrand J: Distribution of fluoride in saliva and plaque fluid after a 0.048 mol/l NaF rinse. J Dent Res 1992;71:1553–1557.

50 Rose RK, Shellis RP, Lee AR: The role of cation bridging in microbial fluoride binding. Caries Res 1996;30:458–464.

51 McNee SG, Geddes DA, Main C, Gillespie FC: Measurements of the diffusion coefficient of NaF in human dental plaque in vitro. Arch Oral Biol 1980;25:819–823.

52 Stewart PS: Diffusion coefficient of fluoride in dental plaque. J Dent Res 2005;84:1087.

53 Watson PS, Pontefract HA, Devine DA, Shore RC, Nattress BR, Kirkham J, Robinson C: Penetration of fluoride into natural plaque biofilms. J Dent Res 2005;84:451–455.

54 Duckworth RM, Morgan SN, Burchell CK: Fluoride in plaque following use of dentifrices containing sodium monofluorophosphate. J Dent Res 1989;68:130–133.

55 Yao K, Gron P: Fluoride concentrations in duct saliva and in whole saliva. Caries Res 1970;4:321–331.

56 Weatherell JA, Strong M, Robinson C, Ralph JP: Fluoride distribution in the mouth after fluoride rinsing. Caries Res 1986;20:111–119.

57 Jacobson APM, Stephen KW, Strang R: Fluoride uptake and clearance from the buccal mucosa following mouthrinsing. Caries Res 1992;26:56–58.

58 Duckworth RM, Stewart D: Effect of mouthwashes of variable NaF concentration but constant NaF content on oral fluoride retention. Caries Res 1994;28:43–47.

59 ten Cate JM: In situ models, physicochemical aspects. Adv Dent Res 1994;8:125–133.

60 Whitford GM, Wasdin JL, Schafer TE, Adair SM: Plaque fluoride concentrations are dependent on plaque calcium concentrations. Caries Res 2002;36:256–265.

61 Whitford GM, Buzalaf MA, Bijella MF, Waller JL: Plaque fluoride concentrations in a community without water fluoridation: effects of calcium and use of a fluoride or placebo dentifrice. Caries Res 2005;39:100–107.

62 Nakashima S, Yoshie M, Sano H, Bahar A: Effect of a test dentifrice containing nano-sized calcium carbonate on remineralization of enamel lesions in vitro. J Oral Sci 2009;51:69–77.

63 Duckworth RM, Gao XJ: Plaque as a reservoir for active ingredients; in Duckworth RM (ed): The Teeth and Their Environment. Monogr Oral Sci. Basel, Karger, 2005, vol 19, pp 132–149.

64 Cochrane NJ, Cai F, Huq NL, Burrow MF, Reynolds EC: New approaches to enhanced remineralization of tooth enamel. J Dent Res 2010;89:1187–1197.

65 Gilbert RJ: The oral clearance of zinc and triclosan from a dentifrice. Pharm Pharmacol 1987;39:480–483.

66 Afflitto J, Fakhry-Smith S, Gaffar A: Salivary and plaque triclosan levels after brushing with a 0.3% triclosan/copolymer/NaF dentifrice. Am J Dent 1989;2:207–210.

67 Goodson JM: Pharmacokinetic principles controlling efficacy of oral therapy. J Dent Res 1989;68:1625–1632.

68 Gilbert RJ, Williams PEO: The oral retention and antiplaque efficacy of triclosan in human volunteers. Br J Clin Pharmacol 1987;23:579–583.

69 Creeth JE, Abraham PJ, Barlow JA, Cummins D: Oral delivery and clearance of antiplaque agents from triclosan-containing dentifrices. Int Dent J 1993;43:387–397.

70 Scott DC, Coggan JW, Cruze CA, He T, Johnson RD: Topical oral cavity pharmacokinetic modelling of a stannous fluoride dentifrice: an unusual two compartment model. J Pharm Sci 2009;98:3862–3870.

71 Ramji N, Baig A, He T, Lawless M, Saletta L, Suszcynsky-Meister E, Coggan J: Sustained antibacterial actions of a new stabilized stannous fluoride dentifrice containing sodium hexametaphosphate. Compend Contin Educ Dent 2005;26:19–28.

72 Gilbert RJ, Ingram GS: The oral disposition of zinc following the use of an anticalculus toothpaste containing 0.5% zinc citrate. J Pharm Pharmacol 1988;40:399–402.

73 Lynch RJM: Zinc in the mouth, its interactions with dental enamel and possible effects on caries: a review of the literature. Int Dent J 2011;61(suppl 3): 46–54.

74 Sreebny LM, Chatterjee R, Kleinberg I: Clearance of glucose and sucrose from the saliva of human subjects. Arch Oral Biol 1985;30:269–274.

75 Lin YJ, Fung KK, Kong BM, DeSalva SJ: Gingival absorption of triclosan following topical mouthrinse application. Am J Dent 1994;7:13–16.

76 Mustafa M, Wondimu B, Hultenby K, Yucel-Lindberg T, Modéer T: Uptake, distribution and release of 14C-triclosan in human gingival fibroblasts. J Pharm Sci 2003;92:1648–1653.

77 Hall PJ, Green AK, Horay CP, de Brabander S, Beesley TJ, Cromwell VJ, Holt JS, Savage DJ: Plaque antibacterial levels following controlled food intake and use of a toothpaste containing 2% zinc citrate and 0.3% triclosan. Int Dent J 2003; 53:379–384.

78 Marsh PD: Plaque as a biofilm: pharmacological principles of drug delivery and action in the sub- and supragingival environment. Oral Dis 2003;9(suppl 1): 16–22.

79 Vlachojannis C, Magora F, Chrubasik S: Rise and fall of oral health products with Canadian bloodroot extract. Phytother Res 2012;26:1423–1426.

80 Zaura-Arite E, van Marle J, ten Cate JM: Confocal microscopy study of undisturbed and chlorhexidine-treated dental biofilm. J Dent Res 2001;80: 1436–1440.

81 Marsh PD: Controlling the oral biofilm with antimicrobials. J Dent 2010; 38(suppl 1):S11–S15.

Dr. Ralph M. Duckworth
45, Kelsborrow Way
Kelsall, Tarporley
Cheshire CW6 0NP (UK)
E-Mail ralph.duckworth@virgin.net

van Loveren C (ed): Toothpastes. Monogr Oral Sci. Basel, Karger, 2013, vol 23, pp 140–153
DOI: 10.1159/000350480

After-Brush Rinsing Protocols, Frequency of Toothpaste Use: Fluoride and Other Active Ingredients

C. Parnell · D. O'Mullane

Oral Health Services Research Centre, Cork, Ireland

Abstract

The intra-oral retention or substantivity of active ingredients in toothpastes is important for their effectiveness, and this is influenced by product-related and user-related factors. Product-related factors include the formulation and the compatibility of active and other agents in the toothpaste and the concentration of the active ingredient. User-related factors include biological aspects such as salivary flow and salivary clearance, and behavioural aspects, such as frequency and duration of brushing, amount of toothpaste used and post-brushing rinsing behaviour. To date, product-related factors have dominated the research agenda for toothpastes, but user-related factors have the potential to significantly enhance or reduce the effectiveness of toothpaste. In this chapter, we will focus on two of the user-related factors that have been most widely studied: (1) frequency of toothbrushing and (2) post-brushing rinsing behaviour. We will then provide an overview of how evidence on these two behaviours has been used to produce guidance both for the profession and for the public, and make suggestions for the future direction of research in this area.

The advent of modern toothpastes in the 20th century and the evolution of therapeutic toothpastes containing fluoride and other active ingredients from the 1950s onwards has transformed toothpaste into a product that is acceptable and pleasant to use, and benefits oral health. Toothpastes now do more than just clean our teeth: they reduce caries, promote remineralisation, combat erosion, reduce sensitivity, improve gum health and make our teeth whiter – sometimes all in the one product. A summary of the principal active agents in modern toothpastes is presented in table 1.

Of all the active ingredients in toothpaste, the greatest body of evidence exists for fluoride. Several systematic reviews have established the caries-preventive effect of fluoride toothpaste [1, 2], reporting reductions of approximately 24% in caries increment in the permanent dentition for children and adolescents using fluoride toothpaste compared to placebo or no treatment. A Cochrane review of 79 trials involving 73,000 children found that a significant reduction in

Agent	Effect
Fluoride, Remin systems e.g. CCP-ACP	Anti-caries
Triclosan/copolymer (Gantrez)	Anti-plaque/anti-calculus
Chlorhexidine	Anti-plaque/anti-gingivitis
Metal salts (tin and zinc, strontium)	Anti-caries/anti-plaque/anti-calculus/ desensitising
Pyrophosphates	Anti-calculus
Enzymes, peroxide, sodium hexameta-phosphate, sodium tripolyphosphate	Whitening agents
Potassium nitrate/citrate/chloride, arginine/calcium carbonate, calcium sodium phosphosilicate	Desensitising

Adapted from Davies et al. [9].

caries was only seen with toothpastes containing 1,000 ppm F or more compared to placebo. The review also found evidence of a dose-response effect, with caries increment reductions of 23% for toothpastes with fluoride concentrations between 1,000 and 1,250 ppm and reductions of 36% for toothpastes with fluoride concentrations between 2,400 and 2,800 ppm when compared with placebo [3]. Other systematic reviews, drawing on a relatively smaller evidence base, support the anti-plaque and anti-gingivitis effectiveness of toothpastes containing 3% triclosan and 2% Gantrez copolymer and an anti-gingivitis effect for stannous fluoride [4; Sanz et al., this vol.]. No clear evidence was found in support of potassium-containing toothpastes for dentine hypersensitivity [5; Addy, this vol.]. There is a lack of systematic reviews of the effectiveness of other active ingredients in toothpaste.

The intra-oral retention or substantivity of active ingredients is important for their effectiveness [6–8; Duckworth, this vol.], and this is in turn influenced by product-related and user-related factors. Product-related factors include the formulation (e.g. viscosity, pH) and the compatibility of active and other agents in the toothpaste [9] and the concentration of the active ingredient (e.g. NaF, SMFP, SnF) [10–12]. User-related factors include biological aspects such as salivary flow and salivary clearance, and behavioural aspects, such as frequency and duration of brushing, amount of toothpaste used and post-brushing rinsing behaviour. As a product with a predicted global market worth USD 12.6 billion by 2015 and a reported usage by 97% of the population in the developed world [13], product-related factors have dominated the toothpaste research agenda in the quest for new and improved formulations. Recently however, there has been an increased interest in user-related factors and how user behaviours can act to either enhance or reduce the effectiveness of toothpaste. In this chapter, we will focus on two of the user-related factors that have been most widely studied: (1) frequency of toothbrushing and (2) post-brushing rinsing behaviour. We will then provide an overview of how evidence on these two behaviours has been used to produce guidance both for the profession and for the public.

Frequency of Toothbrushing

Daily toothbrushing with toothpaste fulfils two functions: (a) It disturbs the biofilm which is a central aetiological factor in both caries and periodontal disease, and (b) it delivers active ingredients that can help maintain or improve oral health.

The recommendation to brush twice daily with fluoride toothpaste is well established and features in guidelines [14–16] and in educational literature from professional organisations [17]. It even appears on toothpaste packaging. There is strong evidence to support this recommendation: a Cochrane review by Marinho et al. [1] found that brushing twice a day with fluoride toothpaste increased the caries-preventive effect by 14% compared to brushing once a day. Epidemiological data however, show that compliance by the public with the recommended frequency of brushing is not ideal.

Health Behaviour in School-aged Children is a cross-national research study conducted every 4 years in collaboration with the WHO, and involving children aged 11, 13 and 15 from countries in Europe and North America. One of the health behaviours studied is frequency of toothbrushing. The 2009/2010 survey, which involved over 200,000 children in 43 countries, found that on average, across all three age groups, approximately 2 out of 3 (65%) children brushed more than once a day [18]. Although social desirability bias may lead to an overreporting of brushing frequency, these figures show that at least one third of children are not obtaining optimal benefit from toothpaste. There was considerable variation by gender and by country in the reported frequency of brushing, with girls brushing more frequently than boys and more affluent north western countries reporting higher frequency of brushing than eastern or southern European countries (fig. 1). The highest rates for brushing more than once a day for both genders were found in Switzerland (90% for girls and 76% for boys) and the lowest were found in Turkey (50% for girls and 26% for boys). Family af-

fluence had a significant positive association with frequency of brushing [18].

Geographic, gender and social differences in brushing frequency have also been reported among adults. National survey data show that the percentage of adults brushing twice a day or more varies from over 80% in Sweden [19], to 75% in the UK (excluding Scotland) [20], 68% in Denmark [21] and 63% in Finland [22]. Brushing frequency among adults tends to decease with increasing age; for example, in Ireland 71% of those in the 35–44 age group reported brushing twice a day, whereas only 52% of dentate adults aged 65 or over brushed twice a day or more [23]. Stark gender differences in brushing frequency have also been found among adults. A survey of over 4,000 adults in Finland reported that 79% of women but only 47% of men brushed twice a day or more, and lower brushing frequency was associated with higher levels of untreated caries (DT) in both genders (RR 1.5, 95% CI 1.3–1.8). Less than daily use of fluoride toothpaste was also significantly associated with DT in men (RR 2.2, 95% CI 1.6–2.6) [22]. Among adults, as with children, brushing twice a day or more is associated with higher socioeconomic status or education level and with regular dental attendance [20, 21].

What is not known with any certainty is whether using fluoride toothpaste more than twice a day confers any additional anti-caries benefit. A recent experimental study by Nordstrom and Birkhed [24] reported higher plaque and salivary fluoride concentration when toothpastes containing 1,450 and 5,000 ppm F were used three times a day compared to twice a day. However, the authors acknowledged that those who need extra fluoride therapy may not be motivated to brush up to three times a day.

Rinsing with Water after Brushing

The use of an agent to clean teeth and freshen breath stretches back to antiquity. The constituents of early 'dentifrices' included various body

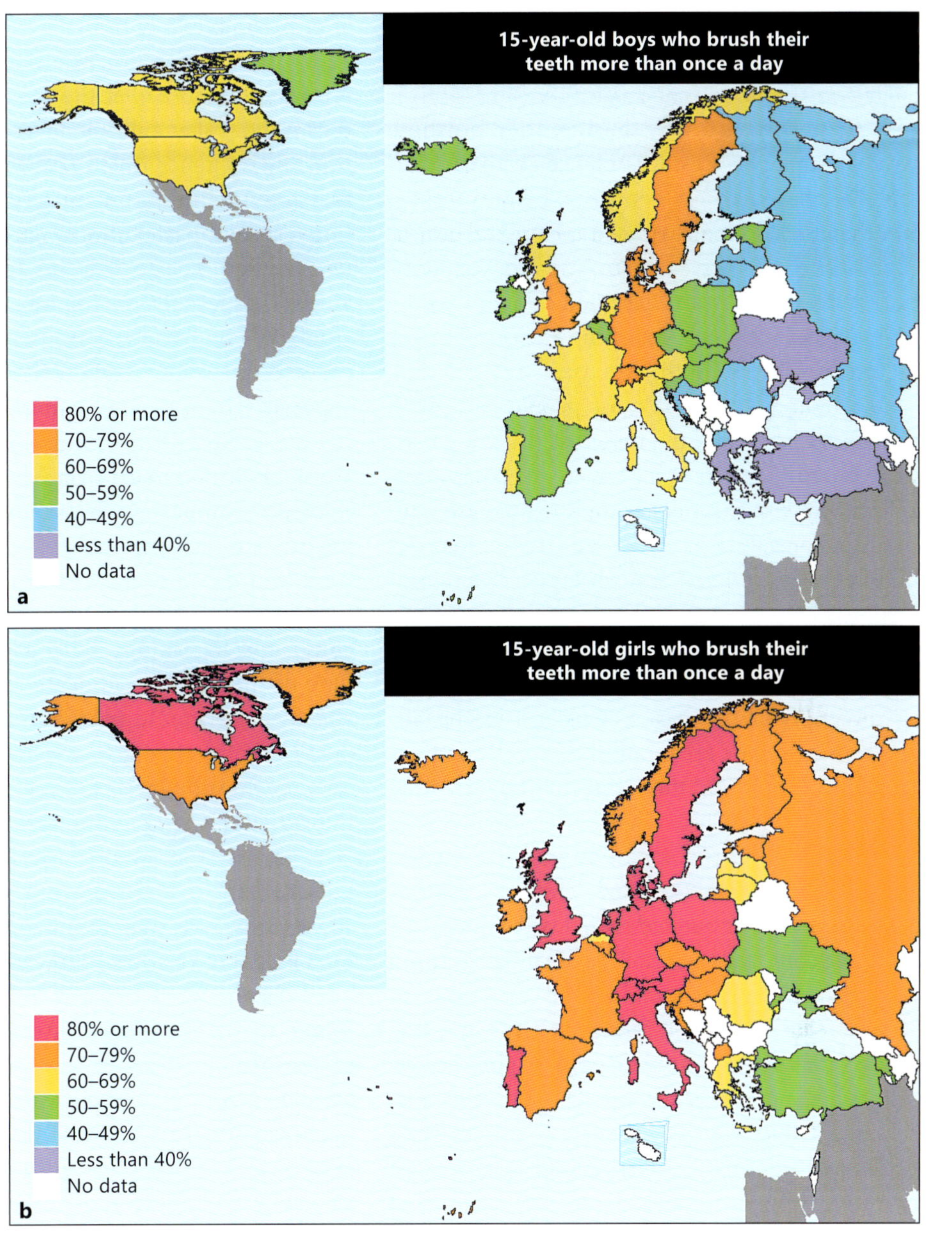

Fig. 1. a Percentage of 15-year-old boys brushing more than once a day. **b** Percentage of 15-year-old girls brushing more than once a day. Reproduced with permission from the World Health Organisation.

parts of rodents, urine, ground stag horn, egg-shells, snail shells and less abrasive components such as herbs, flowers and natural resin [25]. It is easy to understand why rinsing after brushing would become a necessary practice given the contents of these earliest dentifrices! Many toothpastes in the 20th century used calcium carbonate (chalk) as the abrasive system, and most contemporary toothpastes are designed to foam which may explain why post-brushing rinsing remains an integral part of toothpaste use.

It would appear that most people rinse with water after brushing, and that post-brushing rinsing has become such an automatic part of the oral hygiene routine that many people are not aware of their rinsing habits, as evidenced by discrepancies between self-reported and observed rinsing behaviours [26]. The most popular rinsing methods are to use a beaker or glass, cupped hands or the toothbrush to transfer water to the mouth, or to sip directly from the stream of water from the faucet. Rinsing habits are established early: van Loveren et al. [27] found that even children as young as 2.5–3.5 years of age rinsed after brushing. In their study of fluoride ingestion from toothpaste in Irish and Dutch preschool children, 70% of Irish children spat out and rinsed with water after brushing compared to just 27% of Dutch children [27]. A recent cross-sectional survey of 11- to 13-year-olds in England found that rinsing using a glass or beaker was the most popular post-brushing rinsing method, with over 40% of participants rinsing in this way [28]. Differences in rinsing preferences are also seen in adults: A survey of over 2,000 Swedish participants [29] found that over 70% of respondents aged 65 or less used one or two handfuls of water to rinse after brushing, whereas a survey of Irish adults found that using a cupped hand for rinsing was the least popular rinsing method across all age groups, being used by less than 20% of participants [23]. Irish adults under the age of 65 preferred to rinse by sipping water directly from the faucet. There may also be age differences in the preferred method of rinsing after brushing: in both the Swedish and Irish surveys, use of a glass to rinse was most commonly reported by those over the age of 65. These findings suggest that cultural and cohort factors may possibly influence rinsing behaviour. It is notable that few toothpaste manufacturers give instructions on toothpaste tubes or packaging to rinse after using toothpaste, whereas advice is often provided – especially on toothpastes marketed for children – on frequency of use, amount of toothpaste to use, not to swallow the toothpaste and to supervise children while using toothpaste.

Interest in post-brushing rinsing behaviour as a potential moderator of the anti-caries effect of fluoride toothpaste emerged as the understanding of the topical mechanism of action of fluoride grew and the importance of oral fluoride retention following the use of fluoride toothpaste was elucidated [6, 10, 30, 31; Duckworth, this vol.]. One of the earliest publications on the effect of rinsing behaviour tested the effect of five different post-brushing rinsing and spitting procedures on salivary fluoride levels [32]. The highest salivary fluoride levels after 4 min were found when subjects were not allowed to rinse, spit or swallow, but used the paste/saliva mix as a mouthrinse. The lowest levels were found for those who rinsed for 3 s, spat once and swallowed normally. Subsequent short-term experimental studies determined that rinsing with water after brushing reduces intraoral fluoride levels [33–37] and that greater 'wash out' is seen with higher rinse volume (ranging from 5 to 30 ml) and rinse frequency (once or twice) [36–38] and rinse duration [36]. The findings from these experimental studies led authors to suggest that rinsing with water should be minimised to optimise the anti-caries potential of toothpastes.

In all these experimental studies, an intermediate outcome – intra-oral fluoride levels – was used as an indicator of the anti-caries potential of fluoride toothpaste. Few clinical studies have been conducted that measure both post-brushing rinsing habits and the direct outcome of interest

– caries. The most commonly cited studies in this regard are by Chesters et al., [39], O'Mullane et al. [40], Chestnutt et al. [41] and Ashley et al. [42]. All were large-scale, 3-year toothpaste trials in which data on post-brushing rinsing behaviour as well as brushing frequency were collected at each annual examination during the trial (table 2). All four studies found higher 3-year caries increments in children who reported using a beaker of water to rinse after brushing compared to those who used other methods for rinsing. The percentage difference (prevented fraction – PF) in caries increment between beaker and non-beaker users ranged from 9 to 16% across the four studies and was significant in the three studies that tested the result statistically [39, 41, 42]. Brushing once a day or less was also associated with significantly higher caries increment, with PFs ranging from 17 [41] to 27% [42]. Two studies found that the lowest caries increments were seen in children who employed the combination of brushing more frequently and did not use a beaker to rinse [39, 40]. However, none of the four studies measured other potential confounders such as dietary habits or socioeconomic status, or indeed any other user-related factors such as brushing time and amount of toothpaste used that might have explained the association between reported behaviours and caries increment. It is also important to note that although these four studies were randomised and blinded to measure the effectiveness of the fluoride toothpaste being tested, the toothbrushing behaviour element was entirely observational and relied on children's self-reported behaviour. Only one study – a non-randomised prospective study conducted in a high caries population in Lithuania – attempted to test the effect of different rinsing regimens on caries incidence by assigning children to rinse and no-rinse experimental groups as part of a supervised school-based toothbrushing programme with fluoride toothpaste [43]. Children brushed once a day for 3 min using toothpaste containing 1,500 ppm F. The rinse group used a beaker of water (150 ml) and were encouraged to rinse thoroughly. The no-rinse group spat out once after brushing. Fluoride toothpaste was also provided for home use, but children were not given specific rinsing instructions to be carried out at home. At the end of 3 years, the mean caries increment (DMFS) in the no rinse group was 6.2 and in the rinse group was 6.8, a statistically non-significant difference of 0.6 (95% CI –1.6 to 2.8). However, the study was underpowered to show this difference, and the fact that children's rinse methods were uncontrolled at home may have undermined any difference that may have been observed during the supervised brushing and rinsing programme at school.

A modified toothpaste technique has been suggested as a way to increase intra-oral fluoride and to prolong fluoride retention in order to maximise the anti-caries effect of toothpaste [44]. The technique involves 4 steps as follows:

1 Apply 1 g (1 cm) of toothpaste to a wet toothbrush, spread evenly on the teeth and brush for approximately 2 min using the Bass technique.

2 Spit out no more than necessary during brushing.

3 Take a sip of water (approximately 10 ml) and with the remaining toothpaste foam in the mouth, use the toothpaste slurry as a mouthrinse and filter it between the teeth by active cheek movements for 1 min before carefully spitting out.

4 No further rinsing afterwards, and no eating or drinking for 2 h after brushing. (An earlier study by Sjögren and Birkhed [37] showed that eating or drinking immediately after brushing reduced the salivary fluoride level by 12–15 times.)

Reductions of 26% in caries incidence on approximal surfaces of primary molars in preschool children (age 4 at the start of the trial) have been reported with the use of this modified technique compared to children who received no specific instructions on how to use toothpaste or how to rinse [44]. However, only those who complied with

Table 2. Clinical studies measuring effect of post-brushing rinsing and brushing frequency on caries

Reference	Study characteristics	Recording rinse method	Percent using different rinse methods	Caries results				
Chesters [39] Toothpaste SMFP 1,000 ppm F 1,500 2,500 Each ± Zn citrate	Location: Scotland Design: randomised, double-blind toothpaste trial Duration: 3 years n = 2,279 Mean age: 12.5 years	At each examination, informal interview with participant using images of different rinse methods. Participant selected image that most closely resembled how he/she usually rinsed. Rinse method reported at final examination was used in analysis	53% beaker 16% brush 24% head under faucet 7% cupped hand 2 subjects did not rinse 58% of girls and 48% of boys used a beaker		Beaker	Other	Brush ≤1/day	Brush ≥2/day
				Mean DMFS Δ	6.87	5.77	6.95	5.39
				Difference	1.1 (p < 0.001)		1.57 (p < 0.001)	
				PF	16%		23%	
O'Mullane [40] Toothpaste NaF 1,000 1,500 Each ± 3% Na TMP	Location: North Wales Design: Randomised toothpaste trial Duration: 3 years n = 3,467 Age: 11–12 years	Based on Chesters method Categorisation into beaker/non-beaker users was based on participant response at 2 follow-up exams	35.5% beaker 65% non-beaker		Beaker	Other	Brush 1/day	Brush ≥2/day
				Mean DMFS Δ	4.46	3.85	4.20	3.39
				Difference	0.61		0.89	
				PF	14%		21%	
				Statistical significance not reported.				
Chestnutt [41] Toothpaste SMFP 1,000, 1,500 NaF 1,000, 1,500 NaF + TMP 1,000, 1,500	Location: Scotland Design: Randomised, double-blind toothpaste trial Duration: 3 years n = 2,621 Age: 11–13 years	Computer-based version of Chesters' images Categorisation into beaker users was based on participant response at 2 follow-up exams and non-beaker user as reporting beaker use at ≤1 exam	NR		Beaker	Other	Brush 1/day	Brush ≥2/day
				Mean DMFS Δ	6.84	5.84	6.6	5.5
				Difference	1.0 (p < 0.05)		1.1	
				PF	15%		17%	
				Frequency of brushing (1/day vs. >1/day) explained 48% of variation in DMFS increment. Rinse method (beaker vs. non-beaker) explained 12%.				
Ashley [42]	Location: Manchester Design: not specified Duration: 3 years n = 2,888 Age: 15–16 years	Supervised questionnaire No further details provided	39% beaker 24% brush 35% hand/head under faucet 2% did not rinse		Beaker	Other	Brush ≤1/day	Brush ≥2/day
				Mean DMFS Δ	3.97	3.61	4.79	3.51
				Difference	0.36 (p = 0.012)		1.28 (p < 0.001)	
				PF	9%		27%	
Machiulskiene [43]	Location: Lithuania Design: non-randomised, post-brush rinse methods trial Parallel 'control' group from another study Duration: 3 years n= 276 Age: 11–12 years	Children in one school were assigned to rinse after brushing, children in the second school were instructed to spit out after brushing as part of a supervised, school-based fluoride toothbrushing programme. Participants in both schools were free to rinse as they wished at home.			Rinse	No rinse	No brush 'control'	
				Mean DMFS Δ	6.8	6.2	12.4	
				Difference	0.6 (95% CI −1.6 to 2.8)			
				PF	9% NS			

SMFP = Sodium monofluorophosphate.

the instructions were included in the analysis, which may have inflated the effect size. Dropouts overall were higher in the test groups than in the control group, and the biggest difference was seen for dropout due to 'weak co-operation', which was 3 times higher in the modified toothpaste groups compared to the control (14 vs. 4%). This suggests that the technique may not be completely acceptable to users, although the young age of children in this study may have been a factor. A 2-year trial which tested the modified toothpaste technique in Saudi adults with high caries prevalence recorded impressive reductions of 66 and 44% in the incidence of enamel caries on approximal and buccal/lingual surfaces [45, 46]. Compliance with the modified toothpaste technique may also be a problem for adults since, in spite of 'extreme effort' by the researchers to ensure test group compliance with instructions, some patients had to rinse with a sip of water after brushing because they could not get used to the strong taste of the toothpaste that was left after using the modified technique [45]. Another study which tested the modified toothpaste technique in adolescent orthodontic patients noted that rinsing with the toothpaste slurry 'can cause some oral discomfort and irritation of the oral mucosa' although, in the authors' experience, few of their patients reported any complaints [47].

After-Brushing Rinsing with Mouthrinse

Commercial or over-the-counter mouthrinses are used by the public as an adjunct to toothbrushing, and represent the fastest growing sector of the oral care industry in recent years. In the UK for example, sales of mouthrinse increased by 44% between 2005 and 2010 (http://www.mintel.com). The proportion of adults using mouthrinse varies between 47% in Sweden [48], 31% in the UK [20] and 28% in Ireland [23]. The popularity of mouthrinse spans all social groups [20]. Mouthrinses can be used for delivering additional fluoride over and above that provided by tooth-

paste for high caries risk subjects, or to enhance plaque control and improve gingival health. They also freshen breath. As with toothpastes, many modern mouthrinses are now multi-purpose. A recent study of mouthrinse use by Swedish adults, all of whom were regular dental attenders, found that the top three reasons for using mouthrinse were to avoid tooth decay, to have a 'fresh intra-oral feeling', and to avoid bad breath. Of the 47% of respondents who used mouthrinse, most rinsed daily, and the vast majority (87%) used the mouthrinse directly after brushing. Only 12% rinsed at a different time to brushing [48].

Fluoride Mouthrinse
Although short-term experimental studies have shown that the use of a fluoride mouthrinse after brushing with fluoride toothpaste can maintain [49] or increase [37, 50] intra-oral fluoride levels compared to use of fluoride toothpaste alone, clinical evidence for an enhanced anti-caries effect with the combined use of fluoride toothpaste and mouthrinse is sparse. A Cochrane review of combinations of topical fluoride modalities for preventing caries [51] included 5 clinical trials that compared the combined use of fluoride toothpaste and mouthrinse with fluoride toothpaste and placebo rinse. The pooled effect of these studies showed a small but statistically non-significant effect in favour of the combined fluoride regimen (PF 7%, 95% CI 0–13%, p = 0.06). Twetman et al. [52] questioned the additional anti-caries effect of fluoride mouthrinse for children with daily exposure to fluoride toothpaste, but did find limited evidence for the effectiveness of fluoride mouthrinse for the prevention of root caries in adults.

Non-Fluoride Mouthrinses
Short-term experimental studies have shown that using a non-fluoride mouthrinse after brushing with fluoride toothpaste may adversely affect the anti-caries potential of the toothpaste, by 'washing out' the fluoride delivered by the toothpaste [49, 50]. Furthermore, many non-fluoride mouth-

rinses contain therapeutic cationic agents such as chlorhexidine or cetylpyridinium chloride whose effect may be reduced by interaction with anionic constituents of toothpaste such as sodium lauryl sulphate (SLS) [53, 54]. Barkvoll et al. [53] demonstrated that rinsing with a solution of SLS prior to rinsing with chlorhexidine mouthrinse significantly decreased the anti-plaque effect of chlorhexidine when the interval between exposures was 30 min or less. The inhibitory effect of SLS only disappeared when the interval between exposures was greater than 2 h. In another short-term, non-brushing, cross-over trial, Owens et al. [55] used a dentifrice slurry, rather than an SLS solution, to study the interaction between chlorhexidine and toothpaste. They found that the anti-plaque effect of 0.12% chlorhexidine mouthrinse was significantly reduced when it was used before or directly after exposure to the toothpaste slurry. Van Strydonck et al. [56], in an attempt to replicate the 'real life' application of toothpaste, conducted a series of experimental studies in which one dental arch was randomly assigned as the 'study' arch, and was left unbrushed while the other 'toothpaste' arch was brushed with an SLS-containing fluoride toothpaste. After brushing, the toothpaste foam was expectorated and subjects rinsed their mouth with water before rinsing with 0.2% chlorhexidine rinse. Using this study design, the researchers found no significant difference in plaque accumulation in the 'study' arch when the chlorhexidine rinse was used after brushing compared to use of chlorhexidine rinse without any exposure to toothpaste. The authors concluded that ordinary brushing followed by rinsing with water does not appear to reduce the level of plaque inhibition offered by a post-brushing chlorhexidine rinse [56]. The same research team, using an examiner-blind, parallel group 4-day plaque accumulation trial, went on to demonstrate that the anti-plaque effect of 0.2% chlorhexidine rinse was significantly reduced when it was used immediately after rinsing with a toothpaste slurry but not when toothpaste was applied to the 'toothpaste'

arch followed by rinsing with water before using the chlorhexidine rinse [57]. The mean plaque scores for toothpaste slurry-CHX group was 1.62, which was significantly higher than the 'brushing'-CHX group (mean plaque score 1.14) and for the CHX only group (1.17; p < 0.006). Given the limited evidence base, and the different methodologies and mouthrinse concentrations used, it is not surprising that recommendations on the optimum timing for using anti-plaque/anti-gingivitis mouthrinses are inconsistent, with some authors suggesting that the use of toothpaste and chlorhexidine mouthrinse should be separated by 30–120 min [58, 59] while others suggest that chlorhexidine mouthrinse can be used after toothbrushing, provided the toothpaste is washed out with water prior to using the rinse [57]. In this situation, the mouthrinse should ideally contain fluoride to prevent wash-out of the fluoride from toothpaste.

Recommendations on Post-Brushing Rinsing

Evidence-based practice is the dominant paradigm in modern healthcare. Clinical practice guidelines have been defined as 'systematically developed statements to assist practitioner and patient decisions about appropriate healthcare for specific clinical circumstances' [60], and have become an important tool in translating best research evidence into practice. Evidence-based guidelines are increasingly being developed for oral health, and several have included recommendations on post-brushing rinsing after the use of fluoride toothpaste [14–16, 61–67]. The consistent message emerging from these guidelines is to brush twice a day with fluoride toothpaste and to avoid or minimise rinsing with water. The post-brushing rinsing recommendations were based primarily on the results of the four clinical toothpaste trials [39–42] described in table 2. In spite of using the same evidence, the grading of the level of evidence varies between guidelines. However, there is consistency among the guidelines in recommending the use of fluoride mouthrinse only for high caries risk individuals over the age of 6. Of the four guidelines that considered the timing of the use of fluoride mouthrinse in relation to brushing with fluoride toothpaste, two recommended that it should be used at a different time to brushing [14, 64], and one recommended that mouthrinse could be used either following fluoride toothpaste use or independently of brushing [67]. The fourth guideline considered the risk/harm balance and patient compliance when formulating its statement that 'if people are using mouthrinse, then there was no harm in using it at the same time as brushing' [63].

The recommendations of these guidelines, together with the evidence from experimental and clinical studies on post-brushing rinsing described earlier, were recently reviewed by a panel of experts to develop consensus statements and recommendations on post-brushing rinsing behaviour for the control of dental caries [68]. Because of the lack of the highest quality evidence in this area, the panel was explicit in stating that the recommendations constitute expert opinion. In keeping with existing guidelines, the panel advised against rinsing excessively with water after brushing. Based on fluoride retention studies, it stated that fluoride mouthrinse can be used after brushing and also gave other options for enhancing fluoride retention after brushing, namely 'spit, don't rinse' or rinsing with a slurry of fluoride toothpaste and saliva. With the focus on fluoride retention, the panel also recommended that non-fluoride rinses should preferably be used before brushing or at a different time to brushing. The full set of consensus statements and recommendations of the expert panel are reproduced in table 3.

Few guidelines deal with adult oral health, and consequently there is a lack of guidance on the timing of the use of anti-plaque/anti-gingivitis mouthrinses for periodontal health. A guideline from the UK states that chlorhexidine mouthrinses are very effective when used as an adjunct to toothbrushing, but offers no advice as to when they should be used [14]. A comprehensive Swedish guideline on adult oral health does not recommend daily use of antiseptic mouthrinses for periodontal and peri-implant health [69].

Conclusion

Enormous effort and expense goes into developing new toothpaste formulations to improve oral health, and yet relatively little attention has been paid to understanding precisely how these products are used by the population at large, and how to encourage compliance with optimal use. This paper has shown that while there is widespread acceptance of toothbrushing with toothpaste, there is considerable variation in the frequency of brushing and in post-brushing rinsing habits, which can impact on oral health. Guidelines and consensus recommendations can help in establishing 'best practice' particularly in light of the limited evidence-base available on post-brushing rinsing, but implementation of guideline recommendations can be extremely difficult, particularly if the change involves a habit that may be ingrained in a culture, such as rinsing with water after toothbrushing. A recent survey which recorded toothbrushing behaviours of 11- to 13-year-old children in the UK [28] found that only 9–16% complied with the Department of Health's recommendation to spit out and not rinse after brushing [14], whereas 40% still used a glass or beaker of water to rinse after brushing. The recommendations that fluoride mouthrinse can be used after brushing will certainly help compliance, since that is how most people use mouthrinse anyway. Behaviour change may also be required on the part of the dental team as inconsistencies towards caries prevention, and specifically use of fluoride, have been noted among general dental practitioners in the UK [70]. From a public health perspective, it is likely that investing in strategies to promote twice daily use of fluoride toothpaste has the potential to yield greater oral health benefits than focus-

Table 3. Consensus statements from the expert advisory panel on post-brushing rinsing

Consensus statements
Rinsing with water after brushing with fluoride toothpaste can reduce the benefit of fluoride toothpaste
There is a theoretical benefit in keeping the intra-oral levels of fluoride elevated by replacing a post-brushing water rinse with a fluoride rinse
Non-fluoride rinses should preferably be used before brushing or at a different time to brushing with fluoride toothpaste
Mouthrinses containing fluoride can be used before brushing or at a different time to brushing with fluoride toothpaste
The panel endorsed the promotion of the positive messages from the research by Sjögren et al. [44, 71] concerning use of a slurry of fluoride toothpaste
All three documented methods of increasing post-brushing fluoride retention – (a) 'spit don't rinse'; (b) rinsing with a slurry of fluoride toothpaste and saliva, and (c) rinsing with a mouthrinse containing fluoride – could be beneficial for caries control at the individual level
There is a need to tackle the risk profile for dental caries in populations. To this aim, the panel supported Sir Michael Marmot's strategy of 'proportionate universalism' [72]. This approach advocates improving the oral health of all by flattening the social gradient of disease, with a focus on seeking the greatest improvement in those with highest need while still achieving improvements in other population groups
On the basis of balancing risks and benefits, the panel recommended: For children at high risk of caries: – Rinsing should be supervised until an age where parents/carers are confident that children will not drink the rinse – Mouth rinses should not be used before the age of 6 years. (However, studies in Japan have indicated that 4-5-year-olds can rinse under supervision. In addition, children with newly erupting teeth may gain a long-term benefit from using mouth rinses) [73] – Use 10 ml twice daily of mouthrinse up to 100 ppm fluoride, or 10 ml once daily of mouth rinse up to 226 ppm fluoride – Avoid the risk of approaching the lethal dose of fluoride by using an appropriate bottle size For the general population, including children aged 12 years and above: – Brush twice daily with a fluoride toothpaste; do not rinse excessively with water; use one of the three recognised post-brushing approaches to enhance fluoride retention The panel also encouraged future research with a range of mouthrinse products to explore the effects of the interplay between the frequency of use of mouthrinse agents and fluoride concentration
Taken from Pitts et al. [68].

ing on changing post-brushing rinsing methods. The fact that low-frequency toothbrushing tends to be accompanied by smoking, unhealthy eating patterns and low levels of physical activity suggests that it may be useful to integrate oral disease prevention into general health promotion programmes using a 'common risk factor approach' [18]. It is important to understand the determinants of user-related factors such as frequency of brushing and rinsing behaviours to better target oral health care messages.

References

1 Marinho V, Higgins J, Logan S, Sheiham A: Fluoride toothpastes for preventing dental caries in children and adolescents. Cochrane Database Syst Rev 2003;CD002278.

2 Twetman S, Axelsson S, Dahlgren H, Holm AK, Källestål C, Lagerlöf F, Lingström P, Mejàre I, Nordenram G, Norlund A, et al: Caries-preventive effect of fluoride toothpaste: a systematic review. Acta Odontol Scand 2003;61:347–355.

3 Walsh T, Worthington HV, Glenny AM, Appelbe P, Marinho VC, Shi X: Fluoride toothpastes of different concentrations for preventing dental caries in children and adolescents. Cochrane Database Syst Rev 2010;CD007868.

4 Gunsolley JC: A meta-analysis of six-month studies of antiplaque and antigingivitis agents. J Am Dent Assoc 2006;137:1649–1657.

5 Poulsen S, Errboe M, Lescay Mevil Y, Glenny AM: Potassium containing toothpastes for dentine hypersensitivity. Cochrane Database Syst Rev 2006;CD001476.

6 Duckworth RM, Morgan SN: Oral fluoride retention after use of fluoride dentifrices. Caries Res 1991;25:123–129.

7 Cummins D: Mechanisms of action of clinically proven anti-plaque agents; in Embery C, Rølla G (eds): Clinical and Biological Aspects of Dentifrices. Oxford, Oxford Medical Publications, 1992.

8 Marsh P: Contemporary perspective on plaque control. Br Dent J 2012;212:601–606.

9 Davies R, Scully C, Preston AJ: Dentifrices – an update. Med Oral Patol Oral Cir Bucal 2010;15:e976–e982.

10 Duckworth RM, Morgan SN, Burchell CK: Fluoride in plaque following use of dentifrices containing sodium monofluorophosphate. J Dent Res 1989;68:130–133.

11 Zero DT, Raubertas RF, Fu J, Pedersen AM, Hayes AL, Featherstone JD: Fluoride concentrations in plaque, whole saliva, and ductal saliva after application of home-use topical fluorides. J Dent Res 1992;71:1768–1775, erratum in J Dent Res 1993;72:87.

12 Nordstrom A, Birkhed D: Fluoride retention in proximal plaque and saliva using two NaF dentifrices containing 5,000 and 1,450 ppm F with and without water rinsing. Caries Res 2009;43:64–69.

13 Global Industry Analysts Inc (GIA): Global Toothpaste Market to Reach US$12.6 Billion by 2015, according to New Report by Global Industry Analysts, Inc. 2010. http://www.prweb.com/pdfdownload/4661914.pdf; accessed on 20/08/2012.

14 Department of Health and British Association for the Study of Community Dentistry (BASCD): Delivering Better Oral Health – an evidence-based toolkit for prevention. 2009. http://www.oralhealthplatform.eu/resource/other-resources; accessed on 17/04/2013.

15 Irish Oral Health Services Guideline Initiative: Strategies to prevent dental caries in children and adolescents: evidence-based guidance on identifying high caries risk children and developing preventive strategies for high caries risk children in Ireland. 2009. http://ohsrc.ucc.ie/html/guidelines.html; accessed on 04/09/2012.

16 European Academy of Paediatric Dentistry: Guidelines on the use of fluoride in children: an EAPD policy document. Eur Arch Paediatr Dent 2009;10:129–135.

17 Dos Santos AP, Nadanovsky P, de Oliveira BH: Inconsistencies in recommendations on oral hygiene practices for children by professional dental and paediatric organisations in ten countries. Int J Paediatr Dent 2011;21:223–231.

18 Currie C, Zanotti C, Morgan A, Currie D, de Looze M, Roberts C, Samdal O, Smith ORF, Barnekow V: Social determinants of health and well-being among young people. Health Behaviour in School-aged Children (HBSC) study: international report from the 2009/2010 survey vol (Health Policy for Children and Adolescents, No 6). Copenhagen, WHO Regional Office for Europe, 2012.

19 Hugoson A, Koch G, Göthberg C, Helkimo AN, Lundin SA, Norderyd O, Sjödin B, Sondell K: Oral Health of individuals aged 3–80 years in Jönköping, Sweden during 30 years (1973–2003). 1. Review of findings on dental care habits and knowledge of oral health. Swed Dent J 2005;29:125–138.

20 Chadwick B, White D, Lader D, Pitts N: Preventive behaviour and risks to oral health – a report from the Adult Dental Health Survey 2009, 2011. http://data.gov.uk/dataset/adult_dental_health_survey/resource/bbc274d2-d24c-4e22-a2cc-1a6e4478fe92; accessed on 17/04/2013.

21 Christensen LB, Petersen PE, Krustrup U, Kjøller M: Self-reported oral hygiene practices among adults in Denmark. Community Dent Health 2003;20:229–235.

22 Tseveenjav B, Suominen AL, Hausen H, Vehkalahti MM: The role of sugar, xylitol, toothbrushing frequency, and use of fluoride toothpaste in maintenance of adults' dental health: findings from the Finnish National Health 2000 Survey. Eur J Oral Sci 2011;119:40–47.

23 Whelton H, Crowley E, O'Mullane D, Woods N, Mc Grath C, Kelleher V, Guiney H, Byrtek M: Oral Health of Irish Adults, 2000–2002, 2007. http://www.dohc.ie/publications/pdf/oral_health02.pdf; accessed on 17/04/2013.

24 Nordstrom A, Birkhed D: Effect of a third application of toothpastes (1,450 and 5,000 ppm F), including a 'massage' method on fluoride retention and pH drop in plaque. Acta Odontol Scand 2013;71:50–56.

25 Fischman SL: Hare's teeth to fluorides, historical aspects of dentifrice use; in Embery C, Rølla G (eds): Clinical and Biological Aspects of Dentifrices. Oxford, Oxford Medical Publications, 1992.

26 Albertsson KW, van Dijken JW: Awareness of toothbrushing and dentifrice habits in regularly dental care receiving adults. Swed Dent J 2010;34:71–78.

27 van Loveren C, Ketley CE, Cochran JA, Duckworth RM, O'Mullane DM: Fluoride ingestion from toothpaste: fluoride recovered from the toothbrush, the expectorate and the after-brush rinses. Community Dent Oral Epidemiol 2004;32(suppl 1):54–61.

28 McGrady MG, Ellwood RP, Maguire A, Goodwin M, Boothman N, Pretty IA: The association between social deprivation and the prevalence and severity of dental caries and fluorosis in populations with and without water fluoridation. BMC Public Health 2012;12:1122.

29 Jensen O, Gabre P, Skold UM, Birkhed D: Is the use of fluoride toothpaste optimal? Knowledge, attitudes and behaviour concerning fluoride toothpaste and toothbrushing in different age groups in Sweden. Community Dent Oral Epidemiol 2012;40:175–184.

30 Zero DT, Raubertas RF, Pedersen AM, Fu J, Hayes AL, Featherstone JD: Studies of fluoride retention by oral soft tissues after the application of home-use topical fluorides. J Dent Res 1992;71:1546–1552.

31 Zero DT, Fu J, Espeland MA, Featherstone JD: Comparison of fluoride concentrations in unstimulated whole saliva following the use of a fluoride dentifrice and a fluoride rinse. J Dent Res 1988;67:1257–1262.

32 Collins W, Weetman D, Stephen K, Smalls M: Salivary F⁻ concentrations following toothbrushing (abstract). Caries Res 1984;18:155.

33 Attin T, Hellwig E: Salivary fluoride content after toothbrushing with a sodium fluoride and an amine fluoride dentifrice followed by different mouthrinsing procedures. J Clin Dent 1996;7:6–8.

34 Issa AI, Toumba KJ: Oral fluoride retention in saliva following toothbrushing with child and adult dentifrices with and without water rinsing. Caries Res 2004;38:15–19.

35 Zamataro CB, Tenuta LM, Cury JA: Low-fluoride dentifrice and the effect of postbrushing rinsing on fluoride availability in saliva. Eur Arch Paediatr Dent 2008;9:90–93.

36 Duckworth RM, Knoop DT, Stephen KW: Effect of mouthrinsing after toothbrushing with a fluoride dentifrice on human salivary fluoride levels. Caries Res 1991;25:287–291.

37 Sjögren K, Birkhed D: Effect of various post-brushing activities on salivary fluoride concentration after toothbrushing with a sodium fluoride dentifrice. Caries Res 1994;28:127–131.

38 Sjögren K, Melin NH: The influence of rinsing routines on fluoride retention after toothbrushing. Gerodontology 2001;18:15–20.

39 Chesters RK, Huntington E, Burchell CK, Stephen KW: Effect of oral care habits on caries in adolescents. Caries Res 1992;26:299–304.

40 O'Mullane DM, Kavanagh D, Ellwood RP, Chesters RK, Schafer F, Huntington E, Jones PR: A three-year clinical trial of a combination of trimetaphosphate and sodium fluoride in silica toothpastes. J Dent Res 1997;76:1776–1781.

41 Chestnutt IG, Schafer F, Jacobson AP, Stephen KW: The influence of toothbrushing frequency and post-brushing rinsing on caries experience in a caries clinical trial. Community Dent Oral Epidemiol 1998;26:406–411.

42 Ashley PF, Attrill DC, Ellwood RP, Worthington HV, Davies RM: Toothbrushing habits and caries experience. Caries Res 1999;33:401–402.

43 Machiulskiene V, Richards A, Nyvad B, Baelum V: Prospective study of the effect of post-brushing rinsing behaviour on dental caries. Caries Res 2002;36:301–307.

44 Sjögren K, Birkhed D, Rangmar B: Effect of a modified toothpaste technique on approximal caries in preschool children. Caries Res 1995;29:435–441.

45 Sonbul H, Birkhed D: The preventive effect of a modified fluoride toothpaste technique on approximal caries in adults with high caries prevalence. A 2-year clinical trial. Swed Dent J 2010;34:9–16.

46 Sonbul H, Merdad K, Birkhed D: The effect of a modified fluoride toothpaste technique on buccal enamel caries in adults with high caries prevalence: a 2-year clinical trial. Community Dent Health 2011;28:292–296.

47 Al Mulla AH, Kharsa SA, Birkhed D: Modified fluoride toothpaste technique reduces caries in orthodontic patients: a longitudinal, randomized clinical trial. Am J Orthod Dentofacial Orthop 2010;138:285–291.

48 Särner B, Sundin E, Abdulrahman S, Birkhed D, Lingstrom P: Use of different mouthrinses in an adult Swedish population. Swed Dent J 2012;36:53–60.

49 Duckworth RM, Maguire A, Omid N, Steen IN, McCracken GI, Zohoori FV: Effect of rinsing with mouthwashes after brushing with a fluoridated toothpaste on salivary fluoride concentration. Caries Res 2009;43:391–396.

50 Mystikos C, Yoshino T, Ramberg P, Birkhed D: Effect of post-brushing mouthrinse solutions on salivary fluoride retention. Swed Dent J 2011;35:17–24.

51 Marinho VCC, Higgins JPT, Sheiham A, Logan S: Combinations of topical fluoride (toothpastes, mouthrinses, gels, varnishes) versus single topical fluoride for preventing dental caries in children and adolescents. Cochrane Database Syst Rev 2004;CD002781.

52 Twetman S, Petersson L, Axelsson S, Dahlgren H, Holm AK, Kallestal C, Lagerlof F, Lingstrom P, Mejare I, Nordenram G, et al: Caries preventive effect of sodium fluoride mouthrinses: a systematic review of controlled clinical trials. Acta Odontol Scand 2004;62:223–230.

53 Barkvoll P, Rølla G, Svendsen K: Interaction between chlorhexidine digluconate and sodium lauryl sulfate in vivo. J Clin Periodontol 1989;16:593–595.

54 Sheen S, Eisenburger M, Addy M: Effect of toothpaste on the plaque inhibitory properties of a cetylpyridinium chloride mouth rinse. J Clin Periodontol 2003;30:255–260.

55 Owens J, Addy M, Faulkner J, Lockwood C, Adair R: A short-term clinical study design to investigate the chemical plaque inhibitory properties of mouthrinses when used as adjuncts to toothpastes: applied to chlorhexidine. J Clin Periodontol 1997;24:732–737.

56 Van Strydonck DA, Scale S, Timmerman MF, van der Velden U, van der Weijden GA: Influence of a SLS-containing dentifrice on the anti-plaque efficacy of a chlorhexidine mouthrinse. J Clin Periodontol 2004;31:219–222.

57 Van Strydonck DA, Timmerman MF, Van der Velden U, Van der Weijden GA: Chlorhexidine mouthrinse in combination with an SLS-containing dentifrice and a dentifrice slurry. J Clin Periodontol 2006;33:340–344.

58 Kolahi J, Soolari A: Rinsing with chlorhexidine gluconate solution after brushing and flossing teeth: a systematic review of effectiveness. Quintessence Int 2006;37:605–612.

59 Temmerman A, Dekeyser C, Declerck D, Quirynen M: Dentifrices: évaluation sur base de littérature actuelle. Rev Belge Med Dent 2010;65:60–86.

60 Field MJ, Lohr KN (eds): Clinical Practice Guidelines: Directions for a New Program. Washington, National Academy Press, 1990.

61 Scottish Dental Clinical Effectiveness Programme: Prevention and management of dental caries in children: dental clinical guidance. 2010. http://www.sdcep.org.uk/index.aspx?o=2332; accessed on 17/04/2013.

62 American Academy of Pediatric Dentistry: Guideline on fluoride therapy. Pediatr Dent 2009;32:143–146.

63 New Zealand Guidelines Group: Guidelines for the Use of Fluorides. Wellington, New Zealand Ministry for Health, 2009.

64 Australian Research Centre for Population Oral Health: The use of fluorides in Australia: guidelines. Aust Dent J 2006; 51:195–199.

65 Scottish Intercollegiate Guidelines Network (SIGN): Prevention and Management of Dental Decay in the Preschool Child. 2005. http://www.sign.ac.uk/guidelines/fulltext/83/index.html; accessed on 17/04/2013.

66 Scottish Intercollegiate Guidelines Network (SIGN): Preventing Dental Caries in Children at High Caries Risk. Targeted prevention of dental caries in the permanent teeth of 6–16 year olds presenting for dental care (SIGN 47). 2000. http://www.sign.ac.uk/guidelines/fulltext/47/index.html; accessed on 17/04/2013.

67 Zero DT, Marinho VC, Phantumvanit P: Effective use of self-care fluoride administration in Asia. Adv Dent Res 2012;24: 16–21.

68 Pitts N, Duckworth RM, Marsh P, Mutti B, Parnell C, Zero D: Post-brushing rinsing for the control of dental caries: exploration of the available evidence to establish what advice we should give our patients. Br Dent J 2012;212:315–320.

69 National Board of Health and Welfare (Socialstyrelsen) Sweden: National guidelines for adult dental care in 2011: Scientific basis 2011. http://www.socialstyrelsen.se/tandvardsriktlinjer/sokiriktlinjerna; accessed on 03/07/2012.

70 Threlfall AG, Milsom KM, Hunt CM, Tickle M, Blinkhorn AS: Exploring the content of the advice provided by general dental practitioners to help prevent caries in young children. Br Dent J 2007; 202:E9, discussion 148–149.

71 Sjögren K, Birkhed D, Ruben J, Arends J: Effect of post-brushing water rinsing on caries-like lesions at approximal and buccal sites. Caries Res 1995;29:337–342.

72 Marmot M, Allen J, Goldblatt P, Boyce T, McNeish D, Grady M, Geddes I: Fair Society, Healthy Lives: The Marmot review. Strategic review of health inequalities in England, post 2010. London, Global Health Equity Group, 2010.

73 Kobayashi S, Kishi H, Yoshihara A, Horii K, Tsutsui A, Himeno T, Horowitz AM: Treatment and post-treatment effects of fluoride mouthrinsing after 17 years. J Public Health Dent 1995;55: 229–233.

C. Parnell
Oral Health Services Research Centre
University Dental School
Wilton, Cork (Ireland)
E-Mail c.parnell@ucc.ie

Subject Index